AF556758

Progress in Acetabularia Research

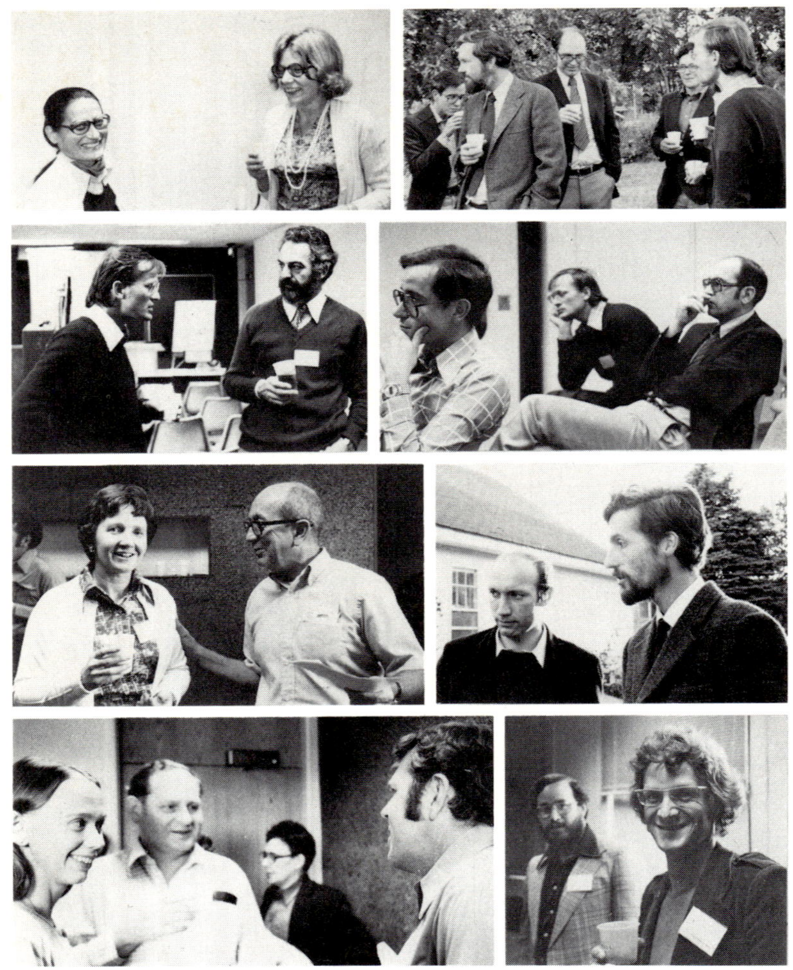

Some of the participants at the 4th International Meeting on Acetabularia, September 2–4 1976, University of Massachusetts, Amherst.
Top row, from left to right: S. Puiseux-Dao, S. Berger, H. Spring, J. D. Palmer, W. W. Franke, G. Richter, W. Herth.
Second row: W. Herth, S. Bonotto, H. Spring, W. Herth, W. W. Franke.
Third row: B. R. Green, A. Gibor, K. Apel, C. L. F. Woodcock.
Botton row: I. Tschismadia, H.-G. Schweiger, G. Richter, F. W. Moore, R. Shoeman, H.-U. Koop.
Photographs courtesy of Dr. Beverly Green.

Progress in Acetabularia Research

Edited by

C. L. F. Woodcock

Department of Zoology
University of Massachusetts
Amherst, Massachusetts

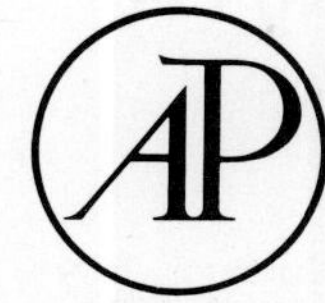

Academic Press

NEW YORK SAN FRANCISCO LONDON 1977

A Subsidiary of Harcourt Brace Jovanovich, Publishers

Academic Press Rapid Manuscript Reproduction

ACADEMIC PRESS, INC.
111 Fifth Avenue, New York, New York 10003

United Kingdom Edition published by
ACADEMIC PRESS, INC. (LONDON) LTD.
24/28 Oval Road, London NW1

LIBRARY OF CONGRESS CATALOG CARD NUMBER: 77-9141

ISBN 0-12-763750-8

PRINTED IN THE UNITED STATES OF AMERICA

Contents

III Chloroplasts

IV Growth and Morphogenesis

V Methodology

List of Contributors

Klaus Apel (137), Biologisches Institut II der Universität, Lehrstuhl für Botanik, Schanzlestr. 9–11, 78 Freiburg, West Germany

P. Baeckelandt (271), Laboratoire de Physiologie et de Physiopathologie, Université Libre de Bruxelles, 2 Rue Evers, 1000 Brussels, Belgium

Friedrich W. Bentrup (249), Abteilung Biophysik der Pflanzen, Institut für Biologie I der Universität, D-7400 Tübingen, West Germany

S. Berger (319), Max-Planck-Institut für Zellbiologie, Anton Dohrn Weg 59, D-2940 Wilhelmshaven, West Germany

Silvano Bonotto (123, 195, 207, 219, 241), Département de Radiobiologie, Centre d'Etude de l'Energie Nucléaire, CEN-SCK, 2400 Mol, Belgium

P. Bourgeois (271), Laboratoire de Physiologie et de Physiopathologie, Université Libre de Bruxelles, 2 Rue Evers, 1000 Brussels, Belgium

W. L. Cairns (331), Max-Planck-Institut für Zellbiologie, Anton Dohrn Weg 59, D-2940 Wilhelmshaven, West Germany

H. Clauss (255), Institut für Pflanzenphysiologie und Zellbiologie, Freie Universität, Königin Luise Str. 12–16a, D-1000 Berlin, West Germany

P. Dehm (319), Max-Planck-Institut für Zellbiologie, Anton Dohrn Weg 59, D-2940 Wilhelmshaven, West Germany

Viviane Delegher (287), Laboratoire de Physiologie Végétale, Université Libre de Bruxelles, 1000 Brussels, Belgium

J. P. Dubacq (175), Laboratoire de Biologie Cellulaire Végétale, Université Paris VII, E. R. A. 325-C. N. R. S., and Laboratoire de Physiologie Cellulaire, Université Paris VI, E. R. A. 323-C. N. R. S., Paris, France

Esther Dujardin (195, 207, 219), Laboratoire de Photobiologie, Départment de Botanique, Université de Liège, Sart-Tilman, Belgium

Bruno Felluga (123), International Institute of Genetics and Biophysics, Consiglio Nazionale delle Ricerche, 80125 Naples, Italy

A. Gibor (231), Department of Biological Sciences, University of California, Santa Barbara, California 93106

Lüder Göke (305), Fachrichtung Feinstrukturforschung und Elektronenmikroskopie and Fachrichtung Biochemie der Pflanzen, Fachbereich Biologie, Freie Universität Berlin, Königin Luise Str. 12-16a, D-1000 Berlin, West Germany

Beverley R. Green (107), Department of Botany, University of British Columbia, Vancouver, B.C. V6T 1W5, Canada

P.-E. Henry (271), Laboratoire de Physiologie et de Physiopathologie, Université Libre de Bruxelles, 2 Rue Evers, 1000 Brussels, Belgium

D. Hoursiangou-Neubrun (175), Laboratoire de Biologie Cellulaire Végétale, Université Paris VII, E. R. A. 325-C. N. R. S., and Laboratoire de Physiologie Cellulaire, Université Paris VI, E. R. A. 323-C. N. R. S., Paris, France

N. Ikehara (33), Max-Planck-Institut für Zellbiologie, Anton Dohrn Weg 59, D-2940 Wilhelmshaven, West Germany

Helga Kersten (39), Institut für Physiologische Chemie der Universität Erlangen-Nurnberg, Wasserturmstrasse 5, D-8520 Erlangen, West Germany

R. Kirchmann (195), Département de Radiobiologie, Centre d'Etude de l'Energie Nucléaire, CEN-SCK, 2400 Mol, Belgium

Klaus Kloppstech (19), Max-Planck-Institut für Zellbiologie, Anton Dohrn Weg 59, D-2940 Wilhelmshaven, West Germany

H.-U. Koop (7), Institut für Pflanzenphysiologie und Zellbiologie, Freie Universität Berlin, Königin Luise Str. 12–16a, D-1000 Berlin, West Germany

F. Legros (271), Laboratoire de Physiologie et de Physiopathologie, Université de Bruxelles, 2 rue Evers, 1000 Brussels, Belgium

T.-Y. Leong (153), Max-Planck-Institut für Zellbiologie, Anton Dohrn Weg 59, D-2940 Wilhelmshaven, West Germany

Antonio Mazza (123), International Institute of Genetics and Biophysics, Consiglio Nazionale delle Ricerche, 80125 Naples, Italy

D. Menzel (69), Fachrichtung Geinstrukturforschung und Elektronenmikroskopie, Frachberiech Biologie, Freie Universität Berlin, Königin Luise Str. 12-16a, D-1000 Berlin, West Germany

Fenton D. Moore (159), Biology Department, John Carroll University, Cleveland, Ohio 44118

Bernice L. Muir (107), Department of Botany, University of British Columbia, Vancouver, B.C. V6T 1W5, Canada

Rainer Niemeyer (95), Institut für Botanik, Technische Universität Hannover, D-3000 Hannover, West Germany

Usha Padmanabhan (107), Department of Botany, University of British Columbia, Vancouver, B.C. V6T 1W5, Canada

M. Paques (207), Laboratoire de Photobiologie, Département de Botanique, Université de Liège, Sart-Tilman, Belgium

H. Hasko Paradies (83, 305), Fachrichtung Feinstrukturforschung und Elektronenmikroskopie and Fachrichtung Biochemie der Pflanzen, Fachbereich Biologie, Freie Universität Berlin, Königin Luise Str. 12–16a, D-1000 Berlin, West Germany

S. Puiseux-Dao (175), Laboratoire de Biologie Cellulaire Végétale, Université Paris VII, E. R. A. 325-C. N. R. S.

Ursula Rahmsdorf (47), Institut für Pflanzenphysiologie und Zellbiologie, Freie Universität Berlin, Königin Luise Str. 12–16a, D-1000 Berlin, West Germany

R. Schmid (255), Institut für Pflanzenphysiologie und Zellbiologie, Freie Universität, Königin Luise Str. 12–16a, D-1000 Berlin, West Germany

Walter Schmidt (39), Institut für Physiologische Chemie der Universität Erlangen-Nurnberg, Wasserturmstrasse 5, D-8520 Erlangen, West Germany

E. Schweiger (331), Max-Planck-Institut für Zellbiologie, Anton Dohrn Weg 59, D-2940 Wilhelmshaven, West Germany

Hans-Georg Schweiger (1, 19, 33, 39, 153, 319, 331), Max-Planck-Institut für Zellbiologie, Anton Dohrn Weg 59, D-2940 Wilhelmshaven, West Germany

Cyrille Sironval (195, 207, 219, 241), Laboratoire de Photobiologie, Département de Botanique, Université de Liège, Sart-Tilman, Belgium

Irene Tschismadia (159), Department of Anatomy, Ohio State University, Columbus, Ohio 43210

Thérèse Vanden Driessche (287), Laboratoire de Cytologie et d'Embyologie Moléculaires, Université Libre de Bruxelles, 1000 Brussels, Belgium

H. G. Wallraff (331), Max-Planck-Institut für Verhaltensphysiologie, D-3131 Seewiesen über Starnberg, West Germany

Günther Werz (83, 305), Fachrichtung Feinstrukturforschung und Elektronenmikroskopie and Fachrichtung Biochemie der Pflanzen, Fachbereich Biologie, Freie Universität Berlin, Königin Luise Str. 12-16a, D-1000 Berlin, West Germany

D. Wolff (331), Max-Planck-Institut für Zellbiologie, Anton Dohrn Weg 59, D-2940 Wilhelmshaven, West Germany

D. O. Woodward (153), Max-Planck-Institut für Zellbiologie, Anton Dohrn Weg 59, D-2940 Wilhelmshaven, West Germany

M. Yamakawa (33), Max-Planck-Institut für Zellbiologie, Anton Dohrn Weg 59, D-2940 Wilhelmshaven, West Germany

Brigitte Zimmer (83), Fachrichtung Feinstrukturforschung und Elektronenmikroskopie and Fachrichtung Biochemie der Pflanzen, Fachbereich Biologie, Freie Universität Berlin, Königin Luise Str. 12-16a, D-1000 Berlin, West Germany

Preface

The Fourth Meeting of the International Research Group on Acetabularia was held on the Amherst Campus of the University of Massachusetts in September 1976. Organized by Lawrence Bogorad and myself, and supported by the U.S. National Science Foundation and the University of Massachusetts Research Council, this symposium was the latest in a series of biennial meetings and reflects the continued need for close communication between investigators using Acetabularia as a research organism.

This volume contains contributions that were presented and discussed at the symposium, together with invited papers from those unable to attend. The result, as discussed in H-G. Schweiger's introductory chapter, is a mirror of the current status and directions of research on Acetabularia.

It is interesting to compare the contents of the proceedings of the first International Symposium on Acetabularia,[1] held in Belgium in 1969, with the present volume. Seven years ago, the analysis of the organism at the subcellular and molecular levels was beginning, and procedures for examining nucleic acids, especially RNA, for determining the capabilities of isolated chloroplasts, and for cataloging the cell at the ultrastructural level predominated. Now, much of the cataloging work has been completed, and the emphasis is split between applying current techniques of cell and molecular biology and returning to the examination of the cell in its entirety.

The basic questions of the interactions and division of labor between nucleus and cytoplasm, for which the Acetabularia cell seems to be the system "par excellence," continue to dominate Acetabularia research. The hunt for the proposed stable "morphogenetic substances" that preprogram the anucleate cell, allowing it to undergo a complex series of changes in form, is now pursued with the latest mRNA technology. The chloroplast, even though it contains more genetic information than those in other plants, nevertheless depends on the nucleus for some of

[1] "Biology of Acetabularia," J. Brachet and S. Bonotto, eds., Academic Press, New York, 1970.

its proteins; further analysis of the molecular composition of the chloroplast components, and the capabilities of isolated organelles continues. The realization that the cell is not a homogenous sac of cytoplasm and organelles, but possess a distinct polarity with apico-basal gradients of many components and functions, has resulted in a number of new lines of research, which may become of increasing importance in the future.

The overall impression is of an active research area, proceeding vigorously on a number of fronts toward a unified goal, with new and exciting developments, such as the isolation of distinct genetic strains, continuing to add to the analytical repertoire.

I am grateful to Dr. John D. Palmer for bringing publisher and symposium together, and to the contributors for their timely submission of manuscripts. I apologize to authors and readers alike for any typographical errors I may have missed in proofreading.

Progress in Acetabularia Research

INTRODUCTION

H. G. Schweiger

Max-Planck-Institut für Zellbiologie
Wilhelmshaven, West Germany

Acetabularia is one of the favorite subjects in modern cell biology. This reputation of *Acetabularia* has existed for the 50 years since Hämmerling found that *Acetabularia*, as opposed to what had been assumed, is a uninuclear alga[1]. The cell nucleus is located in the rhizoid of the cell during the vegetative phase of the life cycle. Therefore, enucleation is a simple process and is easily performed by severing the basal part of the cell which will usually survive the procedure[1]. This simple experiment was logically followed by others which combined the cell nucleus and the cytoplasm[2]. In these experiments, it was most interesting to combine the nucleus and cytoplasm of two cells belonging to different species. Since such experiments can be performed using simple methods and controlled conditions, *Acetabularia* is an extremely useful subject even now when cell fusion is possible between many animal and plant cells.

Based on these two basic experiments, cell biological research on *Acetabularia* underwent a continual and logical development during the past 50 years. During the first phase of this research, the biological principles of nucleocytoplasmic relationships were investigated. After the second World War, biochemical methods for research on *Acetabularia* were introduced both in Brussels[3] and Wilhelmshaven[4] and applied principally to the behavior of anucleate cells.

In the third phase, molecular genetics became prominent, with special attention being paid to the chemical nature of the morphogenetic substances, the stability of messenger RNA in nucleate and anucleate cells, the site of coding of different proteins (nucleus or organelles). Other studies have examined the turnover of several ribonucleic acids and complex particles such as ribosomes[5]. Not all of the questions concerning these problems have been answered.

Recently, another complex series of questions entered the spotlight. This is the behavior of macromolecules when they are in close morphological and functional proximity to higher organized structures. This phase of research, probably most definitively described by the term supramolecular biology, is principally concerned with membranes. It is obvious that chloroplast membranes play an important part. Again, questions concerning the interrelationships of nucleus and cytoplasm are important in this field of investigation and may be answered by using *Acetabularia* as a research subject.

The classical problems for which *Acetabularia* is well-suited are those involving nucleo-cytoplasmic interactions, principally with respect to gene expression[6]. Gene expression in *Acetabularia* is readily monitored since this alga has a distinct species-specific morphogenesis.

Research on *Acetabularia* received new impetus when Jean Brachet, in 1969, invited the scientists involved in research on this alga to Brussels. The result of this meeting was a book edited by Brachet and Bonotto[7]. A second symposium was held in 1972 in Wilhelmshaven[8]. During this conference, the "International Research Group on *Acetabularia*" was founded. A third symposium held at Paris in 1974 [9] was followed by the conference which was held in 1976 in Amherst, Massachusetts. The results of this symposium are summarized in this book. They are extended by the contributions of other scientists who were not able to attend the meeting. The compiled papers of this book in an excellent way reflect the variety of the present directions of research on *Acetabularia*.

A striking step forward in research on *Acetabularia* will be the introduction of a synthetic medium which is at least equivalent to the Erd-Schreiber medium. Therefore, dependence upon sea-water is eliminated and inland laboratories can culture *Acetabularia* without an excessive financial burden. The most striking improvement of using a synthetic medium is the avoidance of the undefined soil extract, the quality of which depends on the soil used. This is especially important with the present increasing pollution. Of equal value are those experiments which result in the first evidence of the potential for genetic investigations on *Acetabularia*. It might well be that the lack of a core of genetic information and mutants prevented many scientists from doing research on this organism.

With the improved chemical and physical techniques, the view of the cell is often restricted to the particular feature of interest. However, the papers concerning cell elongation indicate the value of considering the cell as an entirety. Many fundamental questions arise from this concept.

Several papers presented in this book refer at least indirectly to the particular role of membranes. This includes the contributions concerning hormone-receptors in membranes of *Acetabularia*, electrophysiological investigations and the influence of an auxin-like substance on morphogenesis. Finally, in this connection, the contribution concerning the effects of blue light deserves attention. All these papers concern supramolecular aspects. Molecular biological aspects are featured in the paper on rates in synthesis of poly (A)-RNA with its implications for messenger-type RNA.

On the boundary line between molecular biology and biochemistry are papers such as those concerning the occurrence of methylthioadenosine-nucleosidase, the intracellular distribution of malate dehydrogenase, the investigation of a cell wall protein as well as the electron microscopical localization of catalase and peroxidase.

Cell organelles are especially interesting in the study of nucleocytoplasmic interactions. Therefore, the study of cell organelles, especially the chloroplasts, deserves particular interest. Investigations on those topics include the differentiation and heterogeneity of the chloroplasts as well as biochemical investigations on the D-ribulose-1,5-diphosphate carboxylase, molecular biological investigations on chloroplast DNA, and, finally, a discussion on the supramolecular aspect of the biosynthesis of chloroplast membranes. Logically connected with these topics are the two papers on circadian rhythms, specifically the phase-dependent synthesis of chloroplast membrane proteins and the description of a plotting method for data of circadian periodicity obtained by using the recently developed method for the continuous measurement of oxygen on single cells.

Of course, a composite of papers on *Acetabularia* research as presented in this book cannot be complete. For example, the studies of fine structure of genes of ribosomal RNA had to be omitted[10-12] as well as recent investigations on the regulation of enzyme synthesis in anucleate cells, such as those convincingly demonstrated in previous reports with thymidine kinase[13].

Cell biological research on *Acetabularia* has been performed for 50 years. As opposed to other lines of research, this does not mean the study is becoming stale. In reading this book, one can conclude that the open questions and newly found problems are numerous enough to point to a great future of *Acetabularia* as a subject in science. The unique features of this eukaryote, consisting of a single cell large enough to manipulate and yet showing distinct differentiation and morphogenesis, ensure a special place for it in Cell Biology.

REFERENCES

1. Hämmerling, J. (1931) Biol. Zentralbl. 51, 633-647.
2. Hämmerling, J. (1935) Roux' Arch. Entwicklungsmech. 132, 424-462.
3. Brachet, J., Chantrenne, H. and Vanderhaeghe, F. (1955) Biochim. Biophys. Acta 18, 544-563.
4. Hämmerling, J., Clauss, H., Keck, K., Richter, G. and Werz, G. (1958) Exp. Cell Res. Suppl. 6, 210-226.
5. Schweiger, H. G., Bannwarth, H., Berger, S. and Kloppstech, K. (1975) in Molecular Biology of Nucleocytoplasmic Relationships (Puiseux-Dao, S., ed.), pp. 203-215, Elsevier Scientific Publishing Company, Amsterdam, New York.
6. Schweiger, H. G. (1976) in Handbook of Genetics (King, R. C., ed.), Vol. 5, pp. 451-475, Plenum Press, New York, London.
7. Brachet, J. and Bonotto, S. (1970) Biology of _Acetabularia_. Academic Press, New York, London.
8. Schweiger, H. G. and Berger, S. (1972) Protoplasma 75, 471-492.
9. Puiseux-Dao, S. (1975) Protoplasma 83, 167-183.
10. Berger, S. and Schweiger, H. G. (1975) Protoplasma 83, 41-50.
11. Trendelenburg, M. F., Spring, H., Scheer, U. and Franke, W. W. (1974) Proc. Natl. Acad. Sci. USA 71, 3626-3630.
12. Woodcock, C. L. F., Stanchfield, J. E. and Gould, R. R. (1975) Pl. Sci. Lett. 4, 17-23.
13. Bannwarth, H., Ikehara, N. and Schweiger, H. G. (1977) Proc. R. Soc. Lond., in press.

I GENETICS AND INFORMATION PROCESSING

GENETIC ASPECTS OF *ACETABULARIA MEDITERRANEA*

H.-U. Koop

Institut für Pflanzenphysiologie und Zellbiologie
Freie Universität
Berlin, West Germany

SUMMARY

The fact that meiosis occurs before cyst formation in *Acetabularia*, means that all gametes derived from one single cyst are of the same sex. This, and the ability to induce gametogenesis, makes it possible to perform genetic crosses. *A. mediterranea* cells with a morphological marker involving the arrangement of the cysts in the cap, have been isolated and the frequency of the marker has been studied in three subsequent generations. Crosses between these cells and wild type cells show that the changed morphology is due to a change in the genome. This is the first successfully isolated and cultivated mutant of *Acetabularia* reported to date. The mutant has been used to produce direct biological evidence for the occurence of haploid nuclei in the rhizoid of the cells. The variablity of morphological and physiological characteristics has been studied in clones of *Acetabularia mediterranea*. The data indicate that it might be possible to isolate strains of cells that show a great uniformity and are significantly different from other strains in their morphology and physiology.

INTRODUCTION

Acetabularia is one of the most famous research objects in developmental physiology and cell biology. However, the genetics of this organism, is largely unexplored. This is due to a number of problems that have been discussed very recently in great detail by Green[2]. She pointed out that if an organism is to be studied genetically, it must be possible to make controlled crosses. In *Acetabularia*, crosses can only be made by the combination of two single cysts. It was of some interest, therfore, that we were able to develop a reliable and effective procedure for the induction of gametogenesis in the cysts[3]. Green[2] also discussed the problem of meiosis. If meiosis really occured during gametogenesis, as assumed in general[4,5], gametes of both mating types would be formed in one cyst, and the high probability of selfing would complicate analyses of genetical crosses. By microspectrophotometric measurements of the DNA contents of nuclei from different stages of the development, however, we were able to show[6], that we had to change our hypotheses about the life cycle of *Acetabularia mediterranea* (Fig. 1). We found that all nuclei but the primary nucleus are haploid. The evidence for the occurence of meiosis before cyst formation[7] was confirmed, and one more problem of genetical investigation using *Acetabularia* was solved. Therefore, we thought it would be useful to make a new attempt to do genetical experiments with *Acetabularia*. The experiments, reported here, were designed to find out whether the changed morphology that we had found in some cells of our cultures[8], was due to a change in the genome. The data provide further evidence for the occurence of meiosis during the breakdown of the primary nucleus. Finally, the analysis of the variability in clones of *Acetabularia* is presented, demonstrating that genetics may become very useful in other investigations of *Acetabularia*.

MATERIALS AND METHODS

Cells of *Acetabularia mediterranea* were cultured, following standard procedures[5] in a cycle of 10 hours of light and 14 hours of darkness. Cysts were collected, treated during maturation and induced to form gametes (20° C, in darkness) as reported previously[3]. During gametogenesis we used glass filter discs (diameter 2.5 cm) instead of agar[9]. Crosses were made by collecting single cysts in micropipettes[7] and putting pairs of cysts into test tubes containing culture medium: the cysts were induced to form gametes and collected about 30 hours after the induction, at which time a successful induction was already recognizable[10], but before the first gametes had been released from the cysts. The variability of cap diameters and cell lengths was determined by measuring these characteristics in five independent samples of twenty cells each. The means were calculated and confidence intervals of the means were determined for a confidence coefficient of 1%, using Student's t-distribution.

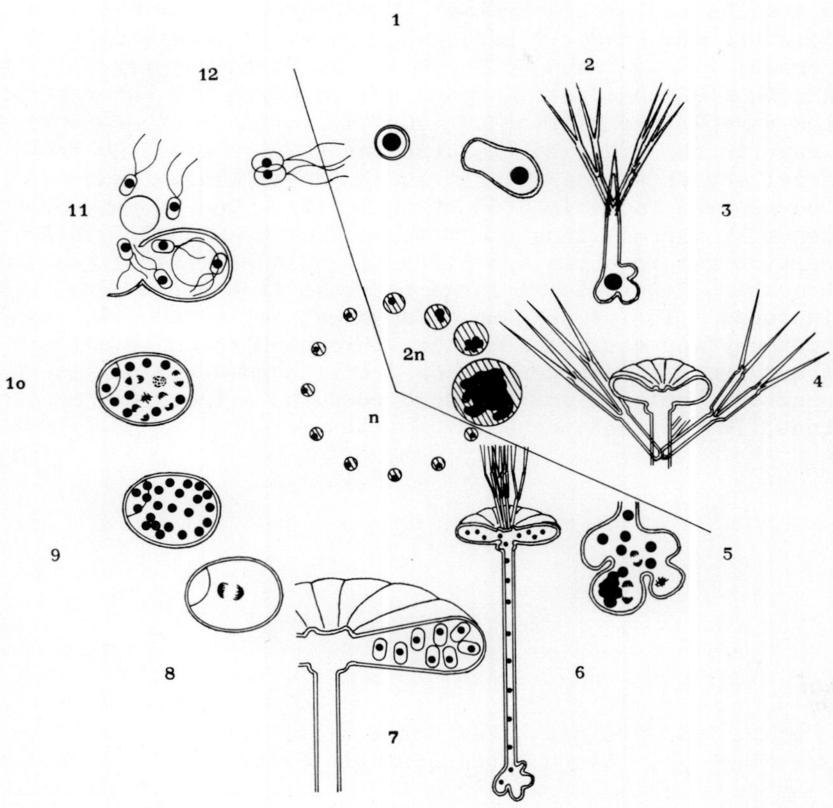

Acetabularia mediterranea: life cycle

1 cygote 2 cygote germination 3 vegetative growth

4 cap formation 5 formation of secondary nuclei 6 transport of secondary nuclei 7 cyst formation 8 cyst maturation

9 cyst dormancy 1o gametogenesis 11 gamete release 12 copulation

Figure 1. Acetabularia mediterranea life cycle. The morphological appearance of the nuclei during the corresponding developmental stages (outer circle) is indicated in the inner circle.

RESULTS

Frequency of the morphological aberration in subsequent generations

The cells that were used for genetical experiments showed a changed arrangement of their cysts in the cap[8]. While cysts are normally arranged in a radial symmetric manner (Fig. 2 a) these cells show a bilateral symmetric arrangement of the cysts. Cysts are found in the outer parts of the rays in one half of the cap and in the central parts of the rays in the other half of the cap (Fig. 2 b). The frequencies are shown in Fig. 3. In the first generation (P) the marker was found in 2.5% of the cells. The progeny of these cells already showed a frequency of about 50%. This proportion was found in two different cultures (F_1, I and II). In the third generation a large increase in the frequency was again found. The proportion of abnormal cells was 74%, when the progeny was derived from the whole population of cells that had shown the marker in the previous generation. In the progeny of single cells, however, we found a frequency of 100% in the five cultures tested.

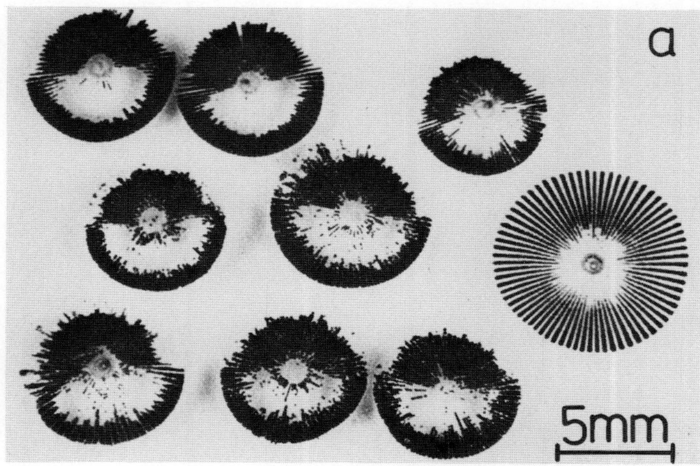

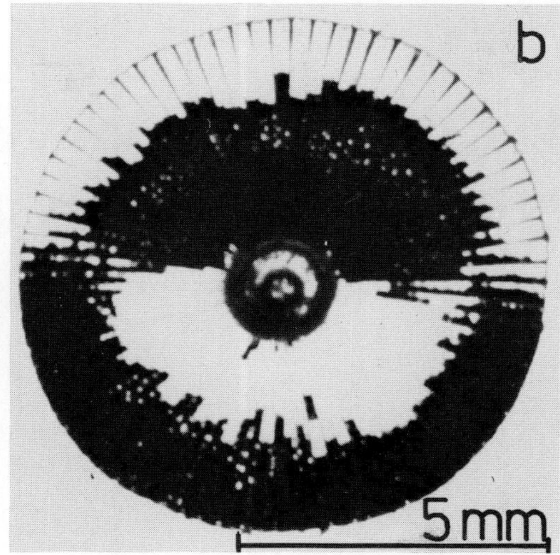

Figure 2.

a. Caps with a bilateral symmetric arrangement of cysts in comparison with one radial symmetric (wild-type) cap

b. Cap with bilateral arrangement of cysts in greater detail.

Generation	Population	Clone	Σ			%
P	I	-	173o	1686	44	2.54
F_1	I	-	519	228	291	56.1
F_1	II	-	6oo	289	311	51.8
F_2	I	-	148	38	116	74.3
F_2	-	I	182	-	182	1oo
F_2	-	II	1o3	-	1o3	1oo
F_2	-	III	189	-	189	1oo
F_2	-	IV	198	-	198	1oo
F_2	-	V	2o7	-	2o7	1oo

Figure 3. Frequencies of the marker "bilateral symmetric arrangement of cysts" in three subsequent generations (for details: see text).

×			×			×		
Nr.			Nr.			Nr.		
1	182	-	7	289	-	14	-	116
2	1o2	-	8	479	-	15	-	123
3	352	-	9	311	-	16	-	136
4	333	-	1o	3o7	-	17	-	27
5	419	-	11	185	-	18	-	67
6	156	-	12	173	-			
			13	225	-			

Figure 4. Crosses of cysts from cells with bilaterl and radial symmetric arrangement of cysts. The genotype of the cysts is given in the first line, the phenotype of the respective progenies in the second line. The data show the number of cells produced by the different crosses.

Crosses

Crosses were performed with cysts of normal cells and cysts of one of the single cells, whose progeny had been found to be uniform in carrying the morphological marker. Test tubes containing pairs of cysts were checked for the formation of germlings three weeks after the inoculation. Twenty-one out of forty-five pairs of cysts had formed germlings, of which three cultures were lost by infection or accident. The frequencies of the marker in the remaining eighteen cultures are given in Fig. 4. All cultures which were derived from the combination of two cysts from normal cells had the normal radial symmetric arrangement of cysts. The same was found in all cells that were produced by the cross of a cyst from a normal cell with a cyst from the cell that showed the marker. All cells of the cultures from two cysts of this abnormal cell, however, showed the bilateral arrangement of cysts. The crosses show the pattern typical for the inheritance of a recessive mutant. It is the first mutant found in *Acetabularia*.

Occurence of the marker in "direct germlings"

Whereas normally the mother cell dies and disintegrates after cyst formation, occasionally new cells may grow out of the old stalk or rhizoid[11]. These cells contain at least one nucleus which is morphologically identical to a primary nucleus but must have derived from secondary nuclei[11]. "Direct germlings" were found in the rhizoids of three different cultures derived from the cross of normal and mutant cysts. Five out of twenty-nine "direct germlings," which have formed cysts, show the mutant phenotype. Since the mutant is a recessive one, hybrid cells show the wild type morphology. The occurence of the mutant phenotype in the "direct germlings" means therefore, that "direct germlings" must have been formed with haploid nuclei. This is a direct biological evidence for the occurence of haploid nuclei in the rhizoid.

Variability in clones of *Acetabularia mediterranea*

The variability of the diameter of caps and length of cells in thirteen different clones in shown in Fig. 5. The means of the diameter of caps (Fig. 5 a) vary from 4.7 to 7.1 mm (clone 1 and clone 13, respectively). The confidence intervals vary from 70% to only 7.8% of the respective means (clone 13 and clone 6, respectively). Four clones have confidence intervals less than 10% of the mean, indicating that the variability is no greater than 5% in either direction. The great uniformity of the diameters of caps in clones is

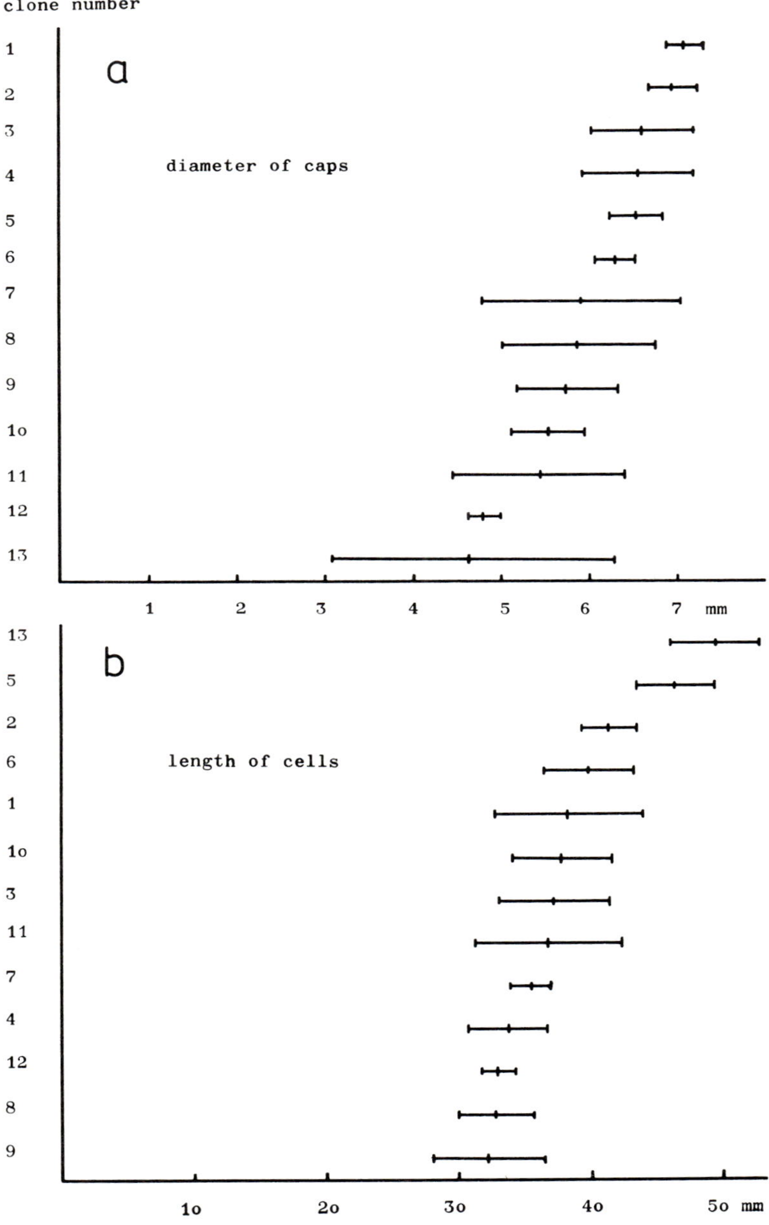
clone number
a
diameter of caps
1
2
3
4
5
6
7
8
9
1o
11
12
13
1 2 3 4 5 6 7 mm
b
length of cells
13
5
2
6
1
1o
3
11
7
4
12
8
9
1o 2o 3o 4o 5o mm

Figure 5 (opposite page). Variability of the diameter of caps and the length of cells in 13 different clones.

a. means and confidence intervals of cap diameters

b. means and confidence intervals of cell lengths.

There is no direct correlation between cap diameter and cell length.

also shown in Fig. 6. Some clones are significantly different from each other, as shown by the confidence intervals in Fig. 5 a.

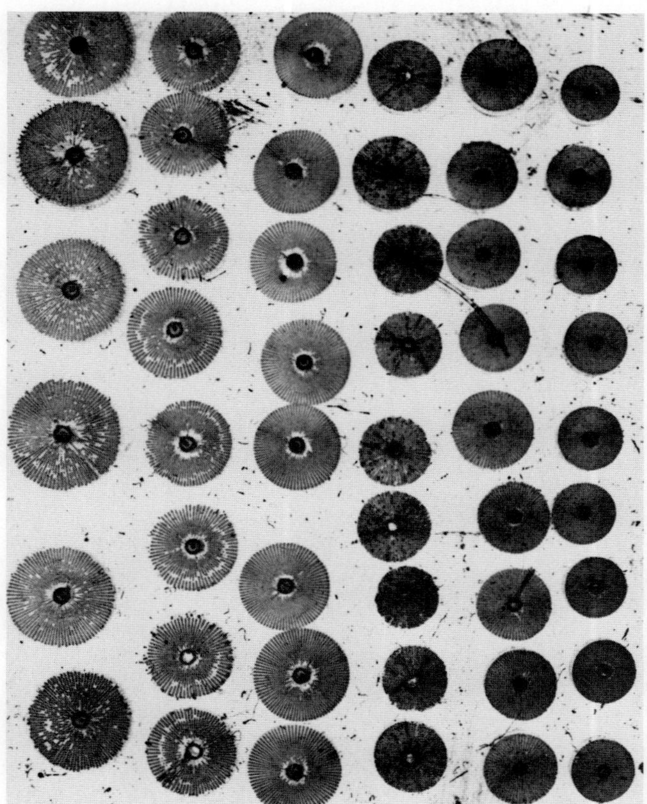

Figure 6. Acetabularia mediterranea: Caps from 6 different clones. Caps derived from one clone are arranged in vertical lines. The clones are identical to clones number (from left to right) 1, 2, 5, 9, 10 and 12, respectively (see Fig. 5).

Similar results are found for the lengths of the cells (Fig. 5 b). The means vary from 32.1 (clone 9) to 49.5 (clone 13), the confidence intervals from 7.7% (clone 12) to 32.4% (clone 11). The differences in cell length are significant in some clones.

More characteristics of the clones are given in Fig. 7. The proportions of cells with morphological aberrations are very different in the clones. Large cysts ("Sammelcysten," Schulze[4]) are found in the range from 0.7% to 100%, irregularly formed caps from 1.1% to 58.9% and split caps from 0% to 28.2%. The time needed to reach the stage of cyst formation, however, is only slightly different in the clones studied so far.

DISCUSSION

The frequency of the marker in three subsequent generations (Fig. 3), especially the frequency of 100% in all progenies of single cells, provides strong evidence for the suggestion that the changed morphology is due to a change in the genome. The crosses (Fig. 4) show the distribution pattern of phenotypes that would be expected from Mendel's laws for recessive mutants. This is the first mutant, found in Acetabularia. Now that the two main difficulties[2], the problems of gametogenesis[3] and of meiosis[6], have been solved, we have demonstrated that it is possible to study the genetics of Acetabularia. The use of mutants is demonstrated by the example of the analysis of "direct germlings." Hämmerling[11] suggested that "direct germlings" were formed from diploid secondary nuclei. The occurence of mutant phenotypes in "direct germlings" of hybrid cells, however, clearly shows that secondary nuclei are haploid. This, together with the evidence presented by Green[7], the discovery of lampbrush chromosomes in the primary nucleus[12] and the microspectrophotometric data[6], corroborates the revised life cycle (Fig. 1). The frequency of the mutant phenotype in the "direct germlings" is very low, compared to a proportion of 50%, which would be expected if there was a normal meiotic distribution of the hybrid genome of the primary nucleus. Since nothing is known, however, about the mechanism which leads to the formation of diploid primary nuclei from haploid secondary nuclei in the "direct germlings," this problem cannot be solved yet. Furthermore, Hammerling[11] found more than one nucleus in almost all of the "direct germlings" he analyzed cytologically. This alone could explain the low proportion of mutant phenotypes in our experiments.

The variability of morphological characteristics was found to be very small in some clones. The surprisingly high degree of uniformity (Fig. 5, Fig. 6) indicates that it might

clone number		1	2	3	4	5	6	7	8	9	1o	11	12	13
cells with large cysts (%)		0.7	63.1	2.6	100	11.6	2.9	89.2	81.6	100	24.5	92.1	91.3	95.3
cells with irregular caps (%)		4.0	1.1	13.4	16.8	16.8	8.3	52.0	58.9	13.0	5.3	36.1	5.0	64.7
cells with split caps (%)		2.5	0	3.6	12.2	1.8	1.7	4.0	6.7	1.2	0.4	2.5	0.8	28.2
time of development : mean age at the time of cyst formation (weeks)		21.1	21.2	20.5	20.1	22.2	19.9	20.5	19.9	21.1	19.9	20.9	20.3	21.4

Figure 7. <u>Acetabularia mediterranea</u>: Frequencies of morphological characteristics and the time of development in 13 different clones.

be possible to isolate strains of great uniformity and with significant differences in morphology and physiology. This would at first mean a higher degree of uniformity in experimental cultures and therefore a smaller variability of experimental data. Secondly, strains of different cell size, for example, could be used for the analysis of the regulation of cell size and related problems. Since genetical analysis has now been added to the methods used in the research on Acetabularia, we hope that it will become a useful tool in this research.

ACKNOWLEDGEMENTS

We wish to thank Mrs. Sabine Artelt for her skilful technical assistance in the experiments.

Some of the data presented in this paper have been published previously[1].

REFERENCES

1. Koop, H.-U. (1976) Ber. dt. bot. Ges. in press.
2. Green, B. R. (1976) The Genetics of Algae, University of California Press, Berkeley, Calif., U.S.A.
3. Koop, H.-U. (1975) Protoplasma 84, 137.
4. Schulze, K. L. (1939) Arch. Protistenkunde 92, 179.
5. Hämmerling, J. (1963) Ann. Rev. Plant Physiol. 14, 65.
6. Koop, H.-U. (1975) Protoplasma 85, 109.
7. Green, B. R. (1973) Phycologia 12, 233.
8. Koop, H.-U. (1976) Protoplasma 89, 197.
9. Koop, H.-U. (1975) Planta 126, 165.
10. Koop, H.-U. (1975) Protoplasma 86, 351.
11. Hämmerling, J. (1955) Biol. Zentralbl. 74, 420.
12. Spring, H., Scheer, U., Franke, W. W. and Trendelenburg, M. F. (1975) Chromosoma 50, 25.

THE RATE OF SYNTHESIS OF POLY(A) RNA IN *ACETABULARIA MEDITERRANEA*

Klaus Kloppstech and Hans-Georg Schweiger

Max-Planck-Institut für Zellbiologie
Wilhelmshaven, West Germany

ABSTRACT

The rate of synthesis of polyadenylated RNA has been estimated in different developmental stages of *Acetabularia mediterranea*. This has been achieved by determination of the specific activity of intracellular UTP and of the rate of incorporation of the labelled precursor uridine into polyadenylated RNA.

The important conclusion is that polyadenylated RNA is transcribed throughout most of the vegetative period, although at a three times higher rate in young than in old cells. Semiquantitative estimations reveal that approximately 7800, 3800 and 2500 genes coding for polyadenylated RNA are simultaneously transcribed in cells of 8, 15 and 35 mm length.

INTRODUCTION

The unicellular and uninuclear alga *Acetabularia* is capable of growing and performing differentiation even in the absence of the nucleus[1]. Detailed analyses at both the morphological[2,3] and the molecular level[4-6] have revealed that removal of the nucleus does not affect the regulation operating during different stages of development, although the information obviously originates in the nucleus. This raises the question of what is the mechanism of the cytoplasmic regulation and one may also ask whether the nucleus when not removed is active at all during these stages of development. Information concerning the latter point is rare and essentially confined to situations where normal development of the cell has been interrupted as for instance by amputation of the cellular apex in regenerating cells[7-9].

Recently we have isolated a poly(A) RNA fraction from

Acetabularia which is synthesized only in nucleate cells[10] and induces peptide synthesis in a cell-free system[11]. In order to elucidate the role of the nucleus during development we studied the synthesis of this poly(A) RNA in different developmental stages of *Acetabularia*. It is shown that the nucleus produces poly(A) RNA throughout the entire vegetative phase although the rate slowly declines as development proceeds.

MATERIAL AND METHODS

Cell cultures

Cells of *Acetabularia mediterranea* were grown in Erd-Schreiber medium (ESM) as described previously[12]. Cells of 8, 15 and 35 mm length were selected for the different experiments.

Preparation of cellular extracts

Depending on their size 100 to 400 cells were frozen in liquid nitrogen and homogenized in 1 ml ice cold 0.6 N perchloric acid, centrifuged at 15,000 xg for 5 min and neutralized with KOH. Precipitated $KClO_4$ was removed by centrifugation. The volume of the supernatant was determined and aliquots corresponding to 3 to 16 cells were added to the polymerase assay together with increasing amounts of a standard UTP solution.

Determination of UTP with RNA polymerase

The determination followed the method of Burgess[13]. The assay contained in 0.26 ml: 10 µmoles Tris/HCl, pH 7.9, 2.5 µmoles $MgCl_2$, 0.025 µmoles EDTA, 0.025 µmoles DTT, 37.5 µmoles KCl, 1 µmole potassium phosphate, pH 7.9, 125 µg bovine serum albumin, 5 µg poly-d {AT}, 0.25 µg {^{14}C} ATP (spec. activity 111 µCi/µmole), 1 unit RNA polymerase in 20 µl buffer (0.05 M Tris/HCl, pH 7.5, 0.1 M $(NH_4)_2SO_4$, 0.01 M DTT, 1 mg/ml bovine serum albumin). Variable amounts of UTP (1.5 to 150 ng) and constant amounts of cell extract were added, the incubation lasted for 2 hours at 37°C. Samples were precipitated with 5% TCA in the presence of 200 µg carrier tRNA from yeast, collected on glass fiber filters, washed 5 times with 5 ml 5% TCA, once with ethanol, dried, and counted in a toluene scintillator (3.64 g PPO and 0.36 g bis MSB per liter toluene).

Determination of the radioactivity of intracellular UTP

One hundred cells were incubated in 10 ml ESM containing 20 µg/ml rifampicin in the presence of 100 µCi{^{3}H} uridine for 1, 3, 5, 16 or 24 hours, washed, and frozen in liquid nitrogen. The cells were homogenized in cold 0.6 N perchloric acid and centrifuged for 5 min at 15,000 xg. The supernatant was neutralized with KOH and again clarified by centrifugation. The extract was supplemented with 2.5 mg UTP and transfered to a Dowex 1X8 column (17 x 230 mm) which had been equilibrated with a solution of 0.5 N NH_4COOH in 4 N HCOOH. After application of the sample the column was washed with 300 ml of the same solution. By this treatment uridine, UMP, UDP, uridinediphosphate sugars, CMP, CDP and CTP were removed. UTP was eluted with a solution of 1.2 N NH_4COOH in 4 N HCOOH. Two ml of each of the 5.6 ml fractions were counted in 10 ml scintillation mix (1.76 l dioxan, 0.2 l methanol, 0.04 l ethylene glycol, 120 g naphtalene, 7.28 g PPO and 0.72 g MSB) with an efficiency of 3.9% as had been determined by the use of {^{3}H} H_2O as internal standard. The radioactivity of the UTP peak was estimated, plotted against incubation time and the average radioactivity of the UTP over a 24 hour incubation period calculated.

Labeling and preparation of poly(A) RNA

Cells were incubated under identical conditions as described above for 24 hours. The cells were washed in ESM and frozen in liquid nitrogen. One hundred cells of 40 mm length were added as carrier cells and poly(A) RNA was extracted[10]. Two ml aliquots of the final oligo(dT) eluate were precipitated with 5% TCA, washed, dried, and counted in toluene scintillator with an efficiency of 28%.

ATP determination

Aliquots of the perchloric acid extracts were added to glass vials which contained in 4 ml: the extract of 1 mg fire-fly abdomens[14], 10 mM $MgSO_4$, 1 mM DTT, 1 mM K_2HAsO_4, and counted for 30 sec. in a liquid scintillation spectrometer at room temperature. At the chosen ATP concentrations the reaction showed linearity.

Material

RNA polymerase, poly-d{AT}, UTP, ATP were products of Boehringer and Söhne, Mannheim. Luciferin-Luciferase was purchased by Serva, Heidelberg. {^{14}C} ATP and {^{3}H} uridine were obtained from Amersham-Buchler, Braunschweig.

List of abbreviations

EDTA	Ethylenediaminetetraacetate
DDT	Dithioerythritol
poly{AU}	Polyadenylic-uridylic acid
poly-d{AT}	Poly-deoxy-adenylic-deoxy-thymidylic acid
PPO	Diphenyloxazole
bis-MSB	p(Bis-(o-methylstyryl))-benzole

RESULTS

The determination of the size of the UTP pool is based on the incorporation of {^{14}C} ATP into poly{AU} in the presence of RNA polymerase and poly-d{AT} where UTP is rate limiting. This method is similar to that which has been developed by Sasvári-Székely et al.[15]. Our system is capable of incorporating labeled ATP into poly{AU} over a period of at least 2 hours. The rate of incorporation is linearly dependent on the amount of UTP present in the reaction mixture (Fig. 1a). However, if a cell extract of *Acetabularia* is added this linear relationship is lost (Figs. 1 b through 1 d). Furthermore, the total incorporation of ATP into poly {AU} is significantly reduced in the presence of the cell extract. This might be due either to the dilution of {^{14}C} ATP by cellular ATP or to the presence of the perchloric acid extract which inhibits the polymerization reaction.

Supposing that the low incorporation of labeled ATP into poly {AU} in the presence of cell extract is caused merely by dilution due to intracellular cold ATP, we obtain values of 220, 710 and 570 ng ATP for a cell of 8, 15 and 35 mm length respectively (for details of the calculation see Sasvári-Székely et al.[15]). Since these values are substantially higher that those reported earlier[16] we estimated the ATP content of the extracts which had been used for the UTP determination by the bioluminescence assay. This method yields 13, 65 and 130 ng ATP per cell of the three stages mentioned above (Table 1). The reliability of these values has been checked by internal standards, which showed that added intracellular ATP was additive and that there is no inhibitory effect of the cell extract on the bioluminescence reaction. Therefore one has to conclude that the apparent inhibitory effect of the cell extract on the formation of poly {AU} by RNA polymerase is not due only to an isotope dilution effect but also to an inhibition of the enzymatic polymerization reaction by the cell extract. This difficulty has been overcome by adding known amounts of UTP as internal standards to the cell extract (Fig. 1 b-d). The incorporation values have been corrected for the cellular UTP. Since there is a more or less linear relationship between the amount of UTP added and the

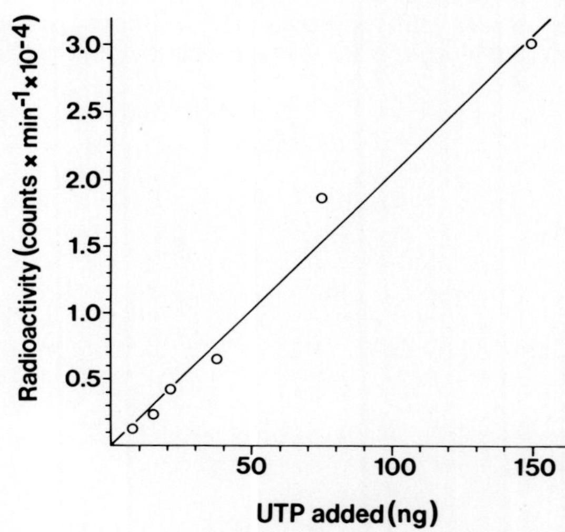

Figure 1 a. Dependence of the formation of poly [AU] on the addition of UTP.

The incorporation has been performed using the conditions described under methods in the absence of cellular perchloric acid extract.

The amount of UTP present in the extract from the indicated number of cells can be read off at that point of the abscissa (total UTP) where no extra UTP (added UTP) is added to the system.

Figure 1 b-d. Dependence of the formation of poly [AU] on the addition of UTP.

The incorporation has been performed using the conditions described under methods:

b) in the presence of perchloric acid extract corresponding to 16.4 cells of the 8 mm stage.

c) 7.25 cells of the 15 mm stage.

d) 3 cells of the 35 mm stage.

The amount of UTP present in the extract from the indicated number of cells can be read off at that point of the abscissa (total UTP) where no extra UTP (added UTP) is added to the system.

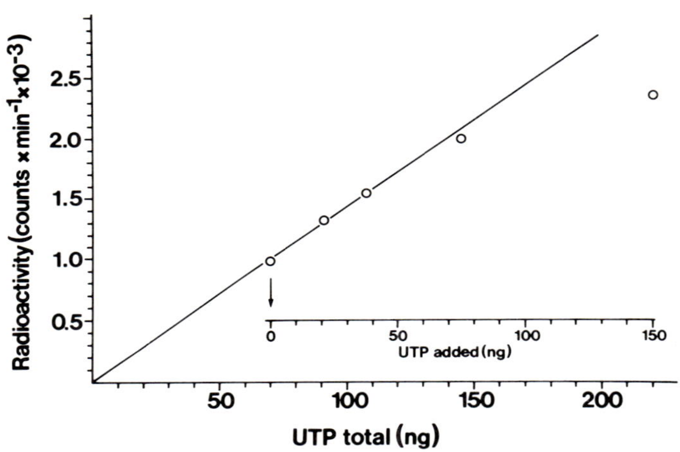

Figure 1 b.

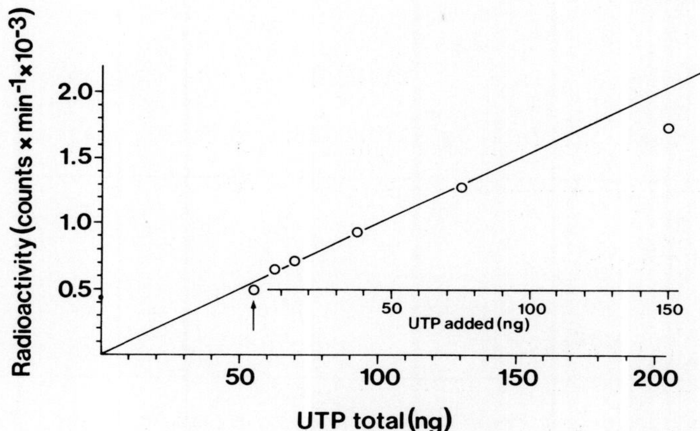

Figure 1 c.

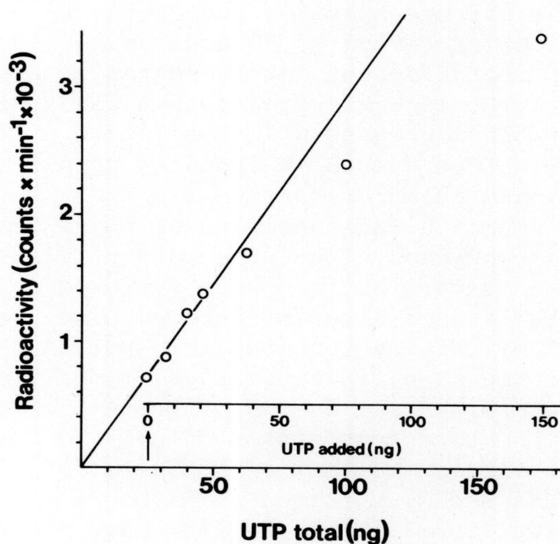

Figure 1 d.

incorporation of labeled ATP at low UTP concentrations it is reasonable to estimate the endogenous UTP content of the cell extract by extrapolation. In this way the cellular UTP content was determined to be 4.3, 7.6 and 8.0 ng per cell of 8, 15 and 35 mm length respectively (Table 2, line 1).

The uptake of labeled uridine into the cellular UTP pool was followed over 24 hours (Fig. 2). After a period of rapid uptake during the first five hours the amount of label remains fairly constant.

TABLE 1

ATP content per cell as a function of developmental stage

stage (mm length)	8	15	35
ATP (ng per cell)	13	65	130

The ATP content has been determined in aliquots taken from the same cellular extracts that have been used for UTP determinations. Experimental details are described under methods.

From this and similar results the average absolute radioactivity and the average specific radioactivity of the UTP during the incubation period of 24 hours have been calculated. A comparison of the different developmental stages under consideration (Table 2, line 2) reveals that the specific radioactivity of the UTP increases with the length of the cells; this increase might be due to an enhanced uptake of uridine through an enlarged cellular surface.

Given the specific radioactivity of the intracellular UTP the rate of incorporation of uridine into poly(A) RNA can be determined. Such determinations were performed on cells of the developmental stages described above. The results show that the amount of UMP incorporated into poly(A) RNA, as calculated from the specific activities of the precursor, declines during growth by a factor of three (Table 2, line 5). Supposing that the base composition of poly(A) RNA in Acetabularia is similar to that of hnRNA[17], 340, 170 and 110 pg of poly(A) RNA are synthesized in 24 hours by single cells at the respective stages (Table 2, line 6). These values represent polymerization rates of 7.8×10^6, 3.8×10^6 and

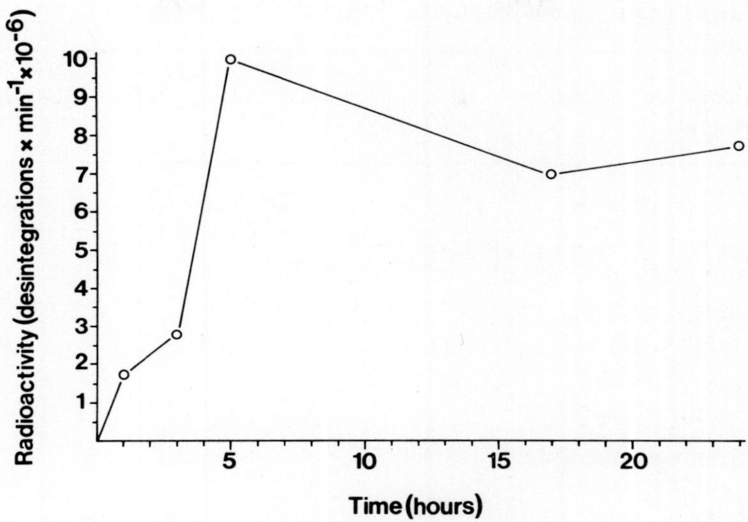

Figure 2. Incorporation of [^{3}H] uridine into cellular UTP as a function of the time of incubation.

Five times one hundred cells of the 35 mm stage have been incubated for the times indicated.

The details for the determination of radioactivity (dpm) are given in the methods section.

2.5 x 10^6 nucleotides per second per cell respectively (Table 2, line 8). Values for cells with maximal caps cannot be given. In this case it was not possible to obtain reliable determinations for the amount of UTP per cell because of the low rates of incorporation into poly {AU}. It is, however, evident that even in this late developmental stage poly(A) RNA is synthesized (Table 2, line 3).

TABLE 2

Calculations of the number of cistrons for poly(A) RNA transcribed in different developmental stages of *A. mediterranea*

Developmental stage (mm length)	8	15	35	cells with maximal caps
UTP per cell*(gram.10^{-9})*	4.3	7.6	8	--
Average specific activity of cellular UTP (dpm.$gram^{-1}$.10^{-12})	3.3	4.4	8	--
Poly(A) RNA synthesized (dpm.$cell^{-1}$.day^{-1})	470	308	371	227
UTP used for polymerization (gram.$cell^{-1}$.day^{-1}.10^{-12})	142	71	47	--
UMP incorporated into poly(A)RNA (gram.$cell^{-1}$.day^{-1}.10^{-12})	95	47	31	--
Nucleotides incorporated into poly(A) RNA (number.$cell^{-1}$.day^{-1}.10^{-11})	6.8	3.4	2.2	--
Nucleotides incorporated into poly(A) RNA (number.$cell^{-1}$.sec^{-1}.10^{-6})	7.8	3.8	2.5	--
Number of RNA polymerases simultaneously transcribing poly(A) RNA per cell (.10^{-5})**	7.8	3.8	2.5	--
Number of polymerase molecules per cistron***	100	100	100	--
Number of cistrons simultaneously transcribed (.10^{-3})	7.8	3.8	2.5	--

* *data of figures 1 b to d.*

** *based on the assumption that 10 nucleotides are polymerized per polymerase molecule per second at 18°C.*

*** *data from* [22].

DISCUSSION

The method introduced by Sasvári-Székely et al.[15] allows precise determinations of UTP even in the presence of perchloric acid extracts. Such extracts may inhibit the RNA polymerase reaction as was also the case in our experiments. Standardization of the assay reaction was achieved by addition of known amounts of UTP to the samples.

It has been shown that the size of the UTP pool doubles during the development from the 8 mm to the 35 mm stage. This is much less than the increase of the ATP content which is about tenfold during the same period. However, one has to take into consideration that this relatively small increase in the UTP pool might be supplemented by surplus increase in the pool of uridine diphosphate-sugars (K. Richter, unpublished results).

Besides the size of the pool, the specific activity of intracellular UTP also increases during the same period of development by a factor of two to three. This increase might be due to an enhanced uptake of uridine by the cell on the basis of an enlarged cellular surface. It is improbable that the uridine added to the medium (80 pg/ml) has an influence on the size of the UTP pools.

The knowledge of the specific activity of the intracellular UTP allowed the determination of the rate of synthesis of polyadenylated RNA. In this calculation the possibility that due to compartmentalization, different UTP pools with different turnover rates might exist in the cell[18], is not taken into account.

Keeping this in mind one may estimate semiquantitatively the number of genes for polyadenylated RNA transcribed at a given time. From the assumption that one RNA polymerase molecule polymerizes 10 nucleotides per second at 18°C[19,20] it can be deduced that 7.8×10^5, 3.8×10^5 and 2.5×10^5 polymerase molecules simultaneously synthesize polyadenylated RNA in the developmental stages under consideration (Table 2, line 9).

Given these data the number of genes transcribed at a distinct time can be derived if the average length of the transcripts and the distance between two polymerase molecules on the cistrons are known.

It is known from electron microscopical studies (S. Berger, unpublished results) that in *Acetabularia*, actively transcribed non-ribosomal RNA cistrons have an average chain length of about 5 µm and therefore may code for an RNA molecule of 5×10^6 daltons. From the cytosol we have obtained polyadenylated RNA with an average molecular weight of 1.5×10^6 daltons[10].

If one denies the possibility that a preferential polyadenylation of the smaller RNA molecules occurs in the nucleus it follows that the polyadenylated RNA in the cytosol should derive from nuclear precursor molecules of the above mentioned molecular weight. If so, the processing of this RNA then would either be rapid in comparison to rRNA processing[21] or polyadenylation would have to take place only after processing, since nuclear precursors of polyadenylated RNA have been obtained neither from whole cells nor from isolated nuclei. Although it seems likely that polyadenylated RNA originates from precursor molecules, these precursors do not substantially contribute to our preparations of polyadenylated RNA.

The following consideration, therefore, has been based on the average molecular weight of polyadenylated RNA especially if we assume that the distance between two RNA polymerase molecules will be the same in those regions of the gene whose transcripts are preserved and those which are lost.

The average distance between two RNA polymerase molecules on non-ribosomal cistrons is 150 nucleotides[22]. If we assume that this distance between two polymerases remains constant during development it then follows that 100 RNA polymerase molecules will be active on those regions of a gene which code for polyadenylated RNA. From this figure and the number of RNA polymerase molecules which simultaneously transcribe polyadenylated RNA in one nucleus, we can conclude that in the developmental stages under consideration 7.8×10^3, 3.8×10^3 and 2.5×10^3 genes for RNA destined to become polyadenylated are transcribed at the same time. That means there is a decrease in the rate of synthesis of polyadenylated RNA by about 70% during the vegetative phase.

Recently, we have shown that in the stage of early cap formation more than 3×10^4 rRNA cistrons are transcribed per nucleus[19]. Accordingly, the number of non-rRNA cistrons transcribed during late developmental stages is roughly one order of magnitude lower than that of the rRNA cistrons. This would still be valid if in *Acetabularia*, as is known from other organisms[23], part of the mRNA is not polyadenylated and therefore cannot be detected by the method of affinity chromatography.

While the rate of synthesis of polyadenylated RNA decreases during the vegetative phase by about 70% the rate of synthesis increases threefold in regenerating cells[9]. One might conclude from this comparison that after amputation of the stalk, the rate of synthesis of polyadenylated RNA is restored in the resulting regenerating cells up to a level which is characteristic of the very young developmental stages.

Of major importance is the proof that polyadenylated RNA is synthesized through at least the greater part of the vegetative phase as was shown in experiments with cells from an early (5mm) and from a late stage (maximal caps). This is a surprising result since cells of 15 mm length have already all the information necessary for complete morphogenesis in their cytoplasm.

Our experiments therefore raise the question as to whether the polyadenylated RNA synthesized in young and in old cells has the same or a different informational content.

ACKNOWLEDGEMENTS

The authors gratefully appreciate helpful discussions with Dr. Bill Cairns. The skilful experimental assistance of Mrs. Ina Hallmann and Mrs. Marion Schimborski is acknowledged.

REFERENCES

1. Hämmerling, J. (1932) Biol. Zentralbl. 52, 42-61.
2. Hämmerling, J. (1934) Roux Arch. Entwicklungsmech. 131, 1-81.
3. Hämmerling, J. (1963) Ann. Rev. Plant Physiol. 14, 65-92.
4. Spencer, T. and Harris, H. (1964) Bioch. J. 91, 282-286.
5. Zetsche, K. (1966) Biochim. Biophys. Acta 124, 332-338.
6. Bannwarth, H. and Schweiger, H. G. (1975) Proc. R. Soc. Lond. B. 188, 203-219.
7. Hämmerling, J. and Hämmerling, Ch. (1959) Planta 52, 516-527.
8. Schweiger, H. G. and Bremer, H. (1960) Exp. Cell Res. 20, 617-618.
9. Kloppstech, K. and Schweiger, H. G. (1973) Differentiation 1, 331-337.
10. Kloppstech, K. and Schweiger, H. G. (1975) Differentiation 4, 115-123.
11. Kloppstech, K. and Schweiger, H. G. (1976) Cytobiologie 13, 394-400.
12. Schweiger, H. G. (1969) Curr. Top. Microbiol. and Immunol. 50, 1-36.
13. Burgess, R. R. (1969) J. Biol. Chem. 244, 6160-6167.
14. Strehler, B. L. and Trotter, J. R. (1954) Methods in Bioch. Analysis 1, 341-356.
15. Sasvári-Székely, M., Vitéz, M., Staub, M. and Antoni, F. (1975) Biochim. Biophys. Acta 395, 221-228.
16. Klitzing, v. L. (1969) Protoplasma 68, 341-350.
17. Darnell, J. (1968) Bact. Rev. 32, 262-290.
18. Wiegers, Ul, Kramer, G., Klapproth, K. and Hilz, H. (1976) Eur. J. Biochem. 64, 535-540.

19. Kloppstech, K. and Schweiger, H. G. (1975) Protoplasma 83, 27-40.
20. Kafatos, F. C. (1972) Curr. Top. Develop. Biol. 7, 125-191.
21. Kloppstech, K., Richter, G. and Schweiger, H. G., submitted for publication.
22. Kloppstech, K., Berger, S. and Schweiger, H. G. (1976) J. Cell Biol. 70, 335a.
23. Milcarik, Ch., Price, R. and Penman, S. (1974) Cell 3, 1-10.

THE OCCURRENCE OF A 5'-METHYLTHIOADENOSINE NUCLEOSIDASE IN ACETABULARIA MEDITERRANEA

M. Yamakawa, N. Ikehara and H. G. Schweiger

Max-Planck-Institut für Zellbiologie
Wilhelmshaven, West Germany

SUMMARY

In *Acetabularia mediterranea*, an enzyme occurs which catalyzes the hydrolytic cleavage of 5'-methylthioadenosine (EC 3.2.2.-). The reaction products were identified as adenine and 5 -methylthioribose.

INTRODUCTION

Since the work of Shapiro and Mather[1] who first demonstrated the enzymatic decomposition of 5'-methylthioadenosine to adenine and 5 -methylthioribose in *Aerobacter aerogenes*, the presence of 5'-methylthioadenosine nucleosidase in other organisms has been reported. Duerre[2] purified this enzyme from *Escherichia coli* and showed that it catalyzes the hydrolytic cleavage of 5'-methylthioadenosine. The phosphate-dependent breakdown of 5'-methylthioadenosine has also been reported in rat ventral prostate[3]. Recently, Ferro et al.[4] have purified this enzyme 220-fold from E. coli. The role of 5'-methylthioadenosine nucleosidase in *Ochromonas malhamesis* has been also discussed by Sugimoto et al.[5].

As far as we know, there is no report of the presence of this enzyme in plant cells with the exception of *Ochromonas*. In preliminary experiments, we found that extracts from the unicellular green alga *Acetabularia mediterranea* contain an enzymatic activity that catalyzes hydrolytic cleavage of 5'-methylthioadenosine. The present paper deals with the occurrence and some properties of 5'-methylthioadenosine nucleosidase in *Acetabularia mediterranea*.

MATERIAL AND METHODS

Cells of Acetabularia mediterranea were grown in Erd-Schreiber medium under previously reported conditions[6-9]. The substrate, 5'-methylthioadenosine, was prepared from S-adenosyl-L-{methyl-^{14}C} methionine (SAM) (specific activity = 59 mCi/mmol) with some modification of the method described by Parks and Schlenk[10]. After incubation of SAM corresponding to 5 μCi in 50 mM phosphate buffer (pH 7.5) at 100° C for 30 min, the mixture was separated by paper chromatography (Whatman No. 1 paper) using an n-butanol: water: formic acid (77:13:10 V/V/V) system. The material of the spot having an Rf of 0.33 was identified as 5'-methylthioadenosine by assay for pentase[11] and sulfur[12,13], spectrophotometry, nuclear magnetic resonance spectroscopy and by mass spectrometry. The spot was cut into small pieces and eluted with water at 4° C for 30 hrs. The eluate was concentrated by lyophilization and used as the enzymatic substrate.

Cytosol, which was obtained by a centrifugation method[14], was used as the source of enzyme. The acidic cytosol was adjusted to pH 8.6 with 0.2 N NaOH, and the protein content was adjusted to 40 μg protein per ml before the enzymatic assay.

The standard reaction mixture consisted of 5 μl of {^{14}C}-5'-methylthioadenosine, 15 μl of enzyme and 45 μl of 50 mM glycine-NaOH buffer, pH 8.6, containing 15 mM mercaptoethanol. The reaction was carried out at 37° C for 15 min and stopped by heating at 100° C for 3 min. Aliquots of 20 μl of the mixture were spotted on the paper and developed by the solvent system described above. Reference samples of 5 -methylthioribose prepared by the method of Shapiro and Mather[1] and adenine were also co-chromatographed. The spot of {^{14}C}-5 -methylthioribose, which was located by a Radio Scanner (Berthold, Varian Aerograph), was excised, and the radioactivity was counted by a liquid scintillation counter (Packard).

Protein content was determined according to the method of Lowry et al.[15].

RESULTS AND DISCUSSION

During the course of studies on the metabolism of S-adenosylmethionine in Acetabularia cells, it was found that crude extracts from A. mediterranea catalyzed enzymatic decomposition of 5'-methylthioadenosine which is one of the degradation products of S-adenosylmethionine. As shown in Fig. 1, 5'-methylthioadenosine disappeared completely during the incubation in the presence of crude extracts from

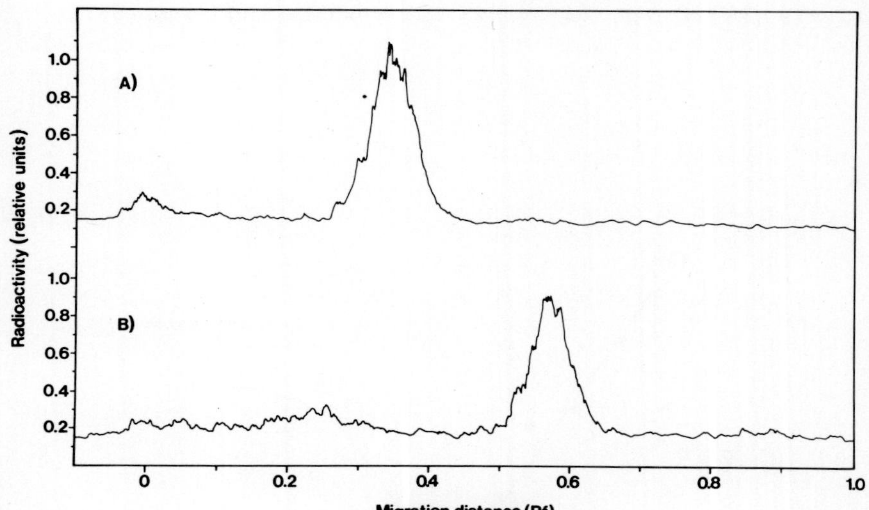

Figure 1. Paper chromatographic separation of 5'-methylthioadenosine and 5 -methylthioribose.

A) 0.04 uCi of [^{14}C] 5'-methylthioadenosine

B) Reaction product (5-methylthioribose) after incubation of [^{14}C] 5'-methylthioadenosine with a homegenate from A. mediterranea.

Acetabularia cells. On the other hand, a new radioactive peak with a Rf value of 0.56 appeared. No conversion of 5'-methylthioadenosine was observed if the extracts were treated at 100° C for 5 min. This indicates the enzymatic nature of conversion.

Since this conversion might be due to microbial contamination, control experiments were performed with axenic cells [16-17] with the same results.

The product of the enzymatic conversion was identified as 5 -methylthioribose by the following criteria:

1. If methyl-labelled 5'-methylthioadenosine was used as substrate, non-labelled adenine was detected as one

product.

2. The labelled product indicated a chromatographic behavior identical with that of chemically prepared 5'methylthio-ribose in paper chromatography using two different solvent systems; n-butanol: water: formic acid and 64% ethanol.
3. The tests for both sulfur and reducing sugar were positive.

The formation of 5'-methylthioribose and the disappearance of 5'-methylthioadenosine during incubation proceeded linearly for 20 min (Fig. 2). The results indicate the

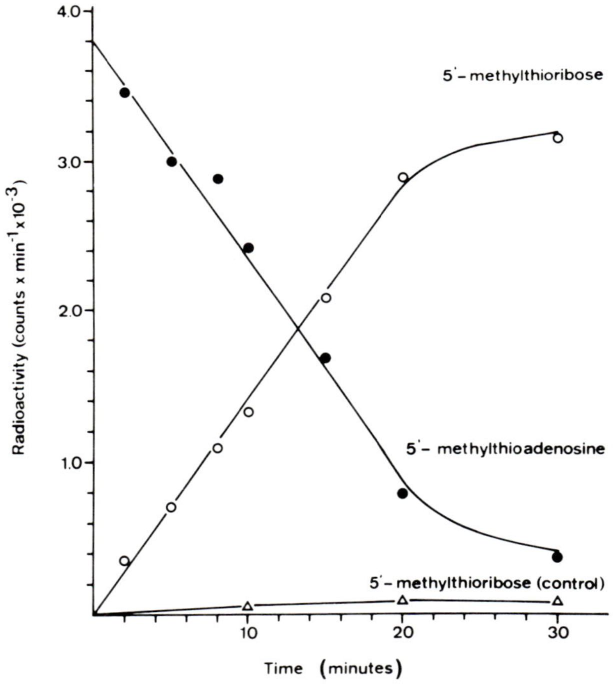

Figure 2. Stoichiometry of the 5'-methylthioadenosine nucleosidase reaction. The reaction mixture contained 80 ul of buffer, 30 ul of [^{14}C]5'-methylthioadenosine (0.059 uCi) and 40 ul of homogenate (3.6 ug protein). Assays were performed in 20 ul aliquots. In the control the enzyme was denatured by heating.

occurrence of 5'-methylthioadenosine nucleosidase in the green alga Acetabularia.

In a number of properties, the enzyme is different from that of other organisms. Although the metabolic pathway of 5 -methylthioribose remains unknown, it has been suggested that the 5'-methylthioadenosine nucleosidase plays a role in the salvage and recycling of adenine[4]. Recently, Sugimoto *et al.*[5] suggested that 5'-methylthioadenosine might be metabolized to S-adenosylmethionine and L-methionine via 5 -methylthioribose. S-adenosylmethionine is considered to be the major donor of methyl groups which may play a role in modifying the bases in RNA, such as those of tRNA, during the development of the cell.

ACKNOWLEDGEMENTS

The authors appreciate the help of Drs. W. Schäfer and J. Sonnenbichler, Martinsried, in identifying 5'-methylthioadenosine and of Dr. D. M. Zellmer in preparing the manuscript.

REFERENCES

1. Schapiro, S. K. and Mather, A. N. (1958) J. Biol. Chem. 233, 631-633.
2. Duerre, J. A. (1962) J. Biol. Chem. 237, 3737-3741.
3. Pegg, A. E. and Williams-Aschman, H. G. (1969) Biochem. J. 115, 241-247.
4. Ferro, A. J., Barrett, A. and Schapiro, S. K. (1976) Biochem. Biophys. Acta 438, 487-494.
5. Sugimoto, Y., Toraya, T. and Fukui, S. (1976) Arch. Microbiol. 108, 175-182.
6. Hämmerling, J. (1931) Biol. Zentralbl. 51, 633-647.
7. Hämmerling, J. (1944) Arch. Prostistenk. 97, 7-56.
8. Beth, K. Z. (1953) Naturforsch. 8b, 334-342.
9. Schweiger, H. G. (1969) Curr. Top. Microbiol. Immunol. 50, 1-36.
10. Parks, L. W. and Schlenk, F. (1958) J. Biol. Chem. 230, 295-305.
11. Mejbaum, W. (1939) Z. physiol. Chem. 258, 117-120.
12. Winegard, H. M. and Toennies, G. (1948) Science 108, 506-507.
13. Toennies, G. and Kolb, J. J. (1951) Anal. Chem. 23, 823-826.
14. Schweiger, H. G. (1966) Planta 68, 247-255.
15. Lowry, O. H., Rosebrough, N. J., Farr, A. L. and Randall, R. J. (1951) J. Biol. Chem. 193, 265-275.

16. Gibor, A. and Izawa, M. (1963) Proc. Natl. Acad. Sci. USA 50, 1164-1169.
17. Berger, S. (1967) Doctoral Thesis, University of Cologne.

BASE ANALYSIS OF tRNA FROM *ACETABULARIA MEDITERRANEA*

Walter Schmidt, Helga Kersten and Hans-Georg Schweiger

Institut für Physiologische Chemie der Universität
Erlangen-Nürnberg
and
Max-Planck-Institut für Zellbiologie
Wilhelmshaven, West Germany

ABSTRACT

The base composition of tRNA from *Acetabularia mediterranea* was analyzed in cells of an early and late stage of development. In the late stage additional nucleosides were found. The percentage of dihydrouridine and ribothymidine was increased more than fourfold.

INTRODUCTION

Differentiation of a cell with a specialized function is characterized by changes in the spectrum of proteins synthesized by the cell. Regulation of translation by tRNA has been proposed (Littauer and Inouye[1]) as one of several regulatory mechanisms which control differential expression of particular groups of genes. The tRNAs from eukaryotic cells, when compared with prokaryotic tRNAs have a higher content of modified nucleosides, e.g. methylated nucleosides, dihydrouridine and pseudouridine. A modulation in the structure of specific tRNAs by modifying enzymes may influence regulatory and functional properties of these molecules at different stages during development.

Here we present the first base analysis of tRNA from *Acetabularia mediterranea* at two defined stages of development.

MATERIALS AND METHODS

Cells of *Acetabularia mediterranea* were grown as described previously[2]. Nucleic acids were extracted by the phenol method from (a) *A. mediterranea* cells, having an average length of 15 mm (without caps) and (b) from cells among which about 20-60% had developed caps. From the nucleic acid extracts tRNAs were purified over DEAE cellulose and by subsequent polyacrylamide gel electrophoresis. The base analysis of tRNA was performed after hydrolysis to nucleosides by the ^{3}H postlabeling-technique and two-dimensional thin-layer chromatography according to Randerath et al.[3].

In some experiments the radioactive labeled nucleoside derivatives were scraped from the plates, eluted and counted in a liquid scintillation spectrometer in order to quantitate the types of bases present.

RESULTS

The digest of tRNA from cells of the early stage of development (no caps) was analysed and the following modified nucleosides, beside the major nucleosides, have been identified on the fluorographic map (Fig. 1a): 1-methyladenosine (m^1A), 5-methylcytosine (m^5C), 1-methylguanosine (m^1G), dihydrouridine (hU), 5-methyluridine = ribothymidine (rT), pseudouridine (ψ), and pseudouridine-degradation product (ψD). Other spots designated as B are background spots; they do not represent compartments of tRNA (Randerath et al.[3]).

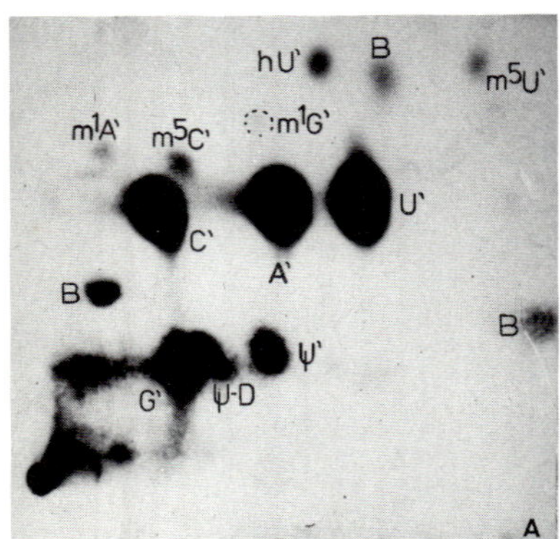

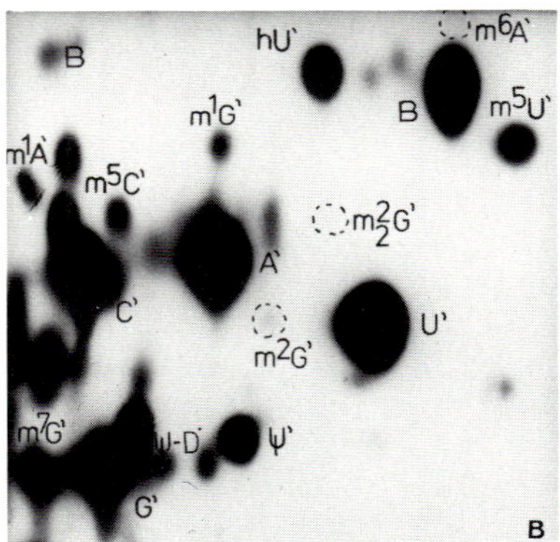

Figure 1. Maps of ^{3}H-labeled digests of A. mediterranea tRNAs on cellulose. The abbreviations for the corresponding modified bases in tRNA are given under results. tRNA was isolated from cells

a. of 15 mm length

b. of the stage of early cap formation.

In addition to the above, other modified nucleosides were detected in the digests of tRNA from the late stage of development (Fig. 1b). These additional nucleosides included 7-methylguanosine (m^7G), 2-methylguanosine (m^2G), 2-dimethylguanosine (m^2_2G) and 6-methyladenosine. The latter two modified nucleosides are clearly visible on the original film (circled areas) but cannot be seen in the photograph.

The results of quantitative measurements are summarized in Table 1. Significant differences were found in the content of ψ, hU and rT from early and late developmental stage tRNAs. In tRNA from cells developing caps the amount of ψ is lower than in undifferentiated cells. On the other hand, hU and rT are at lower levels before and much higher levels after differentiation. m^7G, m^2G, m^5C and m^2_2G, if present in tRNAs from undifferentiated cells, occur in minute amounts below 0.1 mol/% that are not detectable by this method. Since m^1A can undergo rearrangement to m^6A during hydrolysis, it is questionable whether m^6A is indeed a constituent of tRNA from A. mediterranea.

DISCUSSION

Our first results on the base composition of tRNA from A. mediterranea show that the minor components present in tRNA of this organism after development are similar to those found in other eukaryotic tRNAs, e.g. rat liver 4S RNA (Randerath et al.[4]). These results agree well with hitherto known data on the modification of eukaryotic tRNA (Dirheimer et al.[5]). Moreover, the results show that total tRNA from developed cells have higher amounts of hU and of rT than undifferentiated cells. Mitochondrial tRNAs are known to have a rather low content of rT (Randerath et al.[4]). Although cells 15 mm in length contain high amounts of mitochondria the low rT content in total tRNAs of these cells which is only one fifth of that in differentiated cells can hardly be explained solely by contamination of cytosol tRNA with mitochondria tRNA.

Prokaryotic tRNAs have in general one rT located in the tetranucleotide sequence GTψC which occupy positions 24-21 from the 3'-terminus. This sequence was thought to be common to all known tRNAs involved in peptide chain elongation at the ribosome (Dirheimer et al.[6]). It has been shown, however, that the $tRNA^{Glu}_3$ and $tRNA^{Lys}_2$ (Marcu and Dudock[7]) from rabbit liver and $tRNA^{Gly}$ and several $tRNAs^{Thr}$ from wheat embryo are devoid of rT.

The sequence TψCG has been implicated in the binding of tRNA to ribosomes (Ofengand and Henes[8]). It is therefore possible that the modification during development of

TABLE 1

Base analysis of tRNA from A. mediterranea cells
A. cells of 15 mm length
B. cells of the stage of early cap formation

Base	Mole % A	Mole % B
G	27.1	27.7
C	23.2	25.2
A	22.6	20.7
U	24.5	21.2
m^7G	undetectable	0.43
ψ	2.5	1.42
m^2G	undetectable	0.18
m^1A	0.16	0.28
(m^6A)	undetectable	0.24
m^5C	0.20	0.38
m^1G	0.10	0.30
m_2^2G	undetectable	0.16
hU	0.29	1.32
T	0.16	0.84

eukaryotic organisms of the U in the sequence UψCG to rT influences the rate of protein synthesis during different cellular stages of development.

Recently Marcu and Dudock[7] described a tRNA-dependent protein synthesizing system of wheat germ in which the rT lacking tRNAs from wheat germ were used to translate several viral RNAs. The rT lacking tRNAs were found to translate the viral RNA at a much faster rate than the tRNAs in which U had been converted to rT by the S-adenosylmethionine dependent tRNA (uracil-5) methyltransferase from E. coli. Whether the modulation of the structure of tRNA by the methylation of uridine to rT plays a regulatory role in protein synthesis during development has to be clarified by further experiments.

ACKNOWLEDGEMENT

The authors are grateful to Dr. Bill Cairns and Dr. Klaus Kloppstech for valuable discussions. This work was supported by the Deutsche Forschungsgemeinschaft (grant Ke 98/11).

REFERENCES

1. Littauer, U. Z. and Inouye, H. (1973) Ann. Rev. Biochem. 42, 429.
2. Schweiger, H. G. (1969) Curr. Top. Microbiol. Immunol. 50, 1.
3. Randerath, E., Yu, C.-T. and Randerath, K. (1972) Anal. Biochem. 48, 172.
4. Randerath, E., Li-Li, Chia, S. Y., Morris, H. P. and Randerath, K. (1974) Biochem. Biophys. Acta 366, 159.
5. Dirheimer, G., Keith, G., Weissenbach, J. and Martin, R. (1976) Conference on the "Synthesis, Structure and Chemistry of tRNA and their Components," 13-17 Sept. 1976, Dymaczewo near Poznan (Poland).
6. Dirheimer, G., Ebel, J. P., Bonnet, J., Gangloff, J., Keith, G., Krebs, B., Kuntzel, B., Roy, A., Weissenbach, J. and Werner, C. (1972) Biochimie 54, 127.
7. Marcu, K. B. and Dudock, B. S. (1976) Nature 261, 159.
8. Ofengand, J. and Henes, C. (1969) J. Biol. Chem. 244, 6241.

II ENZYMES AND BIOSYNTHETIC PATHWAYS

THE INTRACELLULAR DISTRIBUTION OF MALATE DEHYDROGENASE ISOENZYMES IN ACETABULARIA

Ursula Rahmsdorf

Institut für Pflanzenphysiologie und Zellbiologie
Freie Universität
Berlin, West Germany

SUMMARY

The NADH dependent malate dehydrogenase occurs in *Acetabularia mediterranea* and *Acetabularia cliftonii* in the form of four and three isoenzymes respectively. More than 95% of the total enzyme activity sediment with the particulate fraction of the cell. The chloroplast and the mitochondrial fraction of the cell have different isoenzymes and, in addition, the isoenzyme complements in organelles differ from one species of *Acetabularia* to the other.

INTRODUCTION

Nuclear transplantation experiments yield information on both the influence of the nucleus on the heterologous cytoplasm, and the effects of the cytoplasm on the nucleus. A favorite cell for such transplantation experiments, is *Acetabularia* since the nucleus is localized in a well defined part of the cell and is easily transferred from one cell to another[13,28]. In this organism it has been demonstrated that proteins of chloroplast membranes and of chloroplast ribosomes are encoded in the nuclear genome[1,18].

A prerequisite for a meaningful interpretation of transplantation experiments is a difference of organelle specific proteins in the two investigated species. Because the location of the genes for most of the mitochondrial proteins is unknown, we searched for a mitochondrial protein differing in two species of *Acetabularia*. The NADH-dependent malate dehydrogenase (L-malate: NAD oxidoreductase 1. 1. 1. 37) was chosen for two reasons: i) it is an enzyme of the citric acid cycle and should therefore be localized in the mitochondria,

ii) the isoenzyme patterns of malate dehydrogenase in various species of Acetabularia are quite different[3,27,29].

In this paper we report that indeed the NADH-dependent malate dehydrogenase found in the mitochondria of Acetabularia mediterranea and Acetabularia cliftonii occured in isoenzyme patterns which were species specific. Within the same species, the mitochondria and chloroplasts carried different isoenzymes.

MATERIALS AND METHODS

Cells of Acetabularia mediterranea and Acetabularia cliftonii were grown in "Erdschreiber" medium at 21° C exposing the cells to light of about 2400 lux for 10 hours and to dark for 14 hours[14,28].

Isolation of chloroplasts and mitochondria

The cells were washed several times or brushed and then homogenized in isolation buffer (6.7 mM phosphate, 0.33 M sucrose, 2 mM EDTA, 50 mM 2-(N-morpholino)ethanesulfonic acid, 0.05% β-mercaptoethanol pH 7.1) in a Potter Elvehjem glass homogenizer using a loose pestle[17]. After filtration through 8 layers of gauze the homogenate was centrifuged at 200 g for 90 seconds. Chloroplasts were sedimented at 1000 g for 15 min. The chloroplasts were washed 2-3 times with isolation buffer. The mitochondria were sedimented at 15,000 g for 15 min. and washed twice.

Tests of enzyme activities

NADH dependent malate dehydrogenase. The enzyme activity was measured by following spectrophotometrically the reduction of malate to oxaloacetate[4,22].

NADPH dependent malate dehydrogenase. A measure of enzyme activity was the oxidation of NADPH during the reduction of malate to oxaloacetate. The reaction was followed at 340 mμ[16].

Cytochrome oxidase. The activity of cytochrome oxidase was measured spectrophotometrically according to Wharton and Tzagoloff[32].

Isoenzyme pattern

The separation of the malate dehydrogenase isoenzyme was performed by the polyacrylamide gel electrophoresis technique of Davis[9]. For electrophoresis we used an Ortec electrophoresis equipment operated at 300 V, 45 mA and 300 pulses per second. After electrophoresis, the malate dehydrogenase isoenzymes were stained by the nitro BT technique[11].

Chlorophyll, protein - determination

The chlorophyll was determined according to Arnon[2] and the protein measured by the method of Lowry et al.[20] using crystallized bovine serum albumin as a standard.

RESULTS

1. Isoenzymes of MDH in homogenates of *Acetabularia mediterranea* and *Acetabularia cliftonii*

The NADH dependent MDH activity of *Acetabularia* was resolved into several distinct isoenzymes by polyacrylamide gel electrophoresis (Fig. 1). Cells were homogenized and cell debris sedimented at 200 g for 90 seconds. All MDH activity remained in the supernatant. When the organelles were separated from the supernatant at 15,000 g for 20 minutes, 95% of the MDH activity sedimented with the organelles. The isoenzyme pattern of *Acetabularia* was species specific (Fig. 1). In *Acetabularia mediterranea* four isoenzyme groups were distinguishable (A, B, C and D according to their electrophoretic mobility) whereas *Acetabularia cliftonii* developed three isoenzyme groups (A', B' and C'). The isoenzymes A and B from *Acetabularia mediterranea* corresponded, in their electrophoretic mobility, to the isoenzymes A' and B' from *Acetabularia cliftonii*. C' from *Acetabularia cliftonii* moved faster in the gel than C from *Acetabularia mediterranea*. The isoenzyme D of *Acetabularia mediterranea* was absent in the pattern resolved from extracts of *Acetabularia cliftonii*.

2. Preparative separation of the MDH isoenzymes and biochemical characterization

A purification procedure for two isoenzymes of *Acetabularia mediterranea* is summarized in table 1.

The cell debris of the cell homogenate was spun down and the supernatant was subsequently homogenized in a Yeda pressure cell at 1800 psi. Total protein was precipitated by ammonium sulfate at 0.8 saturation. After extensive dialysis, the protein was chromatographed on DEAE cellulose. With a linear gradient of sodium phosphate (0.02-0.1 M) two peaks with MDH activity were eluted. With higher salt concentrations, no further MDH activity could be eluted. Peak I was eluted at 0.026 M salt, peak II at 0.056 M (Fig. 2 a).

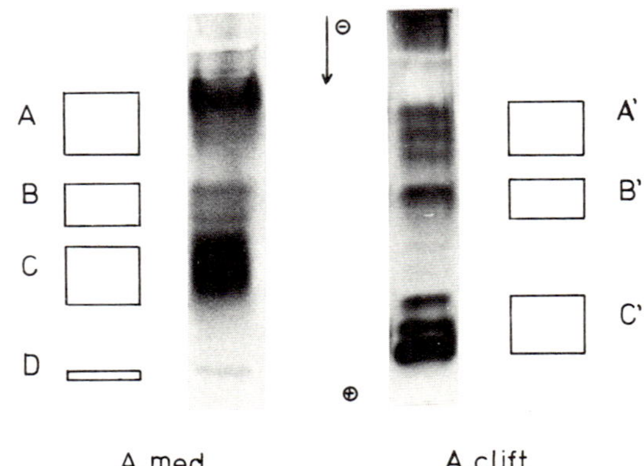

Figure 1. The isoenzyme pattern of NADH dependent malate dehydrogenase from Acetabularia mediterranea and Acetabularia cliftonii.

200 cells each were homogenized in 3 ml isolation buffer, cell debris was sedimented, and 20 ul of the supernatant were analysed by polyacrylamide gel electrophoresis for 1.5 hours at 4° C.

A similar procedure using an extract of Acetabularia cliftonii, resolved three peaks on DEAE cellulose: peak I was eluted at 0.04 M, peak II at 0.095 M and peak III at 0.125 M phosphate (Fig. 2 b).

After DEAE cellulose chromatography, an analysis of the various MDH fractions by polyacrylamide gel electrophoresis revealed that the column chromatography resulted in a separation of the MDH into distinct isoenzymes (Fig. 3). Fraction I from Acetabularia mediterranea contained mainly isoenzyme A and small amounts of isoenzyme B. Fraction II contained isoenzyme C and traces of isoenzyme B.

Fraction I from Acetabularia cliftonii included the isoenzymes A' and B'. In the middle fraction II all three isoenzymes were detectable whereas fraction III contained isoenzyme C' almost exclusively.

After DEAE cellulose chromatography, the MDH activity in fraction I and II from Acetabularia mediterranea was enriched by factors of 56 and 20, respectively, as compared to the activity of the cell homogenate (Table 1).

Figure 2 (overleaf). DEAE cellulose chromatography of NADH dependent malate dehydrogenase from Acetabularia mediterranea (a) and Acetabularia cliftonii (b).

a. 500 cells without cap were homogenized in 20 ml isolation buffer, cell debris removed by centrifugation, and the organelles destroyed by pressure release with 1800 psi in a Yeda pressure cell. The enzyme was precipitated by ammonium sulfate at 0.8 saturation, dissolved in 25 ml 0.005 M sodium phosphate buffer pH 7.1 containing 0.05% mercaptoethanol, and dialysed extensively against this buffer. The enzyme was applied to a DEAE cellulose column (DE 52 Whatman, 1.5 x 12 cm) after which the column was washed with 30 ml sodium phosphate buffer[2] and malate dehydrogenase activity eluted with a gradient of sodium phosphate buffer 250 ml, 0.02-0.1 M). 2.5 ml fractions were collected, and the NADH-MDH activity, the protein content, and the conductivity determined.

b. 750 cells without cap were homogenized in 15 ml isolation buffer and processed as described in 2 a. The elution conditions of the column were: 25 ml volume of enzyme solution applied, followed by 30 ml phosphate buffer, and 250 ml of a sodium phosphate gradient (0.02-0.1 M). In addition, 150 ml of a sodium phosphate gradient (0.1-0.15 M) were used as the last step.

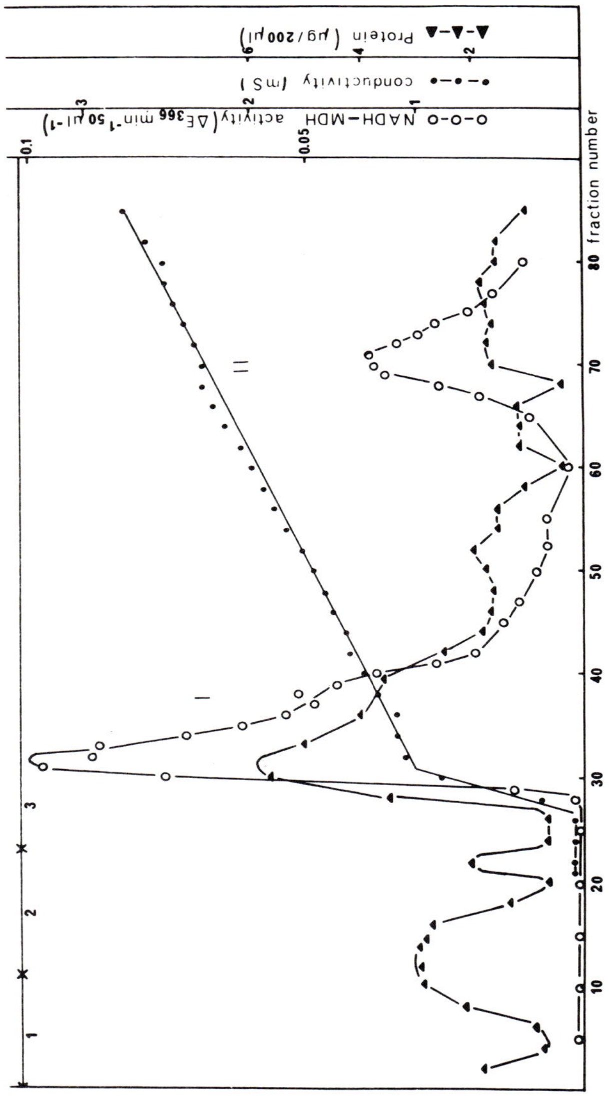

o-o-o NADH-MDH activity (ΔE_{366} min^{-1} 50 µl^{-1})
•-•-• conductivity (mS)
▲-▲-▲ Protein (µg/200µl)
fraction number
I
II

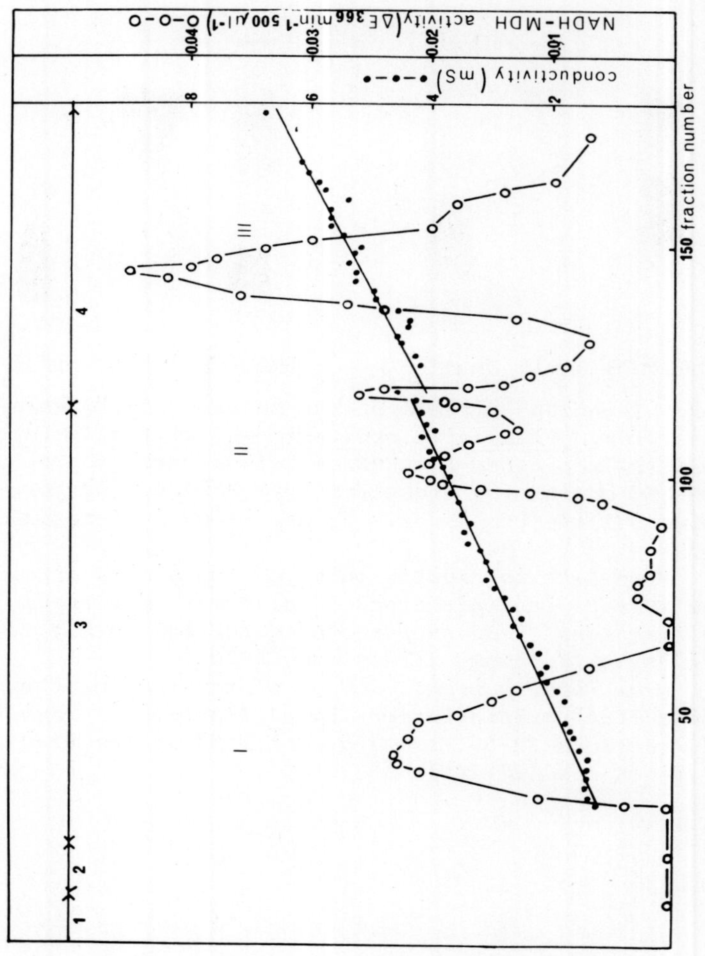

fraction number
50
100
150
conductivity (mS)
2
4
6
8
NADH-MDH activity (ΔE 366 min-1 500 µl-1)
0.01
0.02
0.03
0.040
I
II
III
1
2
3
4

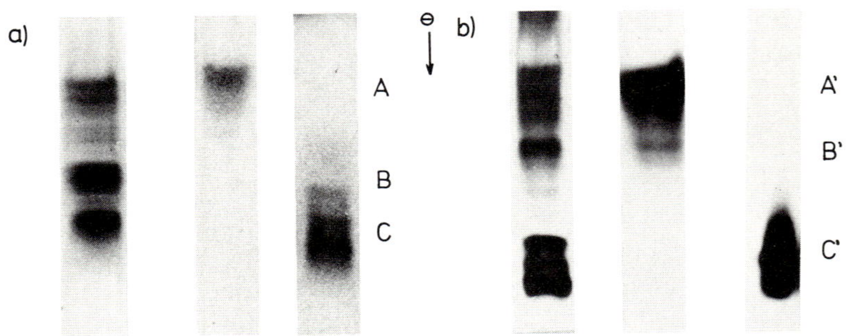

Figure 3. Isoenzyme pattern of the malate dehydrogenase fractions from Acetabularia mediterranea (a) and Acetabularia cliftonii (b) separated by DEAE cellulose chromatography. The NADH-MDH containing fractions were analysed by polyacrylamide gel electrophoresis as described in Materials and Methods.

a. From left to right: 10 ul of the sample after ammonium sulfate precipitation; 50 ul fraction I enzyme (pooled fractions 27-35 prepared as described in Fig. 2 a); 50 ul fraction II enzyme (fractions 66-75).

b. From left to right: 10 ul of the sample after ammonium sulfate precipitation; 50 ul fraction I enzyme (pooled fractions 33-55 from Fig. 2 b); 50 ul fraction III enzyme (fractions 137-160).

TABLE 1

Purification of NADH dependent malate dehydrogenase from Acetabularia mediterranea

Purification procedure	Total NADH-MDH mUnits	Total protein mg	Specific activity mU/mg prot.	Purification factor
1 crude extract	70.990	36	1.970	1
2 $(NH_4)_2SO_4$ precipitation (0-80%)	89.500	33	2.730	1.4
3 dialysis	85.725	9.5	9.190	4.7
4 DEAE cellulose chromatography				
fraction I	3.294	0.03	109.800	56
fraction II	3.148	0.07	43.800	22

500 Acetabularia mediterranea cells without caps were homogenized and processed for malate dehydrogenase purification as described in Fig. 2 a.

The two isoenzymes A and C of *Acetabularia mediterranea* separated by DEAE cellulose chromatography, were characterized biochemically.

Molecular weight. Both isoenzymes had the same molecular weight of 40,000 daltons. This was estimated by chromatography on a Sephadex G 200 column equilibrated with standard proteins (cytochrome c, ovalbumin, and bovine albumin).

pH optimum. The pH optimum for the two fractions was 7 to 7.2.

Stability of the enzymes. Two different experiments were performed to determine the stability of the isoenzymes: the enzymes were preincubated at 30° C for various lengths of time, and then tested for enzyme activity (Fig. 4 a); or the enzymes were preincubated at various temperatures for 10 minutes, and then tested (Fig. 4 b). Both kinds of experiments indicated lower heat stability for enzyme I than for enzyme II.

Substrate affinity. A Lineweaver Burk plot of the reaction velocities of the isoenzymes versus the substrate concentration is shown in Figure 5. The curves indicated no normal Michaelis Menten kinetics. The affinity of the two isoenzymes for oxaloacetate was different.

To summarize, the isoenzymes A and C from *Acetabularia mediterranea* have similar molecular weights and pH optima, but differ in their electrophoretic mobility, in their temperature sensitivity, and in the affinity for their substrate oxaloacetate.

3. Compartmentation of the isoenzymes from *Acetabularia mediterranea* and *Acetabularia cliftonii*

To examine the distribution of the isoenzymes of the NADH dependent malate dehydrogenase within the cell, a separation of the particulate fraction into mitochondria and chloroplasts was attempted.

By differential centrifugation the particulate fraction of the cell homogenate was partially resolved into a fraction enriched with mitochondria and another one enriched with chloroplasts.

After removal of the cell debris a fraction containing most of the chloroplasts was obtained by centrifugation of the homogenate at 1000 g for 15 minutes[26]. From the supernatant the mitochondria were pelleted at 15,000 g for 15 minutes[7].

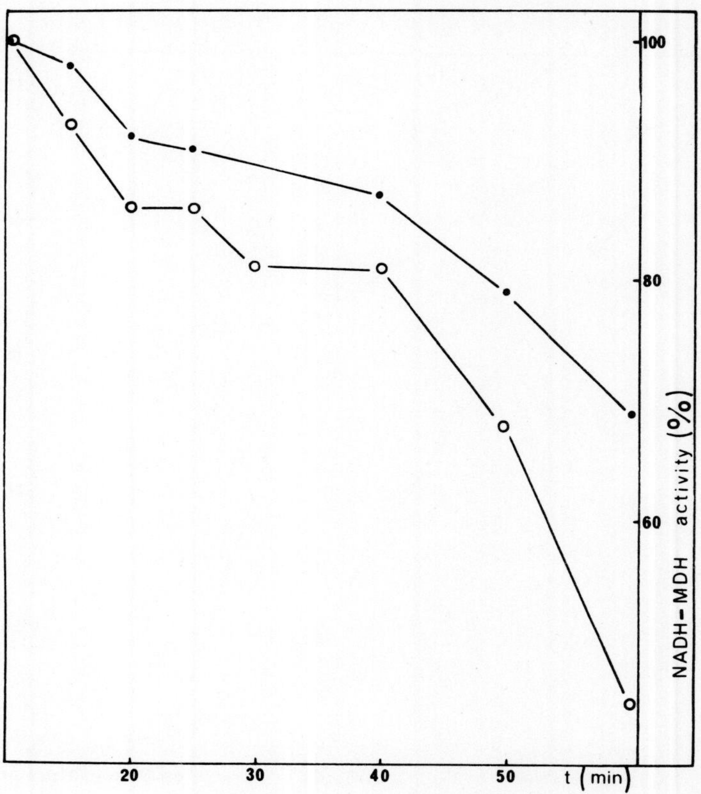

Figure 4 a. Thermal stability of the NADH dependent MDH activity from Acetabularia mediterranea.

Fraction I (· — · — ·) and fraction II (o — o — o) enzyme were prepared as described in Fig. 2 a.

The samples were kept at 30° C for various times as indicated, chilled, and assayed for residual malate dehydrogenase activity at 25° C.

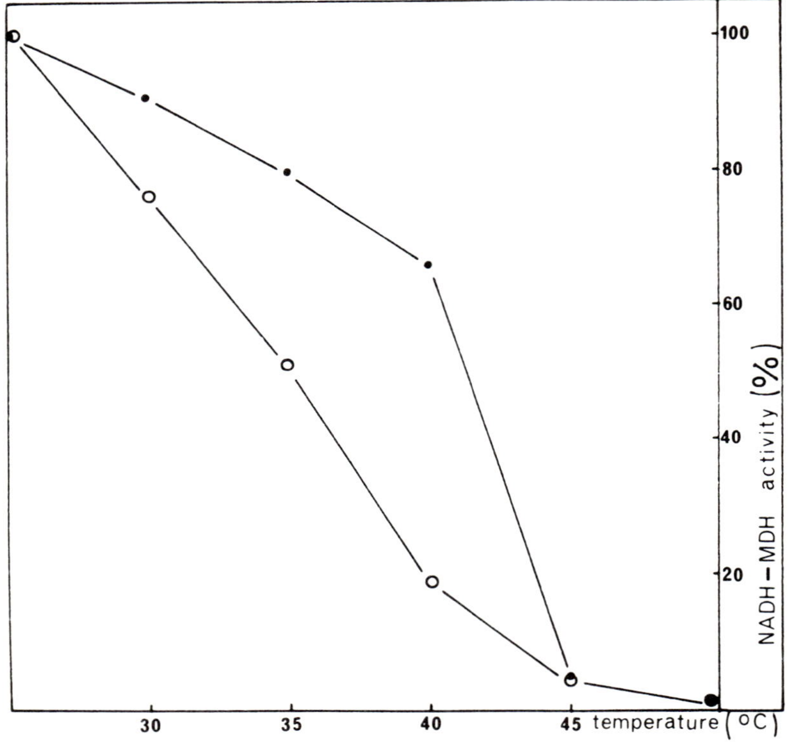

Figure 4 b. Thermal stability of the NADH dependent MDH activity from Acetabularia mediterranea.

Fraction I (· — · — ·) and fraction II (o — o — o) enzyme were prepared as described in Fig. 2 a.

The samples were kept at the temperatures indicated for 10 minutes, chilled, and assayed for residual enzyme activity at 25° C.

The residual enzyme activity is plotted as % of the untreated control.

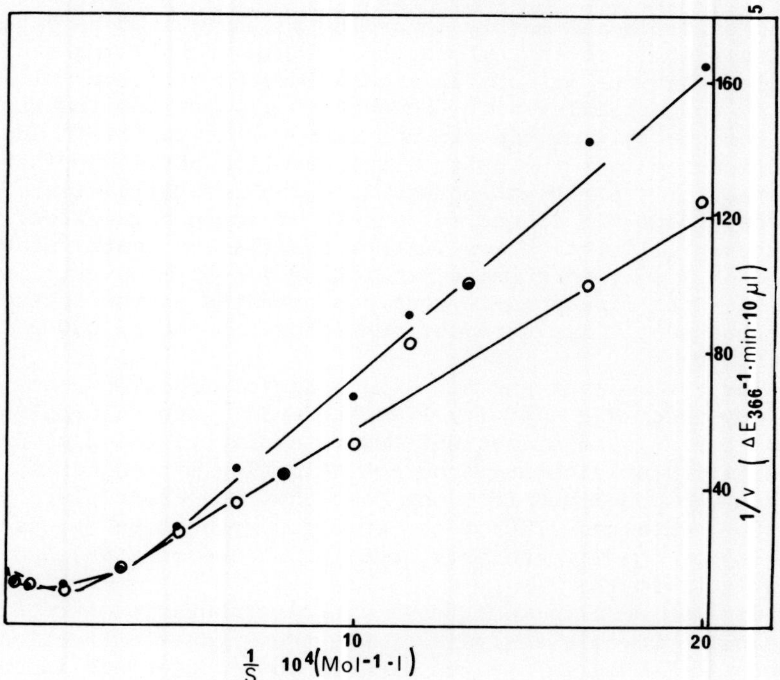

Figure 5. Lineweaver Burk plot.

The velocity of the NADH-MDH reaction was determined under normal assay conditions using various oxaloacetate concentrations. Enzyme fraction I (· — · — ·) and fraction II (o — o — o) were prepared as described in Fig. 2 a.

A characterization of the two fractions according to specific constituents of the cell organelles (chlorophyll and NADPH dependent MDH for the chloroplasts[15,26] and cytochrome oxidase for the mitochondria) is summarized in Table 2.

The mitochondrial fraction was nearly pure, only 3-6% of the cell chloroplasts were found in this fraction. On the other hand the fraction containing the chloroplasts was contaminated considerably with mitochondria varying from 10 to 75% as estimated from the cytochrome oxidase content.

A further purification of the chloroplasts was, therefore, attempted by centrifugation of a cell homogenate on a discontinuous sucrose density gradient (Fig. 6). For example, the chloroplasts of *Acetabularia cliftonii* were separated into four distinct bands mainly according to their starch content[19]. The examination of the cytochrome oxidase in this gradient revealed that the mitochondria cosedimented with the chloroplasts, in particular with the densest chloroplast fractions.

Because this method did not improve the purity to any significant extent the chloroplast fraction obtained after differential centrifugation was used for identification of the NADH dependent MDH isoenzyme pattern of these organelles. The mitochondrial fraction was further purified by centrifugation on a 0.64 M sucrose cushion at 3,800 g for 45 minutes. In this step the mitochondria were concentrated at the interphase and subsequently harvested by centrifugation at 15,000 g for 20 minutes.

The chloroplast and the mitochondrial fraction contained NADH dependent MDH activity (Tables 2, 3). The chloroplast fraction displayed a distinct enzyme activity, in addition to the activity originating from contaminating mitochondria. This may be concluded from the fact that the chloroplast fraction contained 1/10 of the specific cytochrome oxidase activity of the mitochondria, but 1/2 of the malate dehydrogenase activity.

Similar results were found with *Acetabularia cliftonii*. The electrophoretic analysis of the two organelle fractions of both *Acetabularia* species clearly showed distinct isoenzyme patterns which were species specific (Fig. 7). The chloroplasts from *Acetabularia mediterranea* contained the isoenzymes A, B and D whereas in the mitochondrial fraction the most prominent enzyme was C. In *Acetabularia cliftonii* the isoenzyme C' belonged almost exclusively to the chloroplast fraction. The mitochondria of this species were characterized by the isoenzymes A' and B'.

TABLE 2

Enzyme characterization of a chloroplast and of a mitochondrial fraction from *Acetabularia mediterranea*

	Protein mg	Chlorophyll ug	NADPH-MDH mUnits	Specific activity mU/mg	Cyt. oxidase ΔE_{550}/5min	Specific activity ΔE_{550}/5min/mg	NADH-MDH $mU \cdot 10^{-3}$	Specific activity mU/mg
chloroplasts	6.2	546	578	93	0.8	0.13	83	$13.5 \cdot 10^{-3}$
mitochondria	1.2	35	14.5	12	0.25	0.21	17	$14.4 \cdot 10^{-3}$

300 Acetabularia mediterranea cells were homogenized in 5 ml isolation buffer and the subcellular fractions were obtained by differential centrifugation as described in materials and methods. The total protein and chlorophyll content and the activity of NADPH-MDH, cytochrome oxidase, and NADH-MDH were determined.

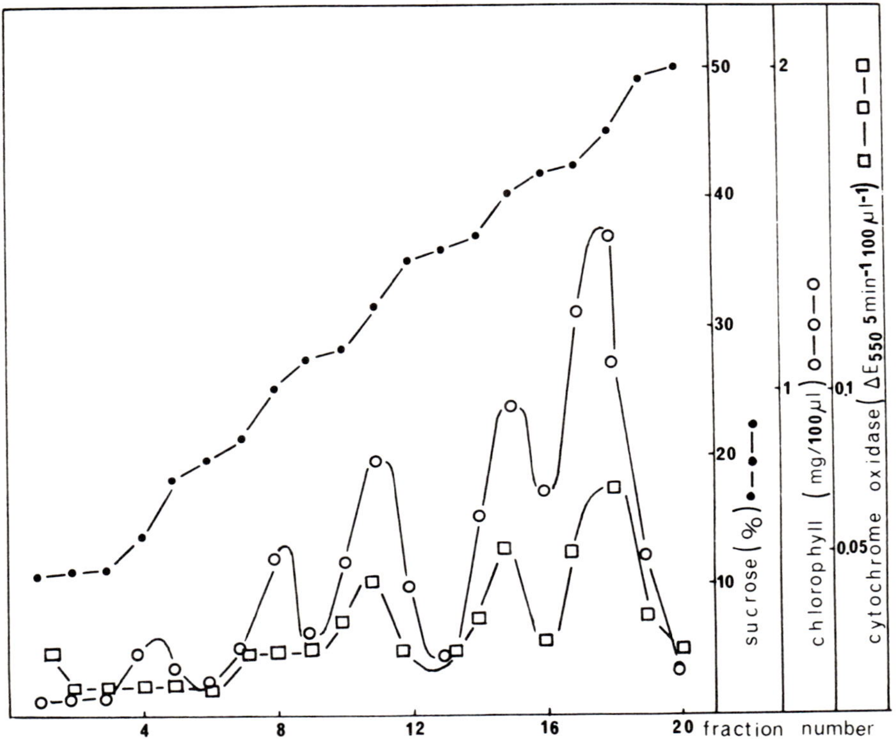

Figure 6. Fractionation of a particulate fraction from *Acetabularia cliftonii by sucrose density centrifugation.*

500 Acetabularia cliftonii cells were homogenized, cell debris sedimented, and the cell organelles harvested by centrifugation at 30,000 g for 20 minutes. The organelles were washed twice, resuspended in 1 ml isolation buffer, and layered on top of a discontinuous sucrose gradient. The gradient consisted of 2 ml cushions of 1.8 M, 1.45 M, 1.2 M, 0.9 M, and 0.6 M sucrose. The centrifugation was carried out at 60,000 g (SW 41) and 4° C for 2 hours. The gradient was fractionated (20 drops), and sucrose concentration, chlorophyll, and cytochrome oxidase determined.

TABLE 3

Comparison of the specific activities of cytochrome oxidase and NADH dependent malate dehydrogenase in a chloroplast and a mitochondrial fraction from Acetabularia mediterranea

	NADH-MDH/protein mU/mg	Cytochrome oxidase/protein ΔE_{550}/5 min/mg
Chloroplasts	1.020	0.03
Mitochondria	2.200	0.29

200 Acetabularia mediterranea cells were homogenized in 6 ml isolation buffer and subcellular fractions obtained by differential centrifugation as described in Materials and Methods. The mitochondrial fraction was further purified by centrifugation on a 0.64 M sucrose cushion at 3800 g for 45 minutes. The mitochondria were harvested from the interphase by centrifugation at 15,000 g for 20 minutes.

DISCUSSION

The NADH dependent malate dehydrogenase activity of both Acetabularia mediterranea and cliftonii, is associated almost completely with the organelle fraction of the cell. The enzyme activity can be resolved into various isoenzymes. The isoenzyme pattern is both species specific and specific for chloroplasts and mitochondria.

Species specificity

In Acetabularia mediterranea four NADH dependent MDH isoenzymes were found which differ markedly in their electrophoretic mobility. Two of these enzymes (A and B) may correspond to enzymes described earlier[29]. Using the same methods, only three isoenzymes were resolved from the extract of Acetabularia cliftonii. Two of these enzymes had electrophoretic mobilities similar to isoenzymes from Acetabularia mediterranea.

Only two percent of the total MDH activity remains in the postmitochondrial supernatant. The isoenzyme pattern of a concentrated supernatant corresponds to the pattern of the

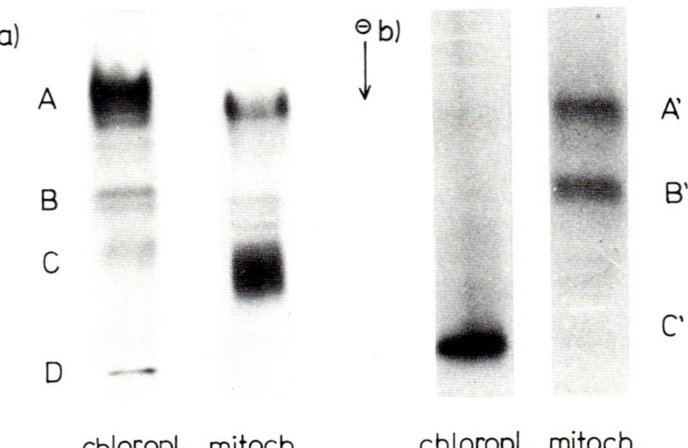

Figure 7. The malate dehydrogenase isoenzyme pattern of organelle fractions from Acetabularia mediterranea (a) and Acetabularia cliftonii (b).

200 cells each (without cap) were homogenized in 3 ml isolation buffer and the subcellular fractions were obtained by differential centrifugation as described in Materials and Methods. Chloroplasts were resuspended in 1.5 ml and mitochondria in 0.5 ml isolation buffer. 20 ul of the suspensions were subjected to electrophoresis as described.

organelle fraction suggesting that the MDH of the supernatant originates from broken organelles. There is no indication of a specific isoenzyme of the cytoplasm. In this respect, Acetabularia differs apparently from other plants where a large portion of the total MDH is found in the postmitochondrial supernatant[10,21,30,33].

Organelle specificity

In order to ascribe with certainty an isoenzyme to either the mitochondria or chloroplasts, two problems must be considered: i) Because of the viscosity of the cytoplasm[8,31] 'cytoplasts'[12] may be formed upon disruption of the cells.

The chloroplast preparation may have been contaminated by 'cytoplasts' (mitochondria plus chloroplasts trapped in an artificially closed piece of plasma membrane). ii) The chloroplasts show a considerable heterogeneity due to their fine structure[5,6,23,24]. This makes separation of chloroplasts and mitochondria by sucrose density centrifugation impossible (Fig. 6).

Therefore the distribution of the isoenzymes in the different organelles was studied after enrichment of the organelles in two fractions after differential centrifugation. Because the mitochondrial fraction was contaminated by chloroplasts to an extent below 5-10%, the isoenzyme bands found in this fraction, could be safely attributed to an activity located in the mitochondria. The mitochondria from _Acetabularia mediterranea_ contained only one isoenzyme band (C), the mitochondria from _Acetabularia cliftonii_ harbored two isoenzymes (A' and B').

Thus, the isoenzyme patterns of the mitochondria of the two _Acetabularia_ species are quite different. The occurence of a specific isoenzyme associated with the chloroplasts is suggested by two facts: (1) There is much more MDH activity in the chloroplast fraction than would correspond to the contaminating mitochondria. (2) The chloroplast fraction shows a specific isoenzyme pattern differing from the mitochondrial fraction. However, it is not yet clear whether the MDH is associated loosely with the surface of the chloroplasts or whether it is an intrinsic part of these organelles.

The MDH isoenzyme pattern of the chloroplasts is species specific: The chloroplasts of _Acetabularia mediterranea_ contain the enzyme A, B, and D, those of _Acetabularia cliftonii_ the enzyme C'. The chloroplast enzymes are coded for by the nucleus[29]. The study presented is the basis for investigating the same question for mitochondria.

ACKNOWLEDGEMENTS

I wish to thank Drs. G. Werz and H. G. Schweiger for valuable discussions and Dr. P. Herrlich for help in preparing the manuscript.

REFERENCES

1. Apel, K. and Schweiger, H. G. (1972) Eur. J. Biochem. 25, 229-238.
2. Arnon, D. J. (1949) Plant Physiol. 24, 1-15.
3. Berger, S., Sandakhchiev, L. and Schweiger, H. G. (1974) J. Microscopie 19, 89-104.

4. Bergmeyer, H. U. and Bernt, E. (1970) in Methoden der enzymatischen Analyse (Bergmeyer, H. U.) Vol. I, p. 575, Verlag Chemie Weinheim/Bergstr.
5. Boloukhère-Presburg, M. (1969) Diss. Université Libre de Bruxelles.
6. Boloukhère, M. (1972) J. Microscopie 13, 401-416.
7. Bonner, W. D. (1967) Meth. Enzymol. (Estabrook, R. W. and Pullman, M. E.) Vol. X, p. 126 Acad. Press, N. Y.
8. Clauss, H. (1968) Protoplasma 65, 49-80.
9. Davis, B. J. (1962) Preprint Disc electrophoresis Dest. Prod. Div. Eastman Kodak Co. Rochester, N. Y.
10. De Jong, D. W. and Olson, A. C. (1972) Biochim. Biophys. Acta 276, 53-62.
11. Fine, J. H. and Costello, L. A. (1963) in Meth. Enzymol. (Colowick, S. P. and Kaplan, N. O.) Vol. VI, p. 958, Acad. Press, N. Y.
12. Gibor, A. (1965) Proc. Nat. Acad. Sci. 54, 1527-1531.
13. Hämmerling, J. (1943) Z. induktive Abstammungs- und Vererbungslehre 81, 84-113.
14. Hämmerling, J. (1963) Ann. Rev. Plant Physiol. 14, 65-92.
15. Hatch, M. D. and Slack, C. R. (1969) Biochem. Biophys. Res. Commun. 34, 589-593.
16. Johnson, H. S. and Hatch, M. D. (1970) Biochem. J. 119, 273-280.
17. Keck, K. (1964) in Meth. Cell Physiol. (Prescott, D. M.) Vol. I, p. 189, N. Y. and London.
18. Kloppstech, K. and Schweiger, H. G. (1973) Exptl. Cell Res. 80, 69-78.
19. Lüttke, A., Rahmsdorf, U. and Schmid, R. (1976) Z. Naturforsch. 31c, 108-110.
20. Lowry, O. H., Rosebrough, N. J., Farr, A. L. and Randall, R. J. (1951) J. Biol. Chem. 193, 265-275.
21. Munkres, K. D. and Richards, F. M. (1965) Arch. Biochem. Biophys. 109, 261-265.
22. Ochoa, S. (1955) in Meth. Enzymol. (Colowick, S. P. and Kaplan, N. O.) Vol. I, p. 735, Acad. Press, N. Y.
23. Puiseux-Dao, S. and Dazy, A. C. (1970) in Biology of Acetabularia (Brachet, J. and Bonotto, S.) p. 111, N. Y. and London.
24. Puiseux-Dao, S., Dazy, A. C., Hoursiangou-Neubrun, D. and Borghi, H. (1972) Protoplasma 75, 484.
25. Rocha, V. and Ting, J. P. (1970) Plant Physiol. 46, 754-756.
26. Rocha, V. and Ting, J. P. (1971) Arch. Biochem. Biophys. 147, 114-122.
27. Sandakhchiev, L., Niemann, R. and Schweiger, H. G. (1973) Protoplasma 76, 403-414.
28. Schweiger, H. G. (1969) Curr. Top. Microbiol. Immunol. 50, 1-36.

29. Schweiger, H. G., Master, R. W. P. and Werz, G. (1967) Nature 216, 554-556.
30. Sulebele, G. and Silverstein, E. (1969) Arch. Biochem. Biophys. 133, 425-435.
31. Tandler, C. J. (1962) Naturwiss. 49, 112.
32. Wharton, D. G. and Tzagoloff, A. (1967) in Meth. Enzymol. (Estabrook, R. W. and Pullman, M. E.) Vol. X, p. 245, Acad. Press, N. Y.
33. Yang, N. S. and Scandalios, J. G. (1975) Biochim. Biophys. Acta 384, 293-306.

ELECTRON MICROSCOPIC STUDIES ON THE LOCALIZATION OF CATALASE AND PEROXIDASE IN *ACETABULARIA* CELLS

D. Menzel

Fachbereich Biologie, Freie Universität
Berlin, Germany

ABSTRACT

Evidence is presented for the localization of catalase in microbodies of *Acetabularia*. Peroxidase is demonstrated in the mitochondrial intermembrane spaces and in the soluble cytoplasm by its cytochemical characteristics which are different from those of catalase. Additionally, in enucleated plants a peroxidase-like activity is located in the plastidal matrix. The occurrence of the two peroxide degrading enzymes in different cell compartments is discussed in relation to certain peroxide producing processes.

INTRODUCTION

The knowledge of metabolic pathways participating in the formation and disintegration of hydrogen peroxide has created an increasing interest in these processes[1,2,3]. Catalase and peroxidase, possibly coupled with superoxide dismutase[4], are known to function in the peroxide breakdown. Accordingly, the physiological role of these enzymes has been a matter of intensive investigations[5,6]. Concerning the localization of peroxide metabolism, catalase is known to occur in microbodies[7] that function as glyoxisomes or peroxisomes in higher plants or algae[8-11]. Peroxidase, on the other hand, exhibits a widespread intracellular localization and a variety of specialized functions[12-16]. In some of the cytochemical studies, the DAB-technique to localize catalase[17] or peroxidase[18] in the cells caused an additional reaction product associated with the mitochondrial membranes that was interpreted as a possible reaction of cytochrome c oxidase[12,17,19]. However, according to recent reports on mitochondrial hydrogen peroxide production[3,20], it seems likely that peroxidase also may be located in the mitochondria.

A positive catalase reaction in the microbodies of *Acetabularia* was reported recently[21], and in the present study, discrimination between peroxidase and catalase is demonstrated.

MATERIALS AND METHODS

Acetabularia mediterranea plants, cultured according to the method described by Hämmerling[22], were chosen at a stage one to two weeks prior to cap formation.

The material was prefixed for 30 min at 4° C in 3% glutaraldehyde in 0.1 M cacodylate buffer at pH 7.0 containing 0.3 M sucrose. During the first minute in the fixative solution the plants were cut twice to improve penetration. After several washings in buffer, preincubation[11] was carried out at 4° C for 1 hour in the same buffer, but containing different inhibitors with the following concentrations: 0.01 M KCN, 0.01 M NaN_3, 0.02 M aminotriazole, and 6 mM Na-pyruvate. The enzyme reactions were carried out without further washings.

Catalase

The localization of catalase was performed as described by Novikoff and Goldfischer[17], modified as described before[21], in a medium composed of 0.1% diaminobenzidine (DAB), 0.003% H_2O_2, 0.1 M Tris-HCl buffer, 0.3 M sucrose, with the final pH adjusted to 9.0. Incubation was carried out in the dark at 37° C for 60-90 min. The incubation medium was usually freshly prepared, handled in dark bottles and filtered before use. Inhibitors were added to the complete reaction mixture as indicated for the preincubation, and controls were made without DAB, without H_2O_2, or without H_2O_2 but containing Na-pyruvate. Moreover, one sample was heated in buffer for 10 min at 50° C just before incubation.

Peroxidase

For peroxidase localization, the pH was lowered to 7.0 and 5.5 with the use of 0.1 M cacodylate buffer, and the temperature was held at 25° C in the dark[28]. Controls and inhibitors were the same as indicated for catalase. Additional enucleated plants were tested for peroxidase. These plants were enucleated 14 days before use and grown under normal conditions.

The incubation was followed by several buffer washings. Thereafter, plants were postfixed at 4° C overnight in 1% OsO_4 in 0.1 M cacodylate buffer, pH 7.0, without sucrose.

Subsequently, the cells were washed again in buffer and dehydrated in a series of ethanol with a last step in propylene oxide and then embedded in Araldite[23] or ERL-4206[24]. After polymerization at 70°C for at least 48 hours, silver sections were cut with glass knives on a Reichert OmU_3 ultramicrotome and transferred to uncoated rhodium/copper grids. Poststaining was performed with a methanolic solution saturated with uranyl acetate and thereafter with lead citrate[25]. Unstained or stained sections were examined in a Jeol T8 electron microscope at 60 kV and photographed on Scientia D23/56 films.

RESULTS

Catalase

a. Microbodies. Incubation of *Acetabularia* plants in the complete reaction mixture at pH 9.0 results in heavy staining of microbodies with osmiophilic reaction product (Fig. 1a). No diffusion of the oxidation product of DAB into the surrounding cytoplasm could be detected. In unstained sections, commonly used to demonstrate DAB-reaction, microbodies could not be distinguished from equally highly contrasted polyphosphate granules, as shown previously[21]. Selective reduction of polyphosphate contrast is possible either by bleaching the sections with peroxide and subsequent staining[21] or by using a methanolic solution of uranyl acetate instead of ethanolic or water solutions (Fig. 1i). The latter method was preferred in this study because of its better presentation of fine structural details.

In ultrathin-sections of untreated plants, poststained in the same manner as indicated above, microbodies appear as spherical profiles with a coarse, granulated, moderately contrasted matrix surrounded by a clearly visible membrane (Fig. 1b). A close relation of microbodies to the endoplasmic reticulum, as found to be typical for higher plant microbodies, can also be demonstrated for *Acetabularia* (Fig. 1c).

The specificity and enzymic nature of the DAB-reaction is shown by the following inhibitor studies: The reaction is blocked by KCN, aminotriazole and heating (Figs. 1d, g, f). Na-pyruvate, which is commonly utilized to destroy endogenous H_2O_2[26] prevented the DAB-oxidation (Fig. 1e). Also when the pH was lowered to 5.5 no reaction was observed in the microbodies (Fig. 1h).

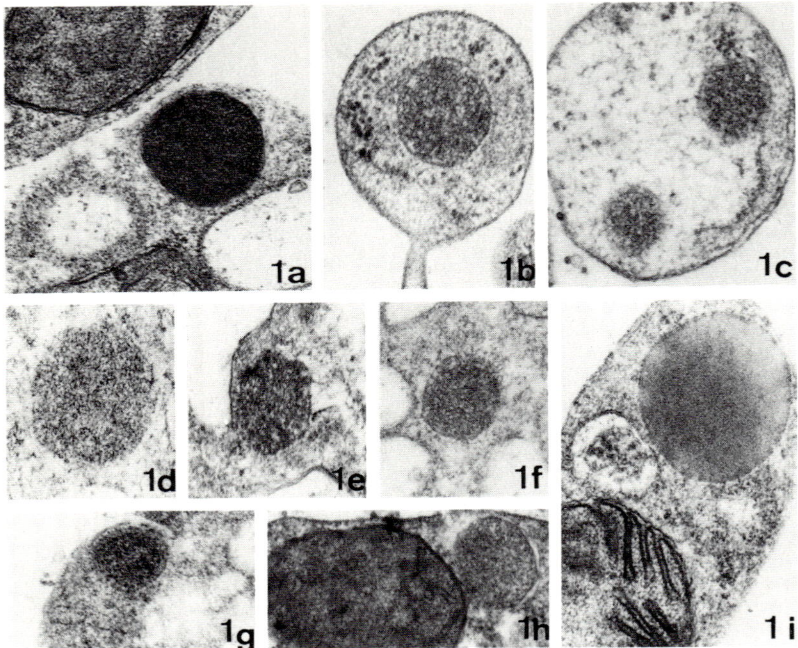

Figure 1. Microbodies of Acetabularia mediterranea incubated for the demonstration of catalase (pH 9.0) and different controls; poststained sections.

a. Complete reaction mixture. Note the heavy, electron dense deposits of reaction product in the matrix of the microbody. 50,000 x.

b. Unincubated plant. The microbody exhibits a coarse, granulated matrix surrounded by a clearly visible, single membrane. 80,000 x.

c. Incubation without DAB. The upper microbody shows a close relation to the endoplasmic reticulum. 80,000 x.

d. Complete reaction mixture with KCN. No reaction product has accumulated in the matrix of the microbody. 50,000 x.

e. Incubation without H_2O_2 but with the addition of Na-pyruvate. The reaction is mostly prevented. 50,000 x.

f. Heat treatment before incubation in the complete reaction mixture. The enzyme is inactivated. 50,000 x.

g. Complete reaction mixture with aminotriazole. The reaction is inhibited. 50,000 x.

h. Complete reaction mixture at pH 5.5. No reaction takes place in the microbody. 50,000 x.

i. Complete reaction mixture, polyphosphate granule with a translucent matrix. The poststaining method allows the distinction of microbodies and polyphosphate granules in the complete reaction mixture. 50,000 x.

b. Mitochondria. Reaction product developed at the mitochondrial membranes. This is demonstrated in unstained sections (Fig. 2a). This reaction is strongly inhibited by KCN (Fig. 2b) but not by aminotriazole (Fig. 2c). It is clearly heat-inactivated (Fig. 2e) and is negative upon destruction of hydrogen peroxide with Na-pyruvate (Fig. 2d).

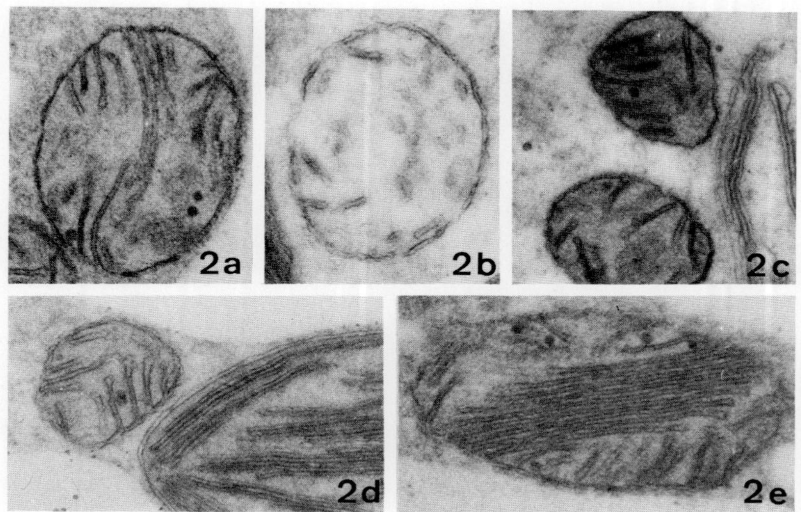

Figure 2. Mitochondria of Acetabularia mediterranea incubated in the catalase medium (pH 9.0) and different controls; not poststained. All 50,000 x.

a. Complete reaction mixture. Osmiophilic reaction product has accumulated partially in the outer compartment of the mitochondria and is associated additionally with some "cisternae."

b. Complete reaction mixture with KCN. The reaction is blocked.

c. Complete reaction mixture with aminotriazole. The reaction product is still visible; no inhibition.

d. Incubation without H_2O_2 but additionally with Na-pyruvate. No reaction takes place.

e. Incubation in the complete reaction mixture after heat treatment. Total inactivation of the enzyme.

Peroxidase

a. Mitochondria. Lowering of the pH to 7.0 and 5.5 causes a marked increase in mitochondrial reaction (Fig. 3a) with an additional cytoplasmic staining at pH 5.5 (Fig. 3b) which, however, is prevented by omitting H_2O_2. Destruction of endogenous peroxide leads to a total inhibition of any reaction at pH 7.0 and 5.5 (Fig. 3d). The inhibitory effect of KCN, aminotriazole and heating was the same as under acidic conditions in the pH 9.0 medium (Figs. 2b, c, e). Additionally tested was NaN_3, which showed a strong inhibitory effect (Fig. 3c).

b. Chloroplasts. In normal plants the chloroplasts exhibit no or only negligible reaction product, but in enucleated portions of Acetabularia incubated in the pH 5.5 medium all chloroplasts are filled with heavy deposits of reaction product (Fig. 3e). The thylakoids appear in a negative-contrast and do not themselves contain reaction product, which would have been typical for light-induced reactions[27]. Also the outer plastidal membrane is free of reaction product. The plastidal matrix in the unincubated, enucleated control plants appears normal and electron translucent, comparable to that of figure 2d. So, the enhanced contrast in the matrix is due only to deposits of reaction product and provides evidence for the presence of enzymes functioning as peroxidases.

Figure 3. Incubation for the demonstration of peroxidase and different controls; not poststained. All 50,000 x.

a. Complete reaction mixture at pH 7.0. The intermembrane spaces of the mitochondria appear filled with osmiophilic reaction product.

b. Complete reaction mixture at pH 5.5. The mitochondria have the same appearance as in the pH 7.0 medium. Additionally, cytoplasmic staining occurs. The lumen of the endoplasmic reticulum and certain vacuoles remain free of reaction product.

c. Complete reaction mixture at pH 5.5 with NaN_3. Cytoplasmic and mitochondrial reaction is prevented.

d. Incubation at pH 5.5 without H_2O_2 but with Na-pyruvate. No reaction occurs in the mitochondria, nor in the cytoplasm.

e. Incubation of enucleated plants in the complete reaction mixture at pH 5.5. The matrix of the chloroplasts shows heavy deposition of reaction product. The chloroplasts of control plants exhibit an electron translucent matrix comparable with that of figure 2d.

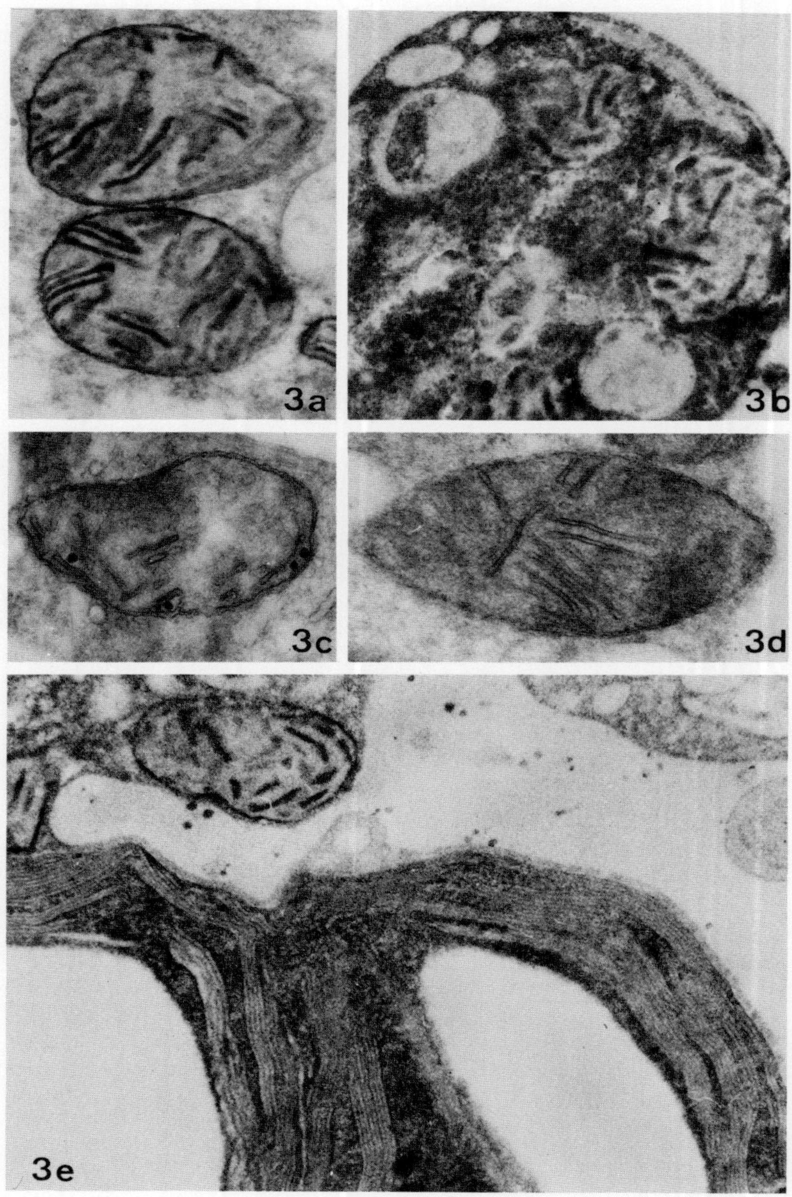
3a
3b
3c
3d
3e

DISCUSSION

Localization of catalase

The best cytochemical technique for localizing catalase at the electron microscopic level is the diaminobenzidine method of Novikoff and Goldfischer[17] with modifications[28,29].

In *Acetabularia*, application of this technique leads to heavy electron dense deposits in the microbodies as identified by the above mentioned poststaining method (Fig. 1a). The enzymic nature of this reaction is demonstrated by heat inactivation (Fig. 1f), while the requirement for hydrogen peroxide can be shown by the use of Na-pyruvate in a peroxide-free medium[26] (Fig. 1e). Both controls prove that no terminal oxidases are involved and, additionally, that no non-specific adsorption of oxidized and pre-polymerized DAB occurred[30,31]. The strong inhibitory effect of KCN (Fig. 1d) indicates that a heme enzyme is involved in the reaction. Finally, aminotriazole which is known as a specific inhibitor of catalase[32], prevents the reaction. So there is no doubt that only catalase reacts with diaminobenzidine in the microbodies of *Acetabularia*.

Additionally, under the same prefixation conditions, but incubated at lower pH, no reaction takes place in the microbodies (Fig. 1h) indicating that the alkaline environment is the most effective for demonstrating positive catalase reactions.

The detection of catalase, the fact that the catalase content decreases in the microbodies of dark grown plants[21], and the presence of a measurable amount of photorespiration in *Acetabularia*[33] resemble the processes found in higher plant microbodies[34,35]. However, the peroxide-producing glycolate oxidase, the key enzyme of the photorespiration pathway[8,34], could not be detected in *Acetabularia*[36] and therefore may not be responsible for the photorespiratory effect. It is therefore possible that these algal microbodies need no catalase[36,37]. However, since other algae possessing glycolate dehydrogenase instead of the oxidase do exhibit catalase in the microbodies[11,38] it is probable that there is a specialized algal type of microbody that is not related to glycolate metabolism[37].

To the author's knowledge, *Acetabularia* is the first alga of siphonous organization to be found with these modified algal microbodies.

Localization of peroxidase

In the catalase medium another type of reaction caused by peroxidase occurs in the mitochondria. This is indicated by several specific characteristics different from those of catalase. The strength of reaction increases greatly by lowering the pH, with a maximum between pH 7.0 and 5.5. It is therefore not dependent on the denaturing conditions of the incubation medium, as is catalase.

In addition, aminotriazole does not inhibit this reaction, supporting the suggestion that catalase cannot be responsible for the positive reaction of the mitochondria. Some investigators who found a similar staining of mitochondrial membranes considered that cytochrome c oxidase was responsible for this reaction[12,17,19] in spite of the unfavorable experimental conditions. In fact, DAB is an excellent cytochemical probe for demonstrating cytochrome c oxidase, but only under well defined conditions[39]. In the presence of peroxide, the apparent presence of cytochrome c oxidase should be treated with caution[30] and a control to exclude the participation of possible peroxidases should be included. Since the endogenous formation of H_2O_2 in glutaraldehyde-fixed tissues is known, the addition of Na-pyruvate to the peroxide-free incubation medium is introduced to destroy any endogenously formed H_2O_2[26,31,40].

In the case of Acetabularia, the DAB-reaction in the mitochondria is negative upon destruction of endogenous peroxide. This implies that an enzymatic reaction of cytochrome c oxidase is not occurring.

However, Hirai[41] reported the possibility of non-enzymatic adsorption of oxidized DAB to cytochrome c, which is prevented by KCN but not by heat inactivation (at 80°C for 20 min). The mitochondrial reaction in Acetabularia, however, is clearly inactivated by heat treatment at even lower temperatures for a shorter period of time (50°C, 10 min). This means that the deposition of reaction product in the mitochondrial membranes under the described conditions is caused by a fully functioning enzyme and not by non-enzymatic processes.

These characteristics are more typical of peroxidase than any other enzyme. Cytochrome c oxidase, therefore, should be demonstrated separately under the defined optimal conditions[39,42,43].

Peroxidase has also been demonstrated by Hirai[44] in Tetrahymena mitochondria. However, since this enzyme is only partially suppressed by KCN, and the inhibition of azide is pH-dependent, it resembles the cytochrome c peroxidase of certain bacteria[45] and of Saccharomyces[46,47]. Therefore, this enzyme may play a role in mitochondrial respiration by substituting for the normal cytochrome c oxidase[44].

A peroxidatic DAB-reaction with unknown physiological function has also been reported to occur in the mitochondrial outer membrane of the parasitic amoeba Hartmanella in the presence of a fully active cytochrome c oxidase system[48].

It is therefore important that peroxidase localization in mitochondria should be viewed in the context of the frequently reported H_2O_2 production in mitochondria and submitochondrial particles[20,49,50]. Recently, Rich et al.[3] reported that the cyanide resistant alternate pathway to a great extent reduced oxygen to H_2O_2, but due to the high level of peroxidase located in the mitochondrial fraction peroxide is effectively destroyed and will not accumulate in the mitochondria.

The occurrence of an alternate pathway seems to be widely distributed in the plant kingdom including the green algae[51,52,53]. However, it does not exclude the simultaneous existence of cytochrome c oxidase[54]. Except for cytochrome c peroxidase[44,46,47], the function of other mitochondrial peroxidases is unknown. It may function not only in protecting the cell against toxic H_2O_2 but also be needed to oxidize endogenous mitochondrial hydrogen donators[3].

In addition to the mitochondrial staining caused by peroxidase, reaction product is dispersed throughout the cytoplasm in the pH 5.5 medium. The cytochemical characteristics are the same as those of the mitochondrial peroxidase reaction and they demonstrate the occurrence of peroxidase in the cytosol of Acetabularia with a more acidic pH optimum.

Beside other localizations in higher plants[12-15] peroxidase is also found to exist in a soluble form in the cytoplasm[16] which seems to be typical in meristematic and developing cells. Although the function of the soluble peroxidases is unknown it may correspond to some H_2O_2-producing processes also located in the cytosol, as shown in animal cells[55].

Only in enucleated Acetabularia cells are the chloroplasts found to be active in peroxide metabolism, producing heavy DAB-deposits in the matrix. This reaction is inconsistent and almost lacking in chloroplasts of nucleated plants. The mechanism involved in this peroxidation reaction has not been studied in detail, but an induction or an increase of a peroxide metabolism in the chloroplasts in the absence of the nucleus seems to be very likely. A similar interrelationship with regard to specific mitochondrial functions has been reported to exist in Neurospora[53].

ACKNOWLEDGEMENTS

I thank Mrs. H. Lehmann for skillful technical assistance and Miss E. Nielsen for the preparation and typing of the English text.

REFERENCES

1. Boveris, A. and Chance, B. (1973) Biochem. J. 134, 707-716.
2. Fridovich, J. (1974) Advances in Enzymology 41, 35-97.
3. Rich, P. R., Boveris, A., Bonner, W. D. and Moore, A. L. (1976) Biochem. Biophys. Res. Commun. 71, 695-703.
4. Halliwell, B. (1974) New Phytol. 73, 1075-1086.
5. de Duve, Ch. (1969) Ann. N. Y. Acad. Sci. 168, 369-381.
6. Yamazaki, I. (1974) in Molecular Mechanisms of Oxygen Activation (Hayaishi, O., ed.), Academic Press, New York, London, pp. 535-554.
7. Vigil, E. L. (1973) Sub-Cell. Biochem. 2, 237-285.
8. Tolbert, N. E. (1971) Ann. Rev. Plant Physiol. 22, 45-75.
9. Richardson, M. (1974) Sci. Prog., Oxf. 61, 41-61.
10. Fredrick, S. E., Gruber, P. J. and Newcomb, E. H. (1975) Protoplasma 84, 1-29.
11. Silverberg, B. A. (1975) Protoplasma 83, 269-295.
12. Oliveira, L. and Bisalputra, T. (1975) Can. J. Bot. 54, 913-922.
13. Hall, J. L. and Sexton, T. (1972) Planta (Berl.) 108, 103-120.
14. Henry, E. W. (1975) J. Ultrastr. Res. 52, 289-299.
15. Oostrom, H., Treurniet, F. E. and Mennes, A. M. (1975) Z. Pflanzenphys. 74, 451-463.
16. Goff, Ch. W. (1975) Amer. J. Bot. 62, 280-291.
17. Novikoff, A. B. and Goldfischer, S. (1969) J. Histochem. Cytochem. 17, 675-680.
18. Graham, R. C. and Karnovsky, M. J. (1966) J. Histochem. Cytochem. 14, 291-302.
19. Beard, M. E. and Novikoff, A. B. (1969) J. Cell Biol. 42, 501-518.
20. Boveris, A., Oshino, N. and Chance, B. (1972) Biochem. J. 128, 617-630.
21. Menzel, D. (1976) Planta (Berl.) 130, 181-184.
22. Hämmerling, J. (1944) Arch. Protistenkunde 97, 7-56.
23. Luft, J. H. (1961) J. Biochem. Biophys. Cytol. 9, 409-414.
24. Spurr, A. R. (1969) J. Ultrastr. Res. 26, 31-43.
25. Venable, J. H. and Coggeshall, R. (1965) J. Cell Biol. 25, 407-408.
26. Fahimi, H. D. (1969) J. Cell Biol. 43, 275-288.
27. Nir, I. and Seligman, A. M. (1970) J. Cell Biol. 46, 617-620.
28. Herzog, V. and Fahimi, H. D. (1976) Histochem. 46, 273-286.
29. Roels, F., Wisse, E., de Prest, B. and van der Meulen, J. (1975) Histochem. 41, 281-312.

30. Seligman, A. M., Shannon, W. A., Hoshino, Y. and Plapinger, R. E. (1973) J. Histochem. Cytochem. 21, 756-758.
31. Nir, I. and Seligman, A. M. (1971) J. Histochem. Cytochem. 19, 611-620.
32. Margoliash, E. and Novogrodsky, A. (1960) Biochem. J. 74, 339-348.
33. Bidwell, R. G. S., Levin, W. B. and Shepard, D. C. (1969) Plant Physiol. 44, 946-954.
34. Tolbert, N. E. (1971) in Photosynthesis and Photorespiration (Hatch, M. D., Osmond, C. D. and Slatyer, R. O., eds.), Wiley-Interscience, New York, London, Sidney, Toronto, pp. 458-471.
35. Tolbert, N. E. (1973) Current Topics in Cellular Regulation 7, 21-50.
36. Nelson, E. B. and Tolbert, N. E. (1970) Arch. Biochem. Biophys. 141, 102-110.
37. Merrett, M. J. and Lord, J. M. (1973) New Phytol. 72, 751-767.
38. Frederick, S. E., Gruber, P. J. and Tolbert, N. E. (1973) Plant Physiol. 52, 318-323.
39. Seligman, A. M., Karnovsky, M. J., Wasserkrug, J. L. and Hanker, J. S. (1968) J. Cell Biol. 38, 1-14.
40. Vigil, E. L. (1970) J. Cell Biol. 46, 435-454.
41. Hirai, K.-I. (1971) J. Histochem. Cytochem. 19, 434-442.
42. Roels, F. (1974) J. Histochem. Cytochem. 22, 442-446.
43. Anderson, W. A., Bara, G. and Seligman, A. M. (1975) J. Histochem. Cytochem. 23; 13-20.
44. Hirai, K.-I. (1974) J. Histochem. Cytochem. 22, 189-202.
45. Lennhoff, H. M. and Kaplan, N. O. (1956) J. Biol. Chem. 220, 967-982.
46. Yonetani, T. and Ray, G. S. (1966) J. Biol. Chem. 241, 700-706.
47. Todd, M. and Vigil, E. L. (1972) J. Histochem. Cytochem. 20, 344-349.
48. Childs, G. E. (1973) J. Histochem. Cytochem. 21, 26-33.
49. Hinckle, P. C., Butow, R. A., Racker, E. F. and Chance, B. (1967) J. Biol. Chem. 242, 5169-5173.
50. Oshino, N., Chance, B., Sies, H. and Bücher, T. (1973) Arch. Biochem. Biophys. 154, 117-131.
51. Sharpless, T. K. and Butow, R. A. (1970) J. Biol. Chem. 245, 50-57.
52. Bendall, D. S. and Bonner, W. D. (1971) Plant Physiol. 47, 236-265.
53. Edwards, D. L. and Rosenberg, E. (1976) Eur. J. Biochem. 62, 217-221.

54. Coleman, J. O. D. and Harley, J. L. (1976) New Phytol. 76, 317-330.
55. Rotilio, G., Calabrese, L. and Finazzi Agro, A. (1973) Biochem. Biophys. Acta 321, 98-102.

ON THE QUATERNARY STRUCTURE OF D-RIBULOSE-1,5-BIPHOSPHATE CARBOXYLASE FROM *DASYCLADUS CLAVAEFORMIS* ROTH (AG.) IN SOLUTION AND IN THE CRYSTALLINE STATE

Brigitte Zimmer, H. Hasko Paradies and Günther Werz

Fachbereich Biologie
Freie Universität Berlin
Berlin, West Germany

ABSTRACT

D-ribulose-1,5-biphosphate from *Dasycladus clavaeformis* Roth (Ag.) was studied by means of small angle X-ray scattering in solution. The enzyme was found to have a molecular weight of 535,000 daltons, a radius of gyration of 45.5 Å, and consist of eight protomers each of molecular weight 64,000 daltons. The protomer consists of a large and a small polypeptide with molecular weights of about 50,000 and about 15,000 daltons, respectively. Single crystals reveal a unit cell spacing of $\underline{a}$ = 315.0 Å with 12 molecules per unit cell, assuming a space group of $I4_132$ or $I432$.

INTRODUCTION

D-ribulose-1,5-biphosphate carboxylase (E.C. 4.1.1.39) plays a key role in photosynthesis. About 50% of the total amount of soluble protein of green plants is made of this enzyme (RuDP-carboxylase). The reason for such a high concentration is still unknown, but it might be important for the kinetic mechanism of the enzyme.

In order to understand the stereochemical mechanism of the function of RuDP-carboxylase, i) size and shape, ii) possible conformational changes due to binding of ligands (activators, inhibitors, substrates and products), and iii) the elucidation of the three dimensional structure at atomic resolution are of considerable interest. Since single crystals of RuDP-carboxylase from tobacco leaves[1,2] and from the green alga *Dasycladus clavaeformis*[3] are available it should be possible to elucidate the three-dimensional structure of this enzyme, although the molecular weight of 535,000 daltons is fairly high. Because the subunit structure of RuDP-carboxylase has been worked out by chemical and physical methods, e.g. small angle X-ray scattering measurements in solution, a structure determination of RuDP-carboxylase crystals is feasible. By applying the rotation function according to Rossman and Blow[4] one should be able to determine with high accuracy the arrangement of the large and small subunits within the enzyme molecule at atomic resolution.

Our investigations of the RuDP-carboxylase from *Dasycladus* have established i) that the *in vivo* formed single crystals (Fig. 1) are identical with the purified RuDP-carboxylase, also in its crystal form, and ii) that the hydrodynamic properties, including small angle X-ray scattering measurements of the enzyme in solution under physiological conditions, are identical with the so-called "fraction I protein." Moreover, in the present study we give evidence for the subunit structure along with the distance distribution, number of subunits and the isometric overall shape of the RuDP-carboxylase in solution.

MATERIALS AND METHODS

RuDP-carboxylase was prepared as described[3] by DEAE-cellulose chromatography with a linear gradient ranging from 0.0-0.2 M NaCl, pH 7.5, and sucrose gradient centrifugation in a SW 41 rotor (Beckman) at 15,000 rpm for 12 hours (Paradies, unpublished results). The small angle X-ray scattering measurements were performed with CuK_α-radiation using a water cooled rotating anode GX 13 (Elliot, U.K.) with Kratky collimation. For dense solutions of RuDP-carboxylase (15 mg/ml) a Franks camera was used with two double bent quartz monochromators, in principle as described[5,6]. The sample-to-receiving-slit distance was 215 mm, the widths of the entrance slit, scatter slit and receiving slit were chosen to be 0.1 mm, 0.3 mm, and 0.1 mm respectively. The measurements were performed at 20° C. Three scattering curves from the protein solution and three blank curves from the buffer solution were recorded by alternating an enzyme run with a buffer run. Data were collected and analyzed as described by Paradies and Franz[7].

Single crystals of RuDP-carboxylase, grown at a protein concentration of 15 mg/ml, pH 7.5, at an ammonium sulfate concentration of 0.5 M, were sealed in a glass capillary (ϕ = 1 mm), at both ends of which were placed a droplet of mother liquor, and raised to a concentration of 1.5 M $(NH_4)_2SO_4$ (Paradies, unpublished). The density of the crystals were determined as described[8].

Still photographs of the single crystals were obtained on a precession camera (Nonius, Eindhoven, Netherlands) with a

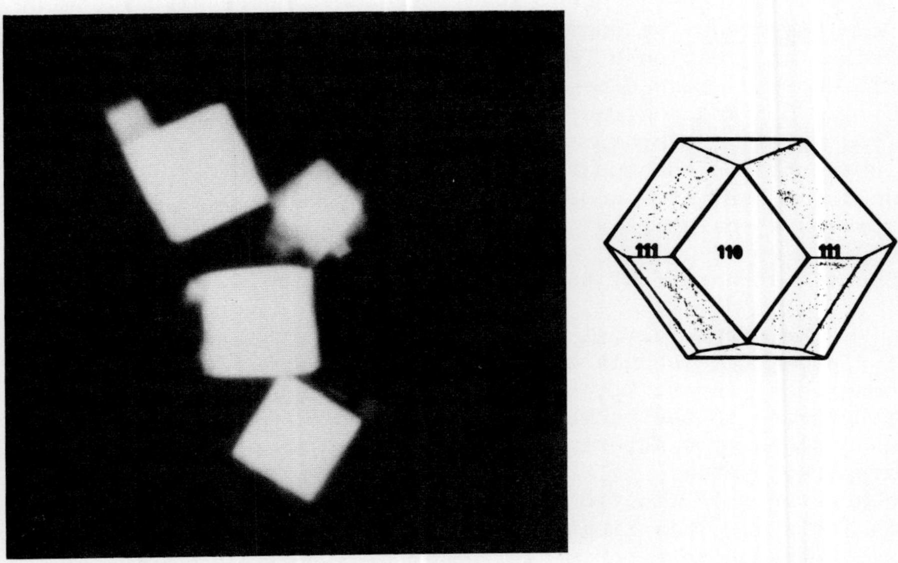

Figure 1.

a. Fluorescence microscopy of single crystals isolated from Dasycladus clavaeformis, stained with 1,8-ANS. Magnification: 260 x.

b. Crystal of RuDP-carboxylase in 0.2 M K_2HPO_4, pH 7.2; certain crystal zone axes are indicated. The [110] zone axis is normal to the diamond shaped face; the [100] zone axis passes through the vertex where four faces meet at the tip of the diamonds; the [111] zone axis passes through the vertex of three faces. The length of the diamond shaped face in this crystal was about 0.15 mm.

film-to-specimen distance of 100 mm. The X-ray beam was monochromatized by two bent quartz monochromators and focussed directly onto the plane of the recording X-ray film. Normally, three degree precession photographs were taken with exposure times ranging from 24 to 48 hours. Electron microscopy was performed on single crystals, on crystals *in situ*, and on isolated enzyme particles in solution[9]. Optical diffraction patterns were obtained from the negative electron micrographs by means of helium-neon laser (λ = 633 nm).

RESULTS

It has already been established that RuDP-carboxylase from Dasycladus belongs to the spherical proteins, having a radius of gyration of R = 45.5 Å, a molecular weight of 535,000 and gross dimensions of a hollow sphere with a diameter of 112.0 Å and a diameter of the inner hole of 24.0 Å[3]. Apart from these morphological parameters, we were considerably interested in the substructure of the oligomeric enzyme in solution for later comparison with the crystalline X-ray structure analysis (Fig. 2).

Subunit structure of the RuDP-carboxylase molecule

The morphological parameters of the enzyme particle including the subunit structure are listed in Table 1. The coherence length, ℓ_c, is analogous to the mean transveral length and to the radius of gyration which are measures of the mean sizes of scattering inhomogeneities in a dilute homodisperse system. All these parameters, determined from the characteristic function H(x), as shown in Figure 3, are listed in Table 1. This cluster-like complex of different spherical subunits has an experimental value of ℓ_c = 84.0 Å which is larger than the theoretical value of 56.2 Å. The physical data found in Table 1 indicate that the enzyme consists of a loosely packed complex of eight subunits.

The scattering function of a particle composed of n spherical subunits can be calculated on the basis of the scattering theory of a molecular gas according to Debye[10,11]. The investigations of the long wave periodicity in the scattering curves at very large angles permit the elucidation of the substructure of the particle. For example, from the position of the minimum in the outer section of the scattering curve (Fig. 2), the size of identical or very similar subunits can be determined. This is easily shown in the characteristic function (Fig. 3) that allows us to determine the mean diameter of the subunits which was found to be 56.4 Å (Table 1). The mean value of the diameter of the subunits of RuDP-carboxylase is determined by means of the break in the distance distribu-function at an X-value of about 58.0-60.0 Å (Fig. 4).

By separating the characteristic function H(x) into two separated terms $H_1(x)$ and $H_2(x)$ $\{H(x) = H_1(x) + H_2(x)\}$, where $H_1(x)$ represents the electronic interaction within the subunits and $H_2(x)$ the interaction of electrons between the subunits, we are able to determine the number of subunits according to

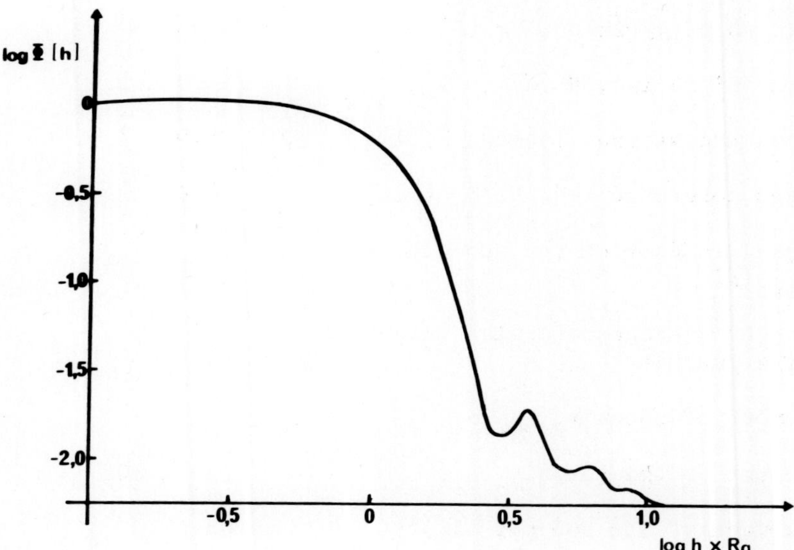

Figure 2. Scattering curve of RuDP-carboxylase in a plot of log Φ(h) versus h; desmeared, monochromatized and normalized $\Phi(h) = I(h)/I_o = 1$ for $h = 0$, where $h = (4\pi/\lambda \sin\theta)$ and $\lambda = 1.54$ Å.

Hosemann[12], since the diameter of the subunits are known through application of the characteristic function. We obtained a value of 8 subunits, each with a radius of a sphere of 26.2 Å and a molecular weight of 64,500 daltons, using a partial specific volume for the subunit of $\nu = 0.730$ ml · g^{-1}. This result would imply that the protomer structure involves one small subunit of a molecular weight of about 15,000 and a large subunit of a molecular weight of about 50,000, yielding one stereochemical subunit in the whole enzymatic complex of about 65,000. It is not clear whether both subunits (15,000

TABLE 1

Morphological parameters and subunit structure of RuDP-carboxylase from Dasycladus

Molecular weight (daltons)	530,000-540,000
Volume (Å^3)	74.0×10^4
Surface (Å^2)	39.0×10^4
Radius of gyration, Rg (Å)	45.5 ± 0.85
Stokes' radius, R (Å)	57.0 ± 1.50
Mean transversal length, $\bar{\ell}$ (Å)	74.9
Mean coherence length, ℓ_c (Å)	84.0
Mean diameter of the subunit, D_{sub}(Å)	56.4
Weight average molecular weight of a subunit	64,500
Number of subunits, n	8
Volume of the subunit (Å^3)	9.3×10^4
Surface of the subunit (Å^2)	95×10^3
f^{13}	1.01

= S, 50,000 = L subunit) are really spheres. Moreover, the fraction of the total mass contributed by the small subunits is so small in comparison to the eight large subunits that molecules of stochiometry like L_8S_8, L_8S_{12} and L_8S_{16} are all compatible with the small angle X-ray scattering results, hence the wide spread of the molecular weights.

However, it is most likely that the stochiometry of the RuDP-carboxylase particle is L_8S_8. Therefore, the binding between all LS-pairs must be equivalent, giving a D_4 (422) symmetry. This is further substantiated by X-ray diffraction patterns of single crystals and by electron microscopy.

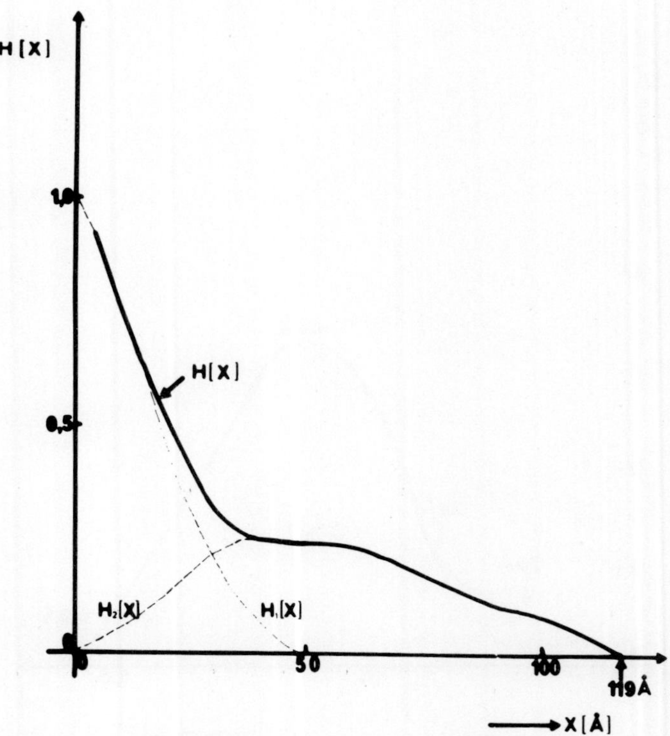

Figure 3. Characteristic function H(x), obtained by a Fourier transformation of the scattered intensity. H(x) gives a maximum diameter of the particle of D = 120 Å and a mean diameter of the subunits of 56.6 Å. H(x) can be separated into two terms, $H_1(x)$ and $H_2(x)$, as indicated in the text.

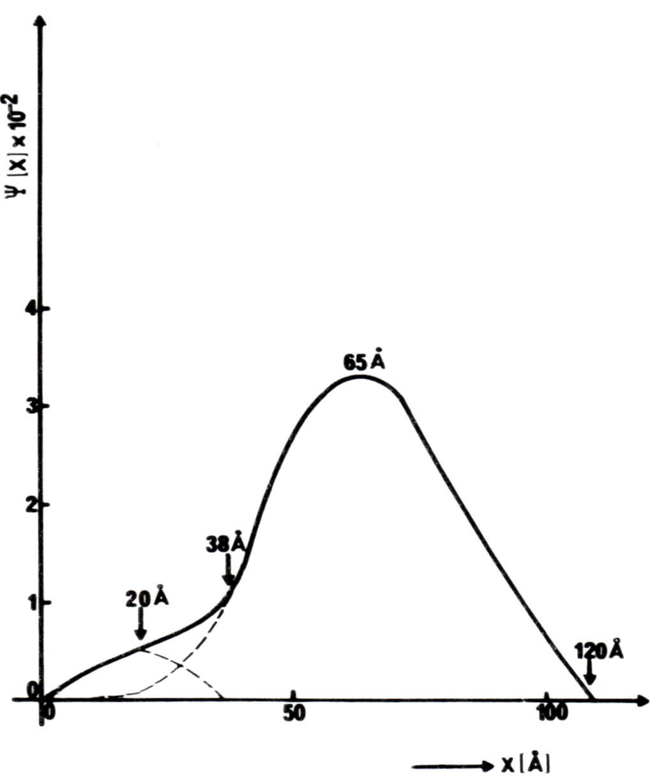

Figure 4. Distance distribution $\Psi(x) = H(x) \cdot x^2$, a measure for the frequency of distances x between scattering centers present in the RuDP-carboxylase. $\Psi(x)$ is separated into two terms, $\Psi_1(x)$ and $\Psi_2(x)$ (see text).

The rhombic dodecahedron crystals with well-defined faces are non-birefringent, highly hydrated, and extremely sensitive to X-rays during long exposures (Fig. 1). The crystallographic characteristics of these crystals are listed in Table 2.

TABLE 2

Characteristics of RuDP-carboxylase crystals

Unit cell spacing	315.0 Å
Crystal density	1.07 ± 0.005 g/ml
Solvent density	1.058 ± 0.005 g/ml
Volume fraction of solvent	0.74 g/ml
Space group	$I4_132$ or $I432$
Unit cell volume	31.26×10^6 $Å^3$
Molecules per unit cell	12
Crystal volume perunit of protein molecular weight, V_M	5.15 $Å^3$/dalton

A section through an RuDP-carboxylase crystal is shown in Figure 5. The corresponding optical diffraction pattern is given in Figure 6 from which cell dimensions of $\underline{a}$ = 315.0 Å were obtained. However, from electron micrographs of positively stained thin sections dimensions of $\underline{a}$ = 300-320 Å of various preparations were determined. The RuDP-carboxylase, therefore, crystallizes in the cubic crystal class with $\underline{a}$ = 305-310 Å. For molecular packing considerations we tried to index the corresponding optical diffraction patterns from the thin sections of RuDP-carboxylase. The patterns normally do not have a very high resolution, only weak reflections of third and fourth order can be seen. The geometry of the diffraction patterns can be interpreted in the sense that we are looking down the three- and four-fold axes of the crystal

Figure 5. Negatively stained thin sections of RuDP-carboxylase crystals.

Figure 6. Optical diffraction pattern of the lattice shown in Figure 5.

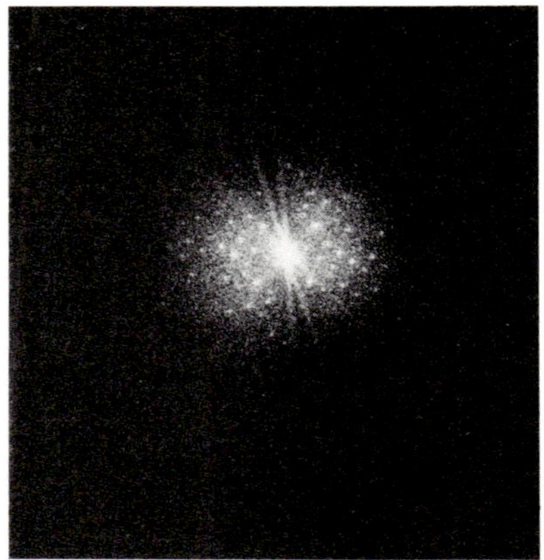

(Fig. 6) which would imply views of the 111 and 100 crystallographic planes of the cubic crystal class. The optical diffraction patterns are compatible with a body-centered, cubic cell with a Laue symmetry of <u>m</u>3<u>m</u> and a possible space group of I432 or $I4_132$. Because of the low resolution and lack of X-ray patterns of high resolution we were not able to insure that the 6,0,0 reflection was extinguished.

However, a very new and important source of structural information that can supplement chemical studies and electron microscopy is X-ray diffraction from concentrated solutions of RuDP-carboxylase. The pattern (Fig. 7) obtained corresponds to the spherically averaged transform of an isolated RuDP-carboxylase particle. The patterns have very distinctive sets of rings of varying intensity, not unlike a powder pattern. The differences in the intensities of the rings in the 1/75 $Å^{-1}$ to 1/50 $Å^{-1}$ regions indicate differences in the structures of the polypeptide chains of the two types of protein subunits that make up the whole particle. This is also true for the 1/10 $Å^{-1}$ to 1/20 $Å^{-1}$ region.

The interpretation of the different rings and their intensity distribution in terms of structural features has not yet been completed since interparticle interference effects must be taken into account.

We are now trying to grow stable crystals of RuDP-carboxylase that give a better resolution to at least 10.0 Å, in order to determine unequivocally the space group according to Fourier's methods. So far, we only can conclude

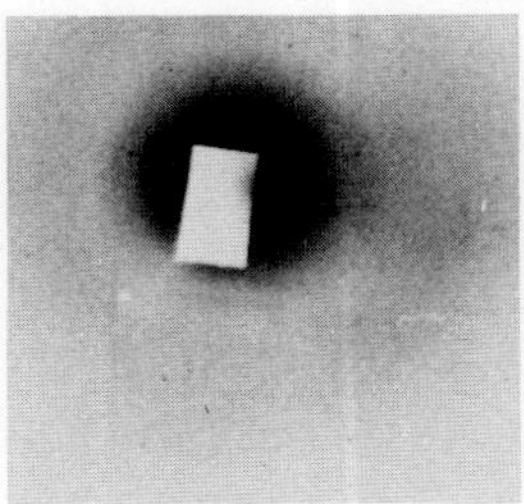

Figure 7. X-ray scattering pattern from a concentrated solution of RuDP-carboxylase. The pictures were taken at 100 mm film to specimen distance with monochromatized CuKα-radiation. Magnification: 2.6 x.

that the enzyme molecule is composed of eight subunits each of a molecular weight of 64,500 daltons and each consisting of one smaller subunit (S) of a molecular weight of about 15,000 daltons and one large one (L) of about 50,000 daltons, apparently with equivalent binding domains of all monomeric LS pairs.

Assuming that the enzyme is of different size, only D_4 symmetry is possible by arranging the subunits at the corners of a cube or of a square antiprism if the binding of all pairs of large and small subunits is equivalent. Moreover, with twelve molecules per unit cell in the possible space group each molecular unit must at least occupy a position of 222-symmetry (D_2).

REFERENCES

1. Buchanan, R. B. and Schürmann, P. (1973) in Current Topics in Cellular Regulation (Horecker, B. L. and Stadtman, E. R., eds.), vol. 7, Academic Press, New York, pp. 1-20.
2. Chan, D. H., Singh, K. S. S. and Wildman, S. G. (1972) Science 176, 1145-1146.
3. Paradies, H. H., Zimmer, B. and Werz, G. (1976) Biochem. Biophys. Res. Commun., in press.
4. Rossmann, M. G. and Blow, D. M. (1961) Acta Crystallograph. 15, 24-39.
5. Clark, B. F. C., Doctor, B. P., Holmes, K. C., Marker, K. A., Morris, S. J., Klug, A. and Paradies, H. H. (1968) Nature 219, 1222-1224.
6. Witz, J. (1969) Acta Crystallograph. A 24, 30-41.
7. Paradies, H. H. and Franz, A. (1976) Eur. J. Biochem. 67, 23-29.
8. Paradies, H. H. (1971) Eur. J. Biochem. 18, 530-535.
9. Zimmer, B., Paradies, H. H. and Werz, G. (1977) Biochem. Biophys. Res. Commun., submitted.
10. Debye, P. (1915) Ann. Physik 46, 809-823.
11. Debye, P. (1930) Physik. Z. 31, 419-428.
12. Hosemann, R. (1970) in Advances in Structure Research by Diffraction Methods (Mason, S. and Hoppe, W., eds.), Vol. 3, Viewig, Braunschweig, pp. 101-172.
13. Kahovec, L., Porod, G. and Ruck, H. (1953) Kolloid-Z. 133, 16-26.

ON THE BIOSYNTHESIS OF CONDENSED PHOSPHATES

Rainer Niemeyer

Institut für Botanik
Technische Universität
Hannover, West Germany

SUMMARY

In order to study the biosynthesis of the condensed inorganic phosphates, it seemed advisable not to fractionate the high-molecular phosphates with strong alkaline or acid, but to separate them in native conditions. After extraction in Tris-HCl buffer with SDS saturated with phenol, the high-molecular phosphates were further separated by means of gel electrophoresis. Four fractions were obtained: the highest molecular weight migrated very slowly, while the others according to their increasing mobility had chain lengths decreasing constantly from "fraction IV" to "fraction I." The results obtained indicate that initially, linear oligo-polyphosphates are synthesized which subsequently condense to high-molecular weight polyphosphates. They partially serve as a phosphate reserve. However, 80% of the radioactivity incorporated can be found in low-molecular weight condensed inorganic phosphates after a short labeling period. A new hypothesis is proposed for the metabolic cycle of the condensed phosphates in the photosynthetic lower organisms *Chlorella* and *Acetabularia*.

INTRODUCTION

Phosphorus is an essential nutrient of all living cells and one of its most readily available sources is the pool of inorganic condensed phosphates. It has been known for a long time that condensed phosphates occur in a number of organisms. These condensed phosphates, however, have always been believed to be only linear condensed polyphosphates. It was not until 1969 that the existence of cyclic condensed metaphosphates in living lower and higher plants could positively be proved.

Soon it became obvious that metaphosphates were synthesized not only by the then studied blue green algae but also by the members of other groups of algae. Eventually they were also found together with polyphosphates in higher plants (Fig. 1).

ORGANISMS WITH POLY- AND METAPHOSPHATES

BACTERIA:	E.COLI
BLUE GREEN ALGAE:	ANACYSTIS NIDULANS, SYNECHOCOCCUS CEDRORUM
GREEN ALGAE:	CHLORELLA PYRENOIDOSA, ACETABULARIA (MED., CREN.)
BROWN ALGAE:	ILEA FASCIA, ECTOCARPUS SILICULOSUS, PYLAIELLA LITORALIS
RED ALGAE:	RHODOMELA CONFERVOIDES, CERAMIUM RUBRUM, C.DESLONGCHAMPSII
FUNGI:	CANDIDA BOIDINII, NEUROSPORA CRASSA
HIGHER PLANTS:	LEMNA GIBBA, L. PERPUSILLA, L. MINOR

Figure 1.

The basic prerequisite for the finding of the metaphosphates seemed to be a careful method of extraction which maintained pH neutrality. Hydrolyzed products could thus be avoided[1,2]. Until now, very little was known about the biosynthesis of the condensed phosphates, although Langen and his co-workers have published some results from yeast[3]. In order to come to a conclusion concerning high-molecular phosphates, it seemed advisable not to fractionate them with strong alkaline or acid (Langen et al.[3]), but to separate them in native conditions. Consequently, we attempted to separate the high-molecular weight fractions further by means of gel electrophoresis.

MATERIALS AND METHODS

Freely suspended cells of Chlorella pyrenoidosa and cells of Acetabularia mediterranea were cultured under sterile conditions in a synthetic liquid medium (Acetabularia was kindly supplied by Prof. H. G. Schweiger and his group in Wilhelmshaven). The conditions for labeling (10-20 μCi/ml of carrier-free$^{32}P_i$), extraction of the condensed phosphates, column chromatography on MAK and the separation of the labeled condensed inorganic phosphates from the nucleic acids on the QAE Sephadex A 50, and the identification of the different inorganic phosphates were described by Niemeyer and Richter[4] and Niemeyer[6].

A two-dimensional thin layer chromatography on cellulose separates the metaphosphates from the oligopolyphosphates up to chains of 8 phosphate acid residues. All condensed phosphates of more than 8 phosphate residues remain at the starting point and have consequently to be regarded only as a fraction on the chromatograms[1].

RESULTS

The mixture of condensed phosphates was concentrated in a 5% acrylamide stacking gel and afterwards separated in a 40% acrylamide running gel. The electrophoretic buffer contained Tris, glycine and SDS, and the samples were electrophoresed at 4 mA for 2.5 days. The mixture was stained with bromophenol blue. During the electrophoresis, differently colored bands can be seen, whose colors vary according to the pH value, and which correspond to certain fractions. The developed flat gels (16.0 x 8.0 x 0.3 cm) were dried and measured in a thin layer scanner from Berthold (Wildbad, G.F.R.).

On the measured gels (Figs. 2-5), 4 fractions can be recognized, which are labeled to a different extent (electrophoresis was from left to right). Point S indicates the transition from the start gel to the running gel. By comparing different labeling times (5, 10, 20, 60 min), it can be seen that the maximum of radioactivity shifts from the high-molecular phosphates to the low-molecular phosphates and is finally in fraction II. The high-molecular phosphates move very slowly in the highly concentrated gel and are named fraction IV. Consequently the length of the chains constantly decreases from fraction III to II and to fraction I.

Apart from the high ^{32}P-activity in the trimetaphosphate on the two-dimensional thin layer chromatograms, the very strong labeling in the area of the inorganic orthophosphate is remarkable. Since the mixture of phosphates was dialysed 20 hours before the separation by means of the thin layer chromatography, the fraction cannot be composed of inorganic orthophosphate. Instead it consists of organic phosphates, which is - according to our latest studies - very likely to be a mixture of inositol phosphates.

Fraction I of all flat gels, which predominantly contains metaphosphates and inositol phosphates, had a constant

Figures 2 - 5. Electrophoresis of the total condensed inorganic phosphates on a slab gel of 40% polyacrylamide after labeling with $^{32}P_i$ for indicated time. Point S indicates the transition from the stacking gel (5%) to the running gel.

Labelling times:

Figure 2: 5 minutes.
Figure 3: 10 minutes.
Figure 4: 20 minutes.
Figure 5: 60 minutes.

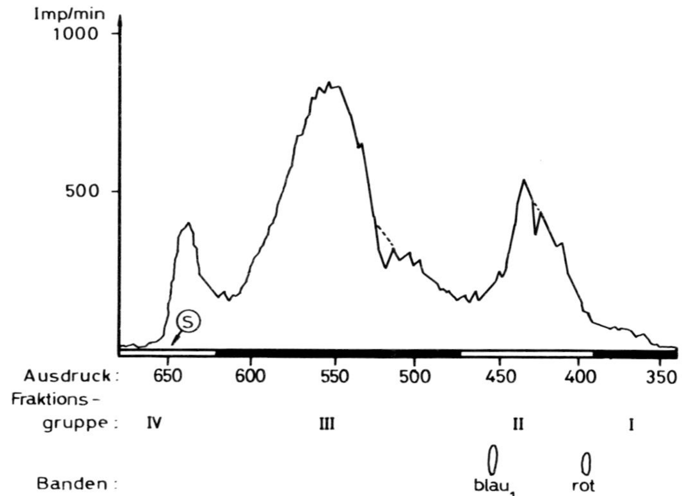

Figure 2.

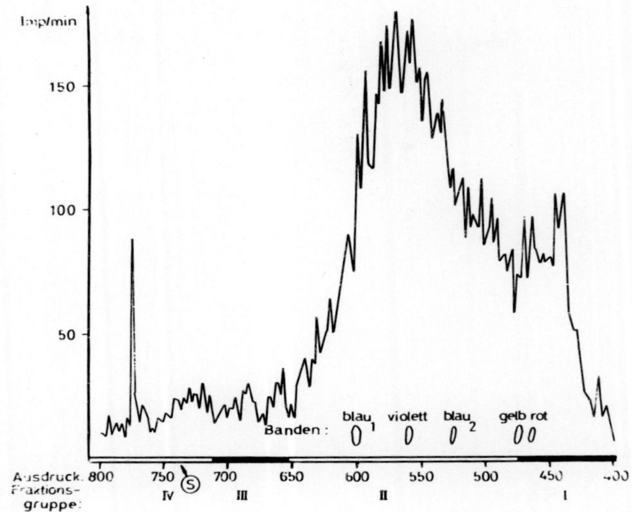

Figure 3.

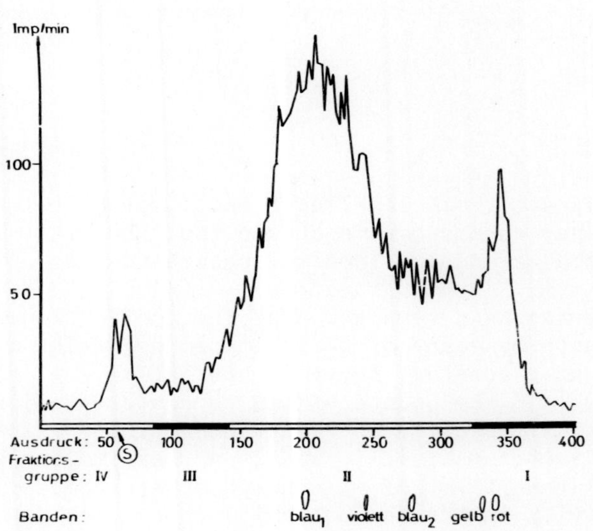

Figure 4.

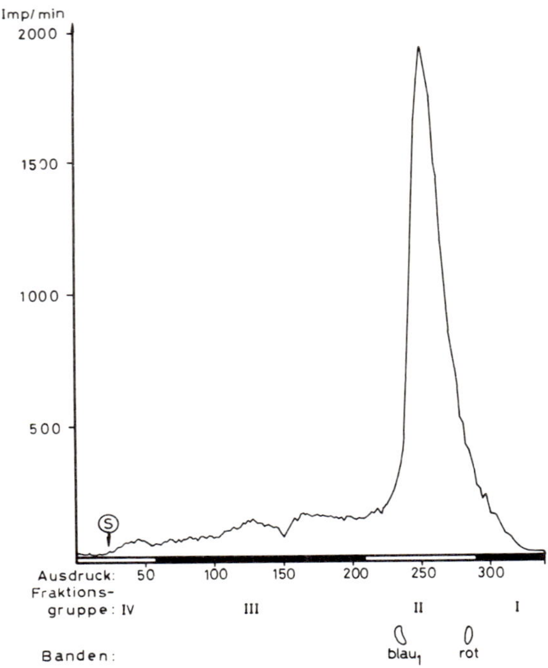

Figure 5.

^{32}P-activity after all labeling times. Moreover the counts of the thin layer chromatograms showed that the ratio between trimetaphosphate and the inositol phosphates was always the same.

This suggests a regulation of the pool of inorganic orthophosphate by means of these compounds, which are obviously kept at a constant level in the cell.

In Figure 6 the counts of the separate fractions are compared after different incubation times. The ^{32}P-activity maxima of fractions II, III, and IV appear in less than 5 min, which means that first of all the phosphate pool is filled. As the activity in the low-molecular phosphates increases, there is an intensified depletion of the high-molecular phosphates as well as a removal of phosphate from the

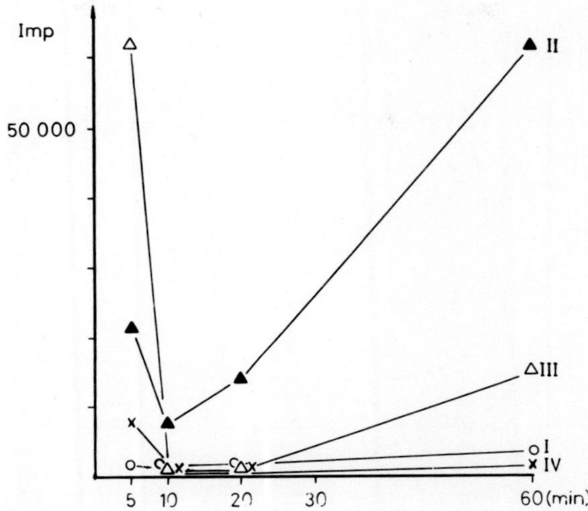

Figure 6. Comparison of the counts of the four separated fractions by gel electrophoresis after different labeling times with $^{32}P_i$.

phosphate pool. This inorganic phosphate is then transferred to other metabolic processes.

In Figure 7 the distribution of radioactivity in the various fractions is shown. The amount of metaphosphate and inositol phosphate (fraction I) reaches its minimum after 5 min. Since here the synthesis of high-molecular phosphates is still dominant, 65% of the activity is in fraction III, whereas after 10 min. 80% of the radioactivity is in fraction II.

These results (Fig. 8) hint at the possibility that at first linear oligopolyphosphates are synthesized, which then condense to high-molecular phosphates. A portion of these high-molecular phosphates is retained as a phosphate reserve, while about 80% of the activity can be found after a short labeling period in low-molecular condensed phosphates, which have about 10-60 phosphate residues. They then form cyclic metaphosphates. The trimetaphosphate either directly regulates the pool of inorganic orthophosphate or the incorporation of the inorganic orthophosphate into the other metabolic processes takes place by means of a system of organic phosphates. Since after a longer incubation in a P-free medium the trimetaphosphate is also rapidly labeled, is is possible

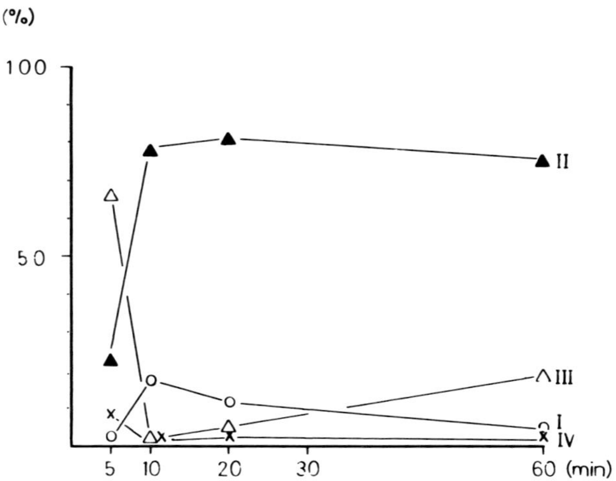

Figure 7. Comparison of the percental distribution of $^{32}P_i$-radioactivity in the various fractions after different labeling times.

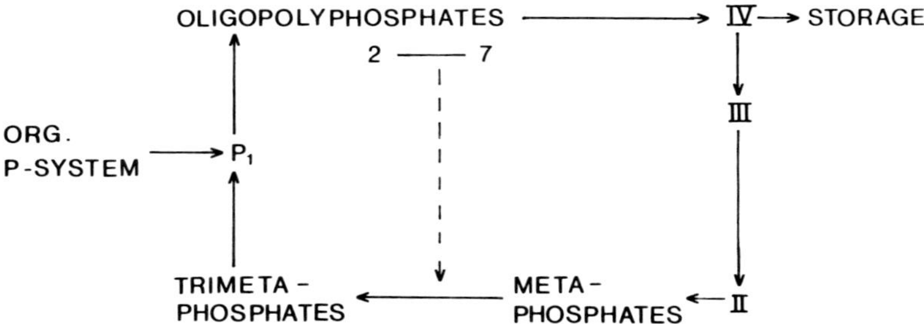

Figure 8. Metabolic cycle of condensed inorganic phosphate in living cells from Chlorella and Acetabularia. II-IV: various fractions of high-molecular condensed phosphates.

that a by-pass in the cycle of condensed phosphates leads from the oligopolyphosphates directly to the metaphosphates.

Fraction IV, which contains the longest chains, is incorporated immediately after phosphate depletion. After that, the labeling decreases and then remains on a constant level. A part of this fraction is likely to be a phosphate reserve or phosphate storage and is identical with the polyphosphate bodies as observed by other authors in electron micrographs[7].

DISCUSSION

As the first product of synthesis of condensed inorganic phosphates, Langen and co-workers[3] could find only high-molecular weight inorganic phosphates in yeast. No low-molecular intermediates, that is oligopolyphosphates were found. The authors could not account for this result. They supposed that ATP transfers inorganic orthophosphate directly to high-molecular phosphate or to a primer. This supposition is certainly not correct, because with the method of extraction without hydrolysis of high-molecular condensed phosphates, labeled oligopolyphosphates were found under all conditions. It is, however, necessary to mention that very long chains consisting of about 260 phosphates can be found even after 15 seconds. Equally questionable is the existence of a poly P_i fraction containing only tetrapolyphosphate.

The activity profiles of the fractions obtained by means of the gel electrophoresis are the same as Langen et al.[3] postulated in their hypothesis of the cycle of inorganic phosphates. It is very likely, however, that no precise figures can be given for the length of the chains in the different fractions. It must be supposed that the transitions between the fractions are labile.

The hexainositol phosphate acid, the so-called phytin acid, is up to now known to occur especially in the seeds of higher plants. It is generally believed that the phytin acid here takes over the function which the condensed phosphates fulfill in lower organisms. Since on the one hand in all organisms which have up to now been studied we could prove the existence of inositol phosphates together with the condensed phosphates and since on the other hand meta- and polyphosphates are to be found also in higher plants, the inositol phosphates cannot exclusively be regarded as a phosphate reserve in higher plants.

Up to now no positive statement is possible about the part which is played by the inositol phosphates, that is to say: by the phytin acid in this context. The ATP-ADP-P_i-system is likely to be in a close connection not only with the condensed phosphates, but also with the metabolism of inositolphosphates.

These studies were supported by the Deutsche Forschungsgemeinschaft.

REFERENCES

1. Niemeyer, R., Richter, G. (1969) Arch. Mikrobiol. 69, 54-59.
2. Niemeyer, R., Richter, G. (1972) In: Biology and Radiobiology of Anucleate Systems. II. Plant Cells (S. Bonotto, R. Goutier, R. Kirchmann, J. R. Maisin, eds.) 225-236, New York, Academic Press.
3. Langen, P., Liss, E., Lohmann, K. (1962) Colloq. Intern. Natl. Rech. Sci. (Paris) 106, 603-612.
4. Niemeyer, R. (1975) Planta 122, 303-305.
5. Inhülsen, D., Niemeyer, R. (1975) Planta 124, 159-167.
6. Niemeyer, R. (1976) Arch. Microbiol. 108, 243-247.
7. Harold, F. M. (1966) Bacteriol. Rev. 30, 772-794.

III CHLOROPLASTS

THE *ACETABULARIA* CHLOROPLAST GENOME: SMALL CIRCLES AND LARGE KINETIC COMPLEXITY

Beverley R. Green, Bernice L. Muir, and Usha Padmanabhan

Department of Botany
University of British Columbia
Vancouver, Canada

SUMMARY

The chloroplast DNAs of *Acetabularia mediterranea*, *A. major*, and *A. cliftonii* have buoyant densities of 1.705, and 1.706 g/cc in CsCl respectively. *A. cliftonii* has a heterogenous profile: when DNA was prepared so as to minimize shear, there was a small, sharp peak at 1.712 g/cc and a shoulder at about 1.700 g/cc in addition to the 1.706 g/cc band. When chloroplasts from axenic cells were lysed and centrifuged to equilibrium in ethidium bromide-CsCl, two bands were formed. The minor, denser band was enriched for the 1.712 g/cc component and contained small circular molecules of average circumference 4.2 µm. No circles 40-45 µm or larger were found in either band. Many attempts to isolate main band DNA without shear gave only linear molecules up to 200 µm long.

It is proposed that the minicircles may represent amplification of the ribosomal cistrons or a chloroplast episome.

A. cliftonii total chloroplast DNA renatured very slowly, with a calculated kinetic complexity of $1.52 \pm 0.26 \times 10^9$ daltons, compared to 0.2×10^9 daltons for *Chlamydomonas* chloroplast DNA and 2.5×10^9 daltons for *E. coli*. The renatured duplexes had very little mismatching (Δ T m = 0.5° C). Similar results were obtained with *A. mediterranea*. The chloroplast genome sizes of *Acetabularia* spp. are therefore considerably larger than those of other organisms, and may reflect the ancient evolutionary history of this genus.

INTRODUCTION

Acetabularia occupies an important position in the history of nucleocytoplasmic interactions. Most of the debate during the 1950's and early 1960's on whether organelles contained DNA resulted from the difficulty of preparing them free of contaminating nuclear material. *Acetabularia* is unique in that this problem can be removed with a pair of scissors before the start of the experiment! In 1963, Gibor showed that chloroplasts prepared from enucleated *A. mediterranea* contained measurable amounts of DNA[1], and thus provided the first rigorous evidence for the existence of a unique chloroplast genome.

In my laboratory, we have been studying *Acetabularia* chloroplast DNA from the point of view of organelle autonomy. An *Acetabularia* cell can continue to grow in the absence of its nucleus, to at least double its mass at the time of enucleation[2]. The chloroplasts continue to increase in number, and incorporate precursors of DNA, RNA, and protein[2, 3]. It has also been shown that isolated chloroplasts can synthesize most of their own amino acids[4], although it is not known whther chloroplast DNA codes for the enzymes involved. All this suggested that, in this organism at least, the chloroplasts might have a considerable degree of genetic autonomy. We therefore investigated the physical properties and conformation of its chloroplast DNA, and determined the appoximate genome size from its kinetic complexity.

MATERIALS AND METHODS

The isolation of chloroplasts, preparation of DNA, ultracentrifugation, and electron microscopy were as described previously[5,6]. The *A. mediterranea* DNA used for renaturation kinetics was isolated using Marmur's method[7]; the *A. cliftonii* DNA was isolated either that way or from eithidium bromide-CsCl gradients of chloroplast lysates[5]. *Chlamydomonas reinhardii* chloroplast DNA was purified from total DNA by two cycles of CsCl centrifugation. It formed a single band at 1.695 g/cc.

Renaturation rates were determined optically on sheared, heat-denatured DNA using a Gilford 2400 recording spectrophotometer. Conditions are given in the legends to Tables 2 and 3. A sample of *E. coli* DNA was renatured as a standard in each experiment. The second order rate constants were corrected to 1.0 M Na [8] and 50% G + C [9], and the kinetic complexities were calculated according to Wetmur and Davidson[10]. Sedimentation rates were determined according to Studier[24].

To determine the amount of DNA per chloroplast, isolated chloroplasts were made up to a known volume and duplicate samples taken for counting with a hemocytometer. Pigments and lipids were extracted from the remaining chloroplasts by the method of Smillie and Krotkov[12]. The air-dried residue was extracted several times with small volumes of 0.5 M $HClO_4$ at 90°. The combined extracts were made up to 200 µl, 400 µl of diphenylamine reagent[13] were added, the mixture shaken, and left at room temperature for 15-20 hours. Deoxyribose and deoxyadenosine heated to 70° for 20 minutes in 0.5 M $HClO_4$ were used as standards. The standard curve was extremely reproducible over a period of months with at least two different batches of diphenylamine reagent. One microgram deoxyribose in 0.6 cc gave an $O.D._{.570} = 0.247 \pm 0.012$.

RESULTS

Characterization

The physical characteristics of chloroplast DNA isolated from enucleated cells of three species of *Acetabularia* are given in Table 1. The base compositions calculated from the buoyant density and T_m of *A. mediterranea* DNA are in good agreement, consistent with the absence of methylated bases. There is a small but significant difference in base composition between *A. mediterranea* and the other two species.

The chloroplast DNA of *A. mediterranea* and *A. major* form single unimodal bands in CsCl [14]. However, a differential plot of the melting curve of the former DNA shows considerable intramolecular heterogeneity (Fig. 1), similar to that reported for the chloroplast DNAs of *Chlamydomonas* and *Chlorella*[15-17]. The chloroplast DNA of a third species, *A. cliftonii*, is noticeably heterogeneous even in a CsCl gradient (Fig. 2 a). In addition to a shoulder at 1.700 g/cc, there is another component at 1.712 g/cc which is visible as a discrete band in high molecular weight preparations.

Conformation

The chloroplast DNAs of *Euglena* and higher plants are in the form of 42-48 µm covalently-closed circles[18-20] which can be detected by centrifuging the DNA in an ethidium bromide-CsCl gradient[19,20]. Covalently closed circles cannot bind as much dye as linear or nicked molecules, and therefore band at a lower position in the gradient. When detergent lysates of *A. cliftonii* chloroplasts were centrifuged in such a gradient, two bands were detected (Fig. 3). The lower band (presumptive circles) made up 5-7% of the total chloroplast DNA.

When lower bands from a number of gradients were pooled and recentrifuged in CsCl without ethidium, it was found that

TABLE 1

Physical Characteristics of *Acetabularia* Chloroplast DNAs

	ρ(g/cm^3)	T_m(^{o}C)	%(G+C)	Conformation
A. mediterranea	1.702		43	linear
		86.7(SSC)	43	
		75.5(0.1xSSC)	42	
A. major	1.705	-	46	-(a)
A. cliftonii				
(a) main band	1.706	-	47	linear
(b) minor band	1.712	-	53	circular (4.2 µm)
(c) shoulder	1.700	-	41	-

(a) *Formed only one band in ethidium bromide-CsCl gradients*

the preparation was enriched for the 1.712 g/cc component (Fig. 2 b). Electron microscopy of this fraction showed the presence of small circular DNA molecules with an average contour length of 4.2 µm. No circles in the 45 µm range or higher were found. This work has been published in more detail elsewhere[5,6].

The main component of *A. cliftonii* chloroplast DNA, removed from the ethidium bromide gradient with minimum shear, contained only linear molecules with no discrete length distribution[5]. Chloroplast lysates from the other two species formed only one band in ethidium bromide-CsCl gradients, indicating the absence of covalently-closed circles. A number of methods were tried in an attempt to get intact chloroplast genomes from *A. mediterranea* chloroplasts, but without success. When chloroplasts lysed very gently with detergent were spread for electron microscopy, only linear molecules of various lengths up to 200 µm were seen[15].

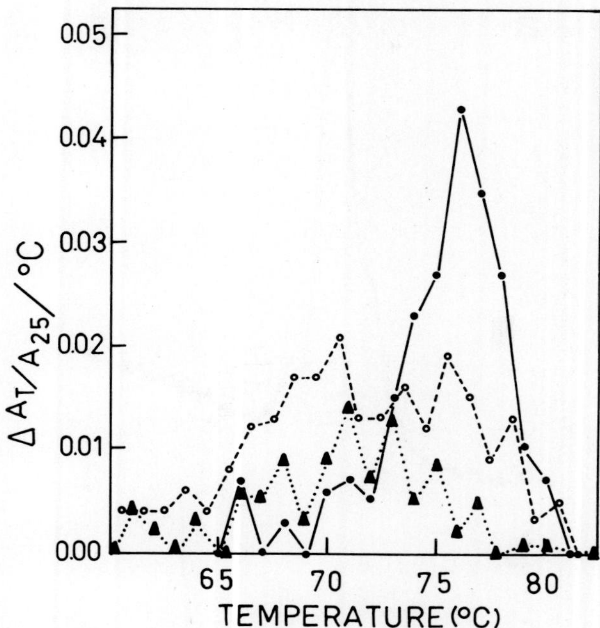

Figure 1. Differential melting curves of DNA in 0.1 x SSC (●———●) E. coli DNA; (o-----o) native Acetabularia chloroplast DNA; (▲.....▲) renatured Acetabularia chloroplast DNA.

Renaturation Kinetics

The first renaturation experiment done on Acetabularia chloroplast DNA had a surprising result: the chloroplast DNA renatured much more slowly than expected. Figure 4 shows a typical renaturation rate plot for A. mediterranea chloroplast DNA along with the E. coli DNA standard for the same experiment. Conditions and concentrations are described in the legend. It is clear that the renaturation rate constants of chloroplast and bacterial DNAs are of the same order of magnitude (Table 2). In order to check the fidelity of the complexes being formed, renatured DNA was dialysed into 0.1 x SSC and remelted. The remelting curve is shown in Figure 5 along with the melting curve for native DNA. The T_m has been

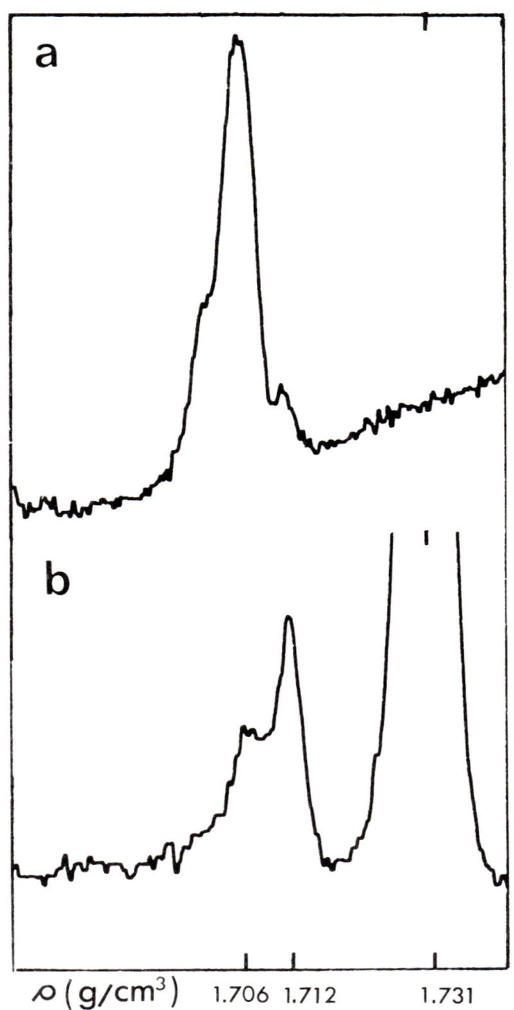

Figure 2. CsCl gradients of A. cliftonii chloroplast DNA.

(a) Total chloroplast DNA.

(b) Pooled lower bands from several ethidium bromide-CsCl gradients, rerun in the absence of dye. DNA at 1.73. g/cm^3 is M. lysodeikticus reference DNA.

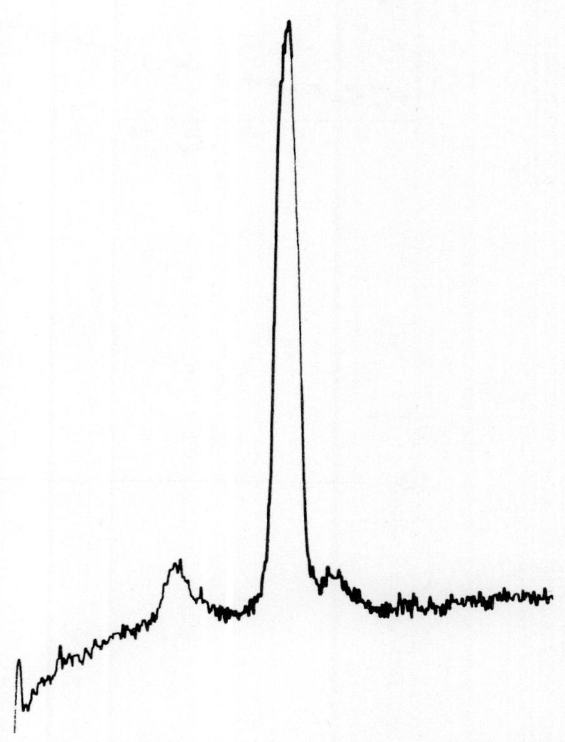

Figure 3. Microdensitometer tracing of photograph of A. cliftonii chloroplast DNA banded in ethidium bromide-CsCl preparative gradient.

lowered by 0.7°, corresponding to approximately 1% mismatching[21]. In addition, a differential plot of the melting curve of the renatured chloroplast DNA (Fig. 1), is essentially identical to that of the native DNA. This shows that there is no preferential renaturation of either GC-rich or AT-rich segments of the genome.

The renaturation rate constants and kinetic complexities calculated for A. mediterranea according to Wetmur and Davidson[10] are given in Table 2. The kinetic complexity of

Figure 4. Renaturation rate plots. Closed circles, A. mediterranea chloroplast DNA, 6 ug/ml. Open circles, E. coli DNA, 13 ug/ml. See Experiment 2, Table 2.

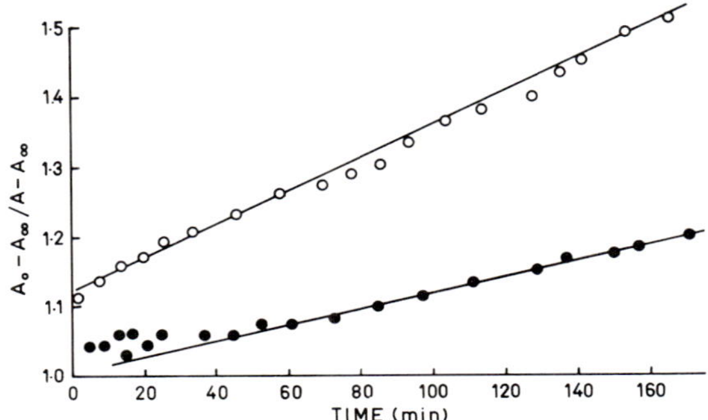

Figure 5. Thermal denaturation of A. mediterranea chloroplast DNA in 0.1 x SSC. Closed circles, native DNA. Open circles, DNA renatured in 2 x SSC, then dialysed into 0.1 x SSC.

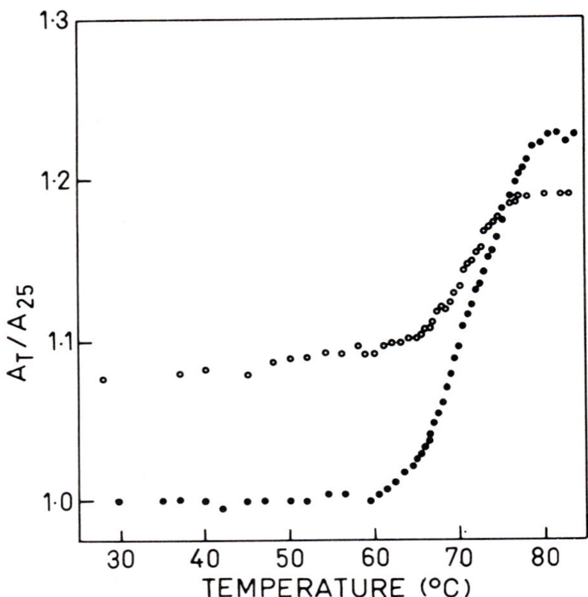

TABLE 2

Renaturation Kinetics of A. mediterranea Chloroplast DNA

Expt. No.	DNA	Conc. μg/ml	k_2 (a)	$S^{pH\ 13}_{20,\ w}$	N_D (c)
1	A. mediterranea chloroplast	15	5.90	6 (b)	8.7×10^8
	E. coli (K - 12)	19	13.57	28	2.6×10^9
2	A. mediterranea chloroplast	6	5.00	9 (b)	1.7×10^9
	E. coli (K - 12)	13	5.31	-	-
3	A. mediterranea chloroplast	10	7.62	7 (b)	8.1×10^8
	E. coli (K -12)	15	6.88	-	-
4	E. coli (K - 12)	19	6.05	13.4	2.3×10^9

(a) *Sheared, heat-denatured DNA was renatured in 2 x SSC at 65° C, and the second-order rate constant (k_2) corrected to 1.0 M Na^+ [8]. The chloroplast DNA was also corrected to 50% G + C according to Laird[9].*

(b) *$S^{pH13}_{20,w}$, s were determined according to Studier[24] on renatured samples and therefore underestimate the molecular weight at the beginning of the experiment.*

(c) *Calculated from the formula[10]:*

$$N_D = \frac{5.5 \times 10^8 \ (S^{13}_{20,w})\ 1.25}{k_2}$$

where N_D = kinetic complexity in daltons.

the E. coli DNA standard was determined to be 2.3-2.6 x 10^9 daltons, in good agreement with the literature value of 2.5 x 10^9 daltons[10,11]. The kinetic complexities of the chloroplast DNA are underestimated, because the $S^{pH13}_{20,w}$ values were determined after the DNA had been partially renatured, and some thermal degradation would have occurred[22]. This was done because of a shortage of material and because it was not realized in time how much the S rates could vary from preparation even under identical conditions of shearing. The actual $S_{20,w}^{pH13}$ values were probably 1.5 to 2.0 times higher at the beginning of the experiment. Using the experimentally determined sedimentation rates, the average kinetic complexity of A. mediterranea chloroplast DNA is 1.1 ± 0.4 x 10^9 daltons. The $S_{20,w}^{pH13}$ values of the E. coli experiments were determined on DNA which had not been renatured.

The kinetic complexities determined for the chloroplast DNA of the other species, A. cliftonii, are given in Table 3. In these experiments, all $S_{20,w}^{pH13}$ values were determined on unrenatured DNA. The kinetic complexities were normalized to give a value of 2.5 x 10^9 daltons for the E. coli standard [10,11]. The average of three determinations gave a genome size of 1.52 ± 0.26 x 10^9 daltons for the A. cliftonii chloroplast.

A renaturation experiment done on Chlamydomonas reinhardi chloroplast DNA under the same conditions (Table 3) gave a genome size of 2.08 x 10^8 daltons, almost too close to the reported values of 1.9-2.0 x 10^8 daltons[15,16,23]! This experiment shows that there is a large difference in rate constant between Chlamydomonas and Acetabularia chloroplasts DNAs and that this difference is easily detected by the methods used. It also shows that reliable results can be obtained by this method even with low concentrations of DNA.

Number of Genomes per Chlorplast

The amount of DNA per chloroplast was determined by the diphenylamine reaction on counted samples of chloroplasts, and the results are given in Table 4. With an average of 1.4 x 10^9 daltons per chloroplast, and a kinetic complexity of at least 1.1 x 10^9 daltons, the A. mediterranea chloroplast has an average of 1.3 or fewer genomes per chloroplast. In contrast, A. cliftonii chloroplasts have about three times as much DNA, giving an average of three genomes per chloroplast. The difference between the two species is unlikely to be due to the stage of growth of the cells, as the two determinations on the latter species were done on cells of about half maximum length (Experiment 1), and full length just prior to cap formation (Experiment 2).

DISCUSSION

The renaturation kinetics method has been very useful in determining the genome sizes of many bacterial and viral species[10,11,25]. When it is applied to higher plant chloroplast DNA, the kinetic complexities of 0.9-1.0 x 10^8 daltons

TABLE 3

Renaturation Kinetics of A. cliftonii and Chlamydomonas reinhardii chloroplast DNAs

Expt. No.	DNA	k_2 (a)	$S_{20,w}^{pH13}$ (b)	N_D (c)
1	Chlamydomonas chloroplast	38.38	8.22	2.08×10^8
	E. coli (K - 12)	4.16	10.11	-
2	A. cliftonii chloroplast	3.787	9.77	1.57×10^9
	E. coli (B - 23)	2.545	10.35	-
3	A. cliftonii chloroplast	4.808	7.75	1.75×10^9
	E. coli (B - 23)	3.349	7.71	-
4	A. cliftonii chloroplast	5.436	7.49	1.23×10^9
	E. coli	3.520	9.34	-

(a) *Sheared, heat-denatured DNA was renatured in 2 x SSC at 66 or 70° C, and the second-order rate constant (k_2) corrected to 1.0 M Na^+* [8]. *The chloroplast DNAs were also corrected to 50% G + C* [9].

(b) *$S_{20,w}^{pH13}$ calculated from the $S_{20,w}^{pH7}$ of heat-denatured DNA according to Studier*[24].

(c) *Calculated as in Table 2 and normalized to an N_D = 2.5 x 10^9 for E. coli*[10,11].

correspond well with the electron microscopic length of 42-48 μm[19]. With the chloroplast DNA of the green alga Chlamydomonas, the situation is not so clear. Three groups of workers have obtained kinetic complexities of 1.9-2.0 x 10^8 daltons[15,16,23], a remarkable degree of unanimity in the Chlamydomonas field. However, Herrmann and his co-workers

TABLE 4

Amount of DNA per Chloroplast

	Expt. No.	Amt. DNA g/chloroplast	Average Analytical Complexity (daltons)	Average Kinetic Complexity (daltons)	No. genomes per chloroplast
A. mediterranea	1	1.7×10^{-15}			
	2	3.0×10^{-15}			
	3	2.1×10^{-15}			
	Average	$(2.3 \pm 0.47) \times 10^{-15}$	1.4×10^{9}	$<1.1 \times 10^{9}$	<1.3
A. cliftonii	1	7.3×10^{-15}			
	2	8.4×10^{-15}			
	Average	$(7.9 \pm 0.79) \times 10^{-15}$	4.7×10^{9}	1.52×10^{9}	3

(pers. comm.) find 63 μm circles in Chlamydomonas DNA preparations, which should give a kinetic complexity of 1.2-1.3 x 10^8 daltons. In addition, Lambowitz et al[26] recently reported that restriction fragments of purified Chlamydomonas chloroplast DNA do not add up to 2.0 x 10^8 daltons. Their results ranged from 0.7 to 1.2 x 10^8 daltons, depending on the enzyme used. It is therefore possible that the renaturation kinetics method may overestimate the genome size by about a factor of two. This is probably largely due to the fact that the kinetic complexity is very sensitive to small changes in $S^{pH13}_{20,w}$, and there is no shearing method which produces fragments of absolutely uniform size.

This does not change the fact that the genome of the Acetabularia chloroplast is as much as eight times larger than that of the Chlamydomonas chloroplast. Since the kinetic complexity of Chlamydomonas chloroplast DNA determined by the methods used here was very close to published values, it shows that comparable kinetic data can be obtained at low concentrations. The remelting of the renatured Acetabularia DNA (Fig. 1 and 5) showed a small proportion of mis-matching and no preferential renaturation of GC-rich parts of the genome. The actual genome size of A. cliftonii chloroplast DNA is therefore between 8 and 15 x 10^8 daltons, and that of the A. mediterranea chloroplast DNA is in the same range. These chloroplast genomes thus have a much higher potential information content than higher plant chloroplast genomes, or the chloroplast genomes of the three algae, Chlamydomonas[15,16,23], Chlorella[17] and Euglena[27]. Their genome sizes are more comparable to those of bacteria[10,11,25]. It should be noted that some of the experiments on A. cliftonii DNA were done with DNA from axenic cells, so the results are not due to bacterial contamination.

What is this enormous genome doing? It does not appear to grant genetic or biochemical autonomy to the chloroplast, since several chloroplast ribosomal proteins[28] and probably some thylakoid membrane proteins[29] are coded for by the nuclear genome and apparently synthesized on cytoplasmic ribosomes. Perhaps Acetabularia and its relatives have been as conservative on the molecular level as they have been on the morphological level. The Dasycladaceae have the most ancient fossil record of any of the green algae, with recognizable members from strata as old as 500 million years[30]. Whether chloroplasts originated from photosynthetic endosymbionts, or from single cells by compartmentalization, there may well have been a stage when they contained more DNA than they do now. Perhaps Acetabularia is a "living fossil" which has not had its chloroplast DNA pruned down by selection or by transfer to the nucleus[31].

The large kinetic complexity explains why no 45 μm

circles were found in the chloroplasts. An intact genome would have to be at least 400 μm long, a length which would be extremely sensitive to shear[32], even the very mild shear associated with spreading in a detergent solution. For the same reason, it cannot be stated that the main component of the chloroplast genome is not circular.

The 4.2 μm minicircles are an interesting puzzle. They are not of bacterial or mitochondrial origin, and have been seen in close association with the chloroplast membrane[5]. Their size and base composition is approximately right to code for two ribosomal cistrons including spacer[6], and it is tempting to speculate that this might be a case of gene amplification. On the other hand, why not a chloroplast episome? A presumptive episome has been reported in yeast[33], and there is no reason why other eukaryotes should not also have them. Unfortunately, the extremely small amount of DNA that can be isolated from thousands of axenic, individually enucleated cells means that further testing of these hypotheses will have to wait until much larger amounts of this DNA can be obtained by cloning.

The amount of DNA per chloroplast is more than an order of magnitude greater than the 10^{-16} g estimated indirectly by earlier workers[1]. Since the genome size is also large, the number of copies of the genome per chloroplast is small. This is in marked contrast with other types of chloroplast, which contain 20 or more copies of a smaller genome[15-17]. In fact, if the average of 1.3 genomes per A. mediterranea chloroplast are distributed randomly according to the Poisson distribution, approximately 27% of the chloroplasts should contain no DNA at all. This may explain why Woodcock and Bogorad[34] could detect no DNA in as many as 60% of the chloroplasts of this species using several different cytochemical methods.

ACKNOWLEDGEMENTS

This research was supported by grants from the National Research Council of Canada. The experiments reported here could not have been done without the dedicated assistance of "The Enucleators": Livia Beck, Margaret Ward, and Valerie Macdonald.

REFERENCES

1. Gibor, A. and Izawa, M. (1963) Proc. Nat. Acad. Sci. U.S. 50, 1164-69.
2. Shepard, D. S. (1965) Exp. Cell Res. 37, 93-110.
3. Shephard, D. S. (1965) Biochim. Biophys. Acta 108, 635-43.

4. Shephard, D. S. and Levin, W. B. (1972) J. Cell Biol. 54, 279-94.
5. Green, B. R. (1976) Biochim. Biophys. Acta 447, 156-166.
6. Green, B. R. (1977) Proc. Colloquium on Nucleic Acids and Protein Synthesis in Plants, C.N.R.S. Paris.
7. Marmur, J. (1961) J. Mol. Biol. 3, 208-218.
8. Britten, R. J. (1970) Problems in Biology: RNA in Development (Hanly, E. W., ed.) p. 187-216. University of Utah Press, Salt Lake City.
9. Laird, C. D. (1971) Chromosoma 32, 378-406.
10. Wetmur, J. G. and Davidson, N. (1968) J. Mol. Biol. 31, 349-370.
11. Gillis, M., DeLey, J. and DeCleene, M. (1970) Eur. J. Bioch. 12, 143-153.
12. Smillie, R. M. and Krotkov, G. (1960) Can. J. Bot. 38, 31-49.
13. Burton, K. (1968) Methods in Enzymology (Grossman, L. and Moldave, K., eds.) Vol. 12 B. Acad. Press, New York.
14. Green, B. R. (1972) Protoplasma 75, 478.
15. Bastia, D., Chiang, K. S., Swift, H. and Siersma, P. (1971) Proc. Nat. Acad. Sci. U.S. 68, 1157-1161.
16. Wells, R. and Sager, R. (1971) J. Mol. Biol. 58, 611-622.
17. Bayen, M. and Rode, A. (1973) Eur. J. Bioch. 39, 413-420.
18. Manning, J. E., Wolstenholme, D. R., Ryan, R. S., Hunter, J. A. and Richards, O. C. (1971) Proc. Nat. Acad. Sci. U.S. 68, 1169-1173.
19. Kolodner, K. and Tewari, K. K. (1975) Biochim. Biophys. Acta 402, 372-390.
20. Herrmann, R. G., Bohnert, H. J., Kowallik, K. V. and Schmitt, J. M. (1974) Biochim. Biophys. Acta 378, 305-317.
21. Hutton, J. R. and Wetmur, J. G. (1973) Biochemistry 12, 558-563.
22. Eigner, J., Boedtker, H. and Michaels, G. (1961) Biochim. Biophys. Acta 51, 165-168.
23. Howell, S. H. and Walker, L. L. (1976) Biochim. Biophys. Acta 418, 249-256.
24. Studier, W. T. (1965) J. Mol. Biol. 11, 373-390.
25. Bak, A. L., Christiansen, C. and Stenderup, A. (1970) J. Gen. Microbiol. 64, 377-380.
26. Lambowitz, A. M., Merril, C. R., Wurtz, E. A., Boynton, J. E. and Gillham, N. W. (1976) J. Cell Biol. 70, 217a.
27. Stutz, E. (1970) FEBS Letters 8, 25-28.
28. Kloppstech, K. and Schweiger, H. G. (1973) Exp. Cell Res. 80, 69-78.
29. Apel, K. and Schweiger, H. G. (1972) Eur. J. Bioch. 25, 229-238.
30. Johnson, J. H. (1961) Quart. Colo. School of Mines 5, #2.

31. Bogorad, L. (1975) Science 188, 891-898.
32. Bowman, R. D. and Davidson, N. (1972) Biopolymers 11, 2601-2624.
33. Guerineau, M., Slonimski, P. and Avner, P. R. (1974) Biochem. Biophys. Res. Comm. 61, 462-469.
34. Woodcock, C. F. L. and Bogorad, L. (1970) J. Cell Biol. 44, 361-375.

ULTRASTRUCTURE OF DNA OF BASAL, MIDDLE AND APICAL CHLOROPLASTS OF INDIVIDUAL *ACETABULARIA MEDITERRANEA* CELLS

Antonio Mazza, Silvano Bonotto, and Bruno Felluga

International Institute of Genetics and Biophysics
Consiglio Nazionale delle Ricerche
Naples, Italy
and
Department of Radiobiology, C.E.N.-S.C.K.
Mol, Belgium

SUMMARY

An original technique has been worked out for the isolation, purification and ultrastructural characterization on a microscale level, of DNA complements of chloroplasts of selected compartments of single *Acetabularia mediterranea* cells. Evidence is obtained of DNA heterogeneity among basal, middle, and apical chloroplasts: apical chloroplasts have the highest DNA content so far observed (up to 2000 µm per chloroplast) and, most likely, the highest transcriptional activity. On the other hand, DNA of middle and basal chloroplasts exhibits a more complex supramolecular organization. These findings extend the concept of the well known apico-basal gradient in *Acetabularia* cells to the chloroplast genome.

INTRODUCTION

The chloroplasts of *Acetabularia mediterranea* are distributed along the stalk of the cell following an apico-basal gradient[1,2]; they are both ultrastructurally[1-5] and functionally[6,7] distinguishable in three different types: apical, middle and basal. Going from the apex to the basis of the cell, they become progressively larger and charged with storage material (starch), which is almost absent in apical chloroplasts[3,5]. Concomitantly, chloroplast multiplication, which is active in apical chloroplasts[1,6], is rare or absent in basal chloroplasts[1,3,6]. Chlorophyll analyses have also shown relevant differences among the three types of chloroplasts[8,9]. Experimental evidence suggests that such a modulation of chloroplast morphology and function requires both the action of morphogenetic substances of nuclear origin[1-3,10,11] and the functional integrity of the chloroplast DNA itself[1,3]. In fact, conversion of apical and middle type chloroplasts into chloroplasts of basal type has been repeatedly observed[1,3,6] in living anucleate halves of _Acetabularia_ cells[12]. Conversely in basal, nucleate, regenerating halves of _Acetabularia_[12], a new population of apical chloroplasts is issued from the basal one at the level of the new apex[3], where substances of nuclear origin are accumulated[13,14]. All these facts are taken as evidence of nuclear control of chloroplast morphology and function[1,3,6]. On the other hand, treatment of normal living _Acetabularia_ cells with ethidium bromide[1,15], which is known to affect only cytoplasmic, i.e. chloroplast and mitochondrial DNA synthesis[15,16], has much the same effect as enucleation on the chloroplast population[1,3,15]. Since ethidium bromide is known to suppress DNA replication[17] and transcription[18], it is reasonable to speculate that both these processes are involved in maintaining the chloroplast apico-basal gradient and that, consequently, heterogeneity of DNA content and/or ultrastructure in the three different types of chloroplasts may be expected. To test this hypothesis, we have worked out a procedure for the electron microscope visualization of the DNA complement of the three types of chloroplasts within individual _Acetabularia_ cells. The following report illustrates the experimental procedure employed and discusses some preliminary findings which suggest genome heterogeneity among the three chloroplast populations.

EXPERIMENTAL PROCEDURE

Growth of axenic algae

One of the major problems in the characterization of cytoplasmic DNAs of _Acetabularia mediterranea_ is the possibility of contamination from DNA of bacterial origin[19]. Methods have been devised to grow practically axenic cells and they consist of either growing _Acetabularia_ in the presence of antibiotics and bacteriocides[16], or frequently renewing the sterile culture medium[16]. Since both theoretical considerations and experimental evidences (16; Bonotto, S., unpublished) argue against the use of antibiotics as sterilizing agents, we decided to follow the second alternative, which proved to be very effective for obtaining sterile cultures of _Acetabularia_ cells[2,20].

Choice and treatment of cells for the experiments

Cells at stage 4 [21] were chosen. At this stage of growth the _Acetabularia_ cell reaches its fully functional maturity but still retains a well-defined cytoplasmic compartmentation[3,21]. All nuclear materials (a possible source of contaminating DNA) reside in one of the branches of the rhizoid[21,22], which can easily be snipped off. This also has the advantage of eliminating the major source of bacterial contamination[19]. Cells were enucleated and repeatedly (2-3 times) brushed in successive changes of large volumes of sterile growth medium[20]. Fragments 5 mm long, were taken from the sub-basal, middle, and sub-apical portions of the stalk. The cytoplasmic content of each fragment was withdrawn with a Pasteur micropipette under a dissecting microscope.

Chloroplast isolation

Each cytoplasmic fraction, corresponding to a volume of 20-40 μl and containing approximately 1 x 10^6 chloroplasts[6], was individually subjected to the Shephard and Levin procedure for isolation and purification of chloroplasts under sterile conditions[23].

Electron microscopy

The Kleinschmidt osmotic shock technique[24] was used. All solutions employed for electron microscope preparations were made with double-distilled water and filtered through Millipore membranes (pore size 0.45 μm). Sterile chloroplast pellets, obtained by the Shephard and Levin procedure[23], were resuspended in 0.02 to 0.2 ml volume of 2 M ammonium acetate and 0.1% cytochrome C (final concentrations). Aliquots of 20-40 μl of the mixture were spread over the 80 cm^2 surface of a double distilled water hypophase. 20 minutes after spreading, the shocked chloroplasts were picked up on formvar carbon-coated 300 mesh copper grids. The samples were stained with uranyl acetate in acetone[25]; some were rotary shadowed with 15 mg Pd, at a distance of 11 cm from the source and an angle of 7°. Best results, both in terms of resolution and visualization of structures were obtained with unshadowed specimens. Electron microscope observations were carried out with a Philips EM 300; a Polaron grating with 2160 lines/mm was used for calibration.

Measurements of contour lengths

These were made with a map ruler on 60,000 x final prints. In order to be able to compare our results with previous findings[26], molecular weights were calculated on the basis of a mass-to-length ratio of 2×10^6 daltons/μm. However there are indications that for DNA prepared by osmotic shock, this figure may exceed 4% [27].

RESULTS

The experimental procedure employed in this work proved to be very effective and highly reproducible for the visualization of the DNA content of fractions of the chloroplast population of single *Acetabularia* cell compartments. By this method, it has been possible to regulate the concentration of chloroplasts per grid, by simply changing the volume of solution used to resuspend the chloroplast pellet, and the area of spreading surface. Our chloroplast preparations showed only typical chloroplast ghosts (Fig. 1); they were devoid of any contaminating material, either of bacterial or cytoplasmic origin. Overlapping of ghosts and associated DNA were avoided by the uniformity of the spreading technique. About 100 chloroplast ghosts were inspected for each region examined. The ghosts either showed attached DNA (Figs. 1-7) or were apparently empty, in the ratio of approximately 50: 50. This ratio was the same for the chloroplasts of the three regions.

Our experimental conditions retained the integrity of the chloroplasts so that the DNA was always observed in form of compact "displays" (in the sense of Green and Burton[26]) made of elementary fibers of 110-120 Å in close contact with ghost remnants (Figs. 1-7); wandering fragments of DNA were never detected. A portion of the DNA of these displays was seen to be closely connected to remnants of the chloroplast ghost, either in the form of laterally synapsed multiple molecules (in the sense of Upadyaya and Grun[28]) (Figs. 2, 3), or of bundles of parallel, individual fibers (Figs. 2, 3, 6). Under favorable conditions, the latter appeared connected to 'knots,' interspersed along linearly oriented DNA fibers (Fig. 2). Twisting of molecules was a common finding (Fig. 4).

Three prominent features enabled the DNAs of the three different populations of chloroplasts examined to be distinguished: (1) DNA content. Apical chloroplasts were, by far, the most homogeneous population. About 90% of them exhibited DNA lengths of 900-2,000 μm (2×10^8 daltons). Of middle and basal chloroplasts, 70% showed DNA lengths of about 500-700 μm (10^9 to 1.4×10^9 daltons); and the remaining 30%, lengths of about 30-200 μm (6×10^7 to 4×10^8 daltons). (2) Spirals,

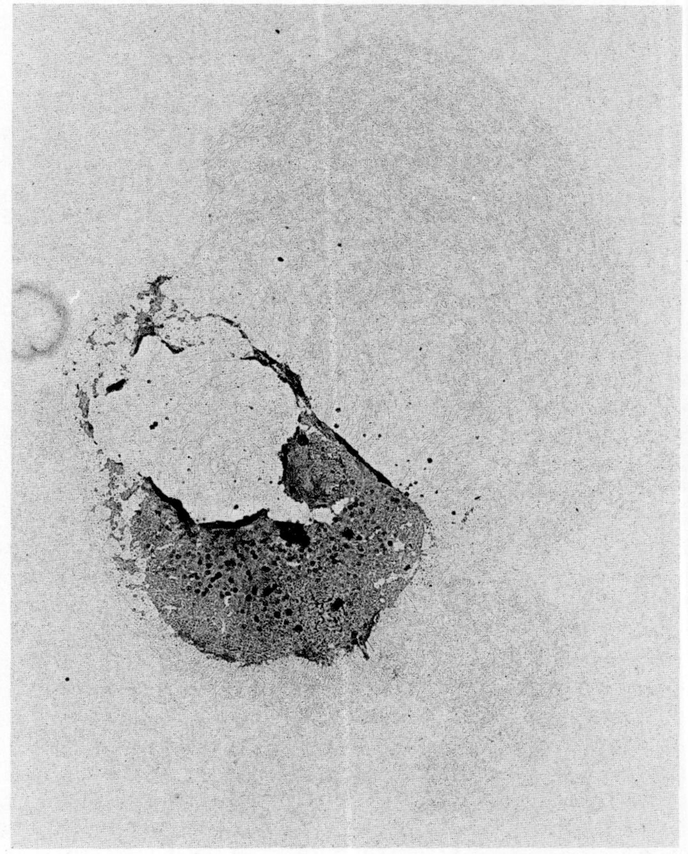

Figure 1. Acetabularia mediterranea apical chloroplast subjected to osmotic shock. Note the compactness of the DNA display, which occupies a large area, and the connections of DNA fibers with the ghost. DNA total length is 918 um. Rotary shadowing. x 14,200.

intermingled with and continuous with very extended linear DNA molecules, have been observed in increasing amounts from apical to basal chloroplasts. While in apical and middle chloroplasts (Figs. 5 and 6) they were found in about 50% of

Figure 2 (opposite page). Portion of a 1,200 um DNA display released from an apical chloroplast, showing laterally synapsed multiple molecules connected to ghost remnants (arrows), spirals, and bundles of parallel individual DNA fibers. Note the organization of the latter in knots, intercalated along linearly oriented DNA fibers (bottom, right). Bushy structures radiate from several linearly oriented fibers (small arrows). Uranyl acetate in acetone. x 42,500.

DNA-containing ghosts, they were observed in 90-100% of the basal chloroplasts (Fig. 7). (3) Bushy structures, either free (Fig. 4) or attached to DNA fibers (Figs. 2, 4) were frequently present in apical chloroplasts and very scanty or absent in both middle and basal chloroplasts. They were more clearly visualized in unshadowed specimens.

DISCUSSION

This work presents a new experimental procedure for the observation of the DNA complements of chloroplast populations of selected compartments of single Acetabularia cells. Over other more commonly used procedures, this method of preselecting particular groups of organelles, offers the possibility of investigating the modifications induced on their DNA complements by the intracellular environment. This is achieved through the examination of the following parameters: total DNA content per chloroplast; DNA topology; DNA transcriptional activity.

Present findings lead to the following comments:

1) As it appears so far, apical chloroplasts of Acetabularia have shown the highest DNA content per chloroplast compared to the middle and basal ones. Although a content of up to 1,000 µm double stranded DNA (dsDNA) has already been shown in Acetabularia mediterranea bulk chloroplasts[29], present observations strongly suggest that these and higher figures, up to 2,000 µm, are restricted to the apical chloroplasts. A correlation of such finding with the observed high multiplication potential of chloroplasts of this region of the cell[1,6] is attractive.

2) According to Woodcock and Bogorad[29], a very high percentage (50-60%) of Acetabularia mediterranea bulk chloroplasts are totally devoid of DNA. On the basis of previous findings on apico-basal gradient[1,2], one would have expected that by far the greatest majority of "empty" chloroplasts should be found among the basal chloroplasts. The experimental procedure employed in this work has shown that this is not the case.

3) That DNA spirals are not spreading artifacts is ruled

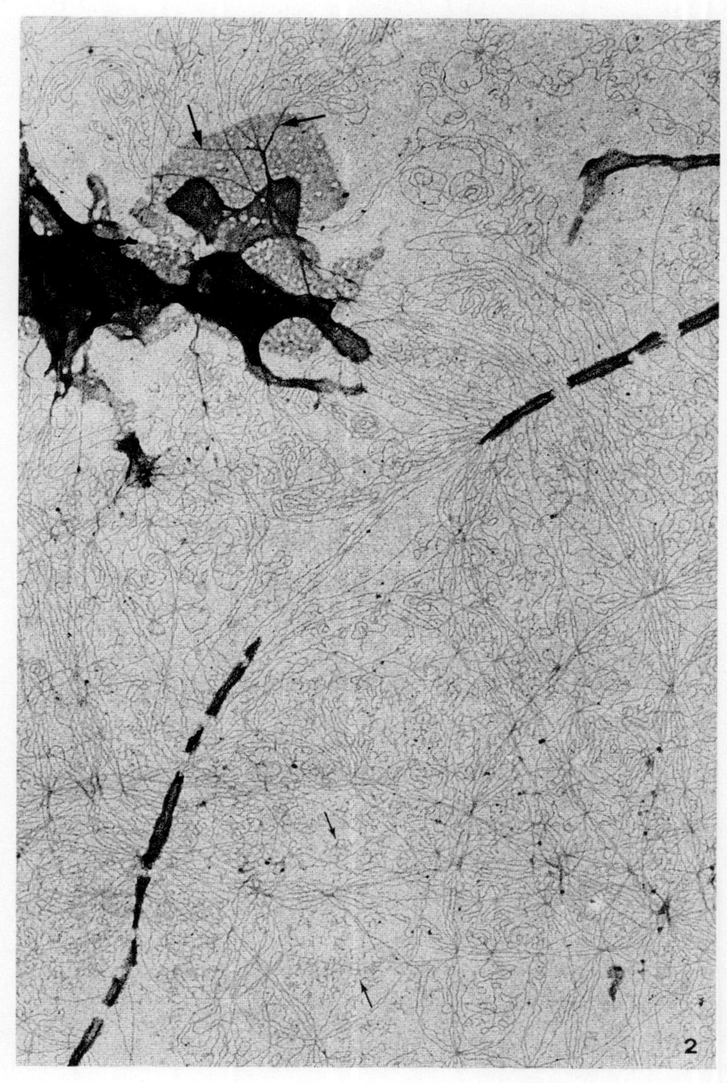
2

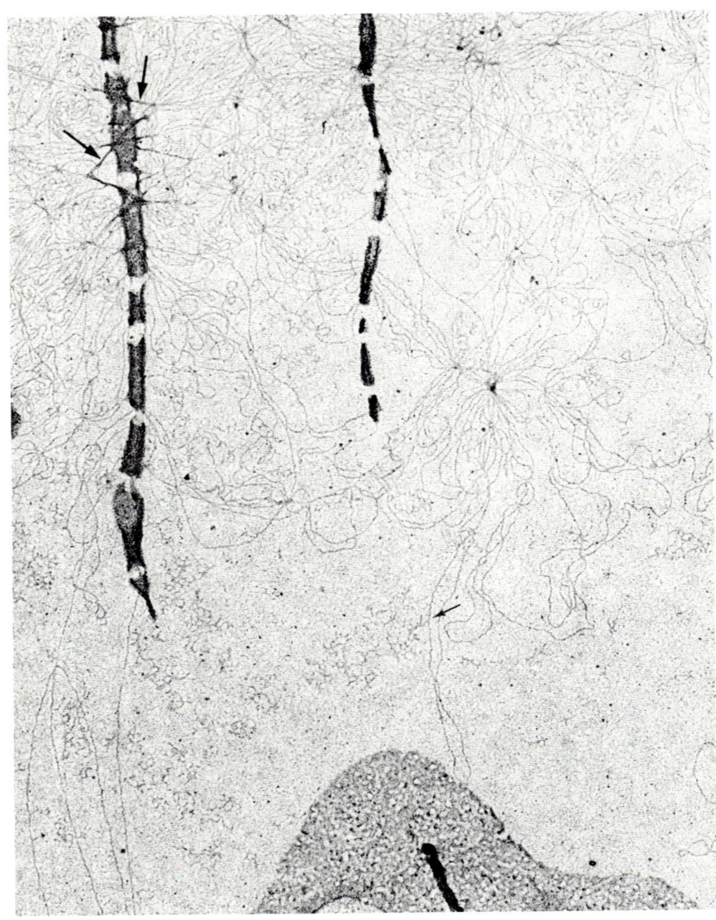

Figure 3. Apical chloroplast. Laterally synapsed multiple molecules connected to linearly oriented ghost structures (arrows). Bushy structures both free and connected to dsDNA molecules (small arrows) are visible. Uranyl stain. x 42,000.

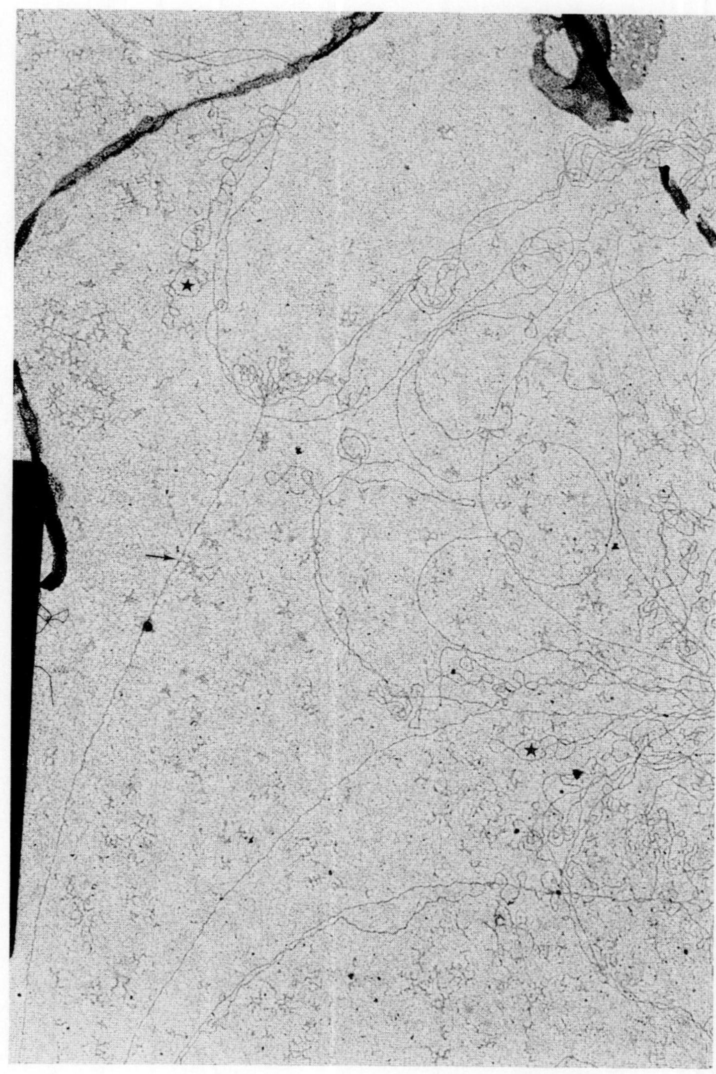

Figure 4. Apical chloroplast. Linear twisted dsDNA molecules suggesting supercoiling (stars), and bushy structures, both free and connected to DNA fibers (arrow). Uranyl stain. x 42,000.

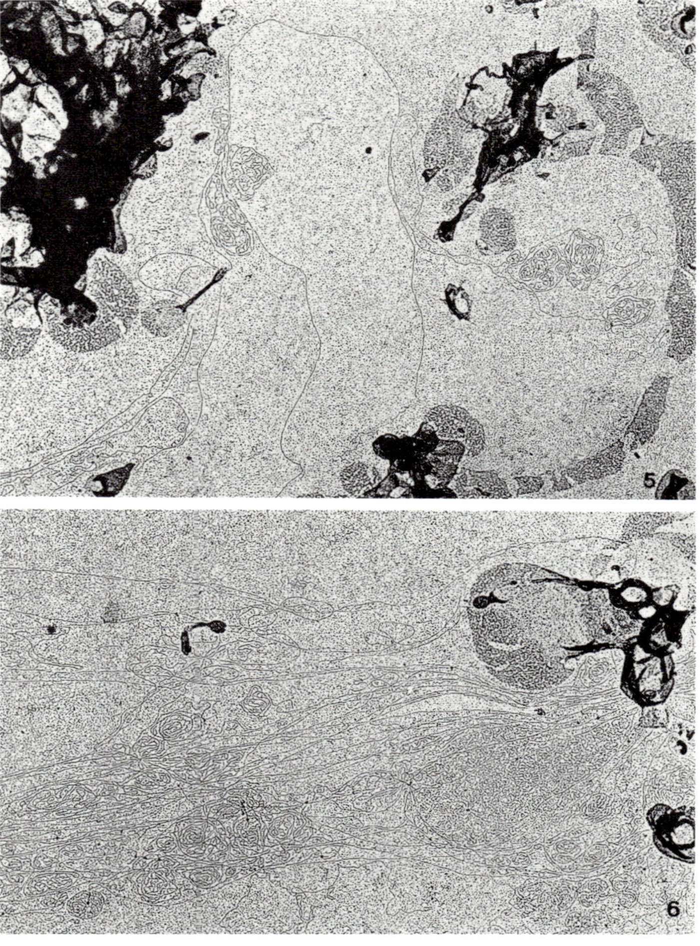

Figures 5 and 6. Middle chloroplasts. DNA spirals and extended DNA fibers, near to ghost remnants. Shadowed specimens. x 16,000.

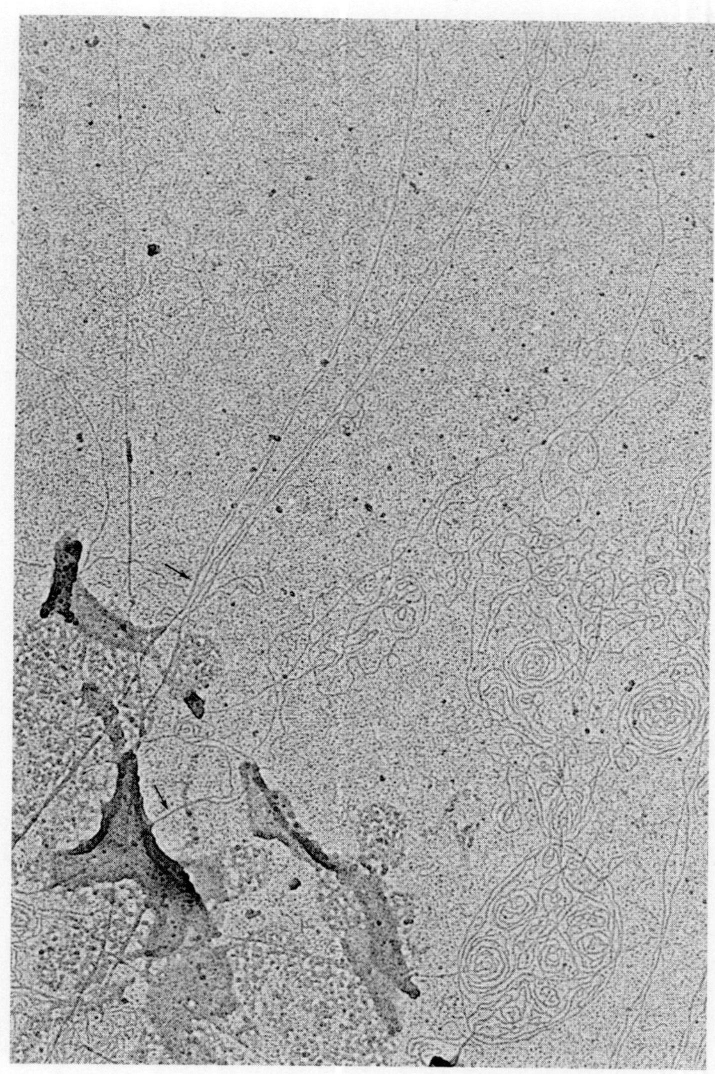

Figure 7. Basal chloroplast. Peripheral ghost region showing laterally synapsed multiple molecules (arrow), elongated fibers and, nearby, spirals of different sizes. Shadowed specimen. x 42,500.

out by their occurrence near linear fibers (Figs. 5, 6). Their presence within the chloroplast genome suggests that some constraints are imposed on the DNA superstructure and that the responsible factors are progressively active toward the base of the cell.

4) The bushy structures here observed may be interpreted as transcribed RNA material on the following grounds: (a) it is known that, under conditions of spreading on water hypophase, only single stranded DNA (ssDNA) and RNA assume the configuration of bushy structures[30]; (b) to our knowledge, ssDNA has not yet been found in Acetabularia chloroplasts; (c) whenever present in chloroplasts, ssDNA has shown a net-like configuration[31]; (d) our bushy structures are frequently seen radiating from linearly oriented dsDNA fibers, and (e) they occur as a gradient of small to larger molecules, as observed in other systems (e.g., 30). Thus, present data strongly suggest that an intense transcription activity occurs on the chloroplastic genome, and is almost exclusively restricted to apical chloroplasts. This is in agreement with recent biochemical findings showing that the highest rates of cytoplasmic (included chloroplast) RNA synthesis in A. mediterranea are localized at the level of the apex[32].

5) In agreement with Green et al.[26], we observed large amounts of supercoiled DNA, but no difference was noticed among the three regions.

ACKNOWLEDGEMENT

We are gratefully indebted to Mrs. A. Casale for her technical assistance. This work has been supported in part by the "Fonds de la Recherche Scientifique Fondamentale Collective," by EMBO and by the NATO Research Grant n° 1027.

REFERENCES

1. Puiseux-Dao, S. and Dazy, A. C. (1970) in Biology of Acetabularia (Brachet, J. and Bonotto, S., eds.), pp. 111-122, Academic Press, New York.
2. Puiseux-Dao, S. (1970) Acetabularia and cell biology, 162 pp. Logos, London.
3. Puiseux-Dao, S., Dazy, A. C., Hoursiangou, D. and Matthys, E. (1972) in Biology and Radiobiology of Anucleate Systems, II. Plant Cells (Bonotto et al., eds.), pp. 101-125, Academic Press, New York and London.
4. Bolouk̀here, M. (1972) J. Microsc. 13, 401-416.
5. Hoursiangou-Neubrun, D. and Puiseux-Dao, S. (1974) Plant Sci. Letters 2, 209-219.
6. Shephard, D. C. (1965) Exp. Cell Res. 37, 93-110.

7. Issinger, O., Maass, I. and Clauss, H. (1971) Planta 101, 360-364.
8. Sironval, C., Bonotto, S., Kirchmann, R., Hoursiangou-Neubrun, D. and Puiseux-Dao, S. (1972) Protoplasma 75, 487.
9. Dujardin, E., Bonotto, S., Sironval, C. and Kirchmann, R. (1975) Plant Sci. Letters 5, 209-216.
10. Puiseux-Dao, S. (1970) C. R. Acad. Sci. Paris 270, 358-361.
11. Hoursiangou-Neubrun, D., Puiseux-Dao, S., Dubacq, J. P. and Borghi, H. (1972) Protoplasma 75, 478-479.
12. Hämmerling, J. (1932) Biol. Zentralbl. 52, 42-61.
13. Puiseux-Dao, S. (1965) Morphologie et morphogenèse chez les Dasycladacées, Travaux dédiés à L. Plantefol, pp. 147-170, Masson, Paris.
14. De Vitry, F. (1965) Bull. Soc. Chim. Biol. 47, 1325-1351.
15. Heilporn, V. and Limbosch, S. (1971) Biochim. Biophys. Acta 240, 94-108.
16. Bonotto, S., Lurquin, P. and Mazza, A. (1976) Adv. mar. Biol. 14, 123-250.
17. Slonimski, P. P., Perrodin, G. and Croft, J. H. (1968) Biochem. Biophys. Res. Commun. 30, 232-239.
18. Nass, M. M. K. (1972) Exp. Cell Res. 72, 211-222.
19. Green, B., Heilporn, V., Limbosch, S., Boloukhère, M. and Brachet, J. (1967) Proc. Nat. Acad. Sci. 58, 1351-1358.
20. Lateur, L. and Bonotto, S. (1973) Bull. Soc. Roy. Bot. Belg. 106, 17-38.
21. Bonotto, S. and Kirchmann, R. (1970) Bull. Soc. Roy. Bot. Belg. 103, 255-272.
22. Hämmerling, J. (1931) Biol. Zentralbl. 51, 633-647.
23. Shephard, D. C. and Levin, W. B. (1972) J. Cell. Biol. 54, 279-294.
24. Kleinschmidt, A. K. K.,Lang, D., Jacherts, D. and Zahn, R. K. (1962) Biochim. Biophys. Acta 61, 857-864.
25. Gordon, C. N. and Kleinschmidt, A. K. K. (1968) Bioch. Biophys. Acta 155, 305-307.
26. Green, B. R., Burton, H., Heilporn, V. and Libosch, S. (1970) in Biology of Acetabularia (Brachet, J. and Bonotto, S., eds.), pp. 35-59, Academic Press, New York.
27. Wellauer, P., Weber, R. and Wyler, T. (1973) J. Ultrastr. Res. 42, 377-393.
28. Upadyaya, K. C. and Grun, P. (1975) Proc. Symp. Structural and Functional Aspects of Chromosomes, pp. 26-46, Bhabha Atom. Res. Centre, Bombay.
29. Woodcock, C. L. F. and Bogorad, L. (1970) J. Cell Biol. 44, 361-375.

30. Aloni, Y. and Attardi, G. (1972) J. Mol. Biol. 70, 363-373.
31. Woodcock, C. L. F. and Fernandez-Moran, H. (1968) J. Mol. Biol. 31, 627-631.
32. Naumova, L. P., Pressman, E. K. and Sandakchiev, L. S. (1976) Plant Sci. Letters 6, 231-235.

ACETABULARIA: A MODEL SYSTEM FOR STUDYING THE BIOSYNTHESIS OF CHLOROPLAST MEMBRANES

Klaus Apel

Lehrstuhl für Botanik
Freiburg, West Germany

SUMMARY

The two major chloroplast membrane components, the chlorophyll-protein complexes of 125,000 and 67,000 daltons were isolated from the chloroplasts of *Acetabularia mediterranea* and their polypeptide components identified. The 67,000 dalton complex contained two different subunits of 23,000 and 21,500 daltons. The 125,000 dalton chlorophyll-protein complex could be dissociated into free chlorophyll and a major polypeptide of 79,000 daltons. The localization of these polypeptides inside the thylakoid membrane was determined by fractionating the chloroplast membrane with EDTA and Triton X-100, by using pronase treatment and by labelling the surface-exposed proteins with ^{125}I. The 125,000 dalton chlorophyll protein complex seems to be buried inside the lipid layer. The 23,000 dalton subunit of the 67,000 dalton complex is largely exposed to the membrane surface and only the chlorophyll-binding subunit of 21,500 daltons is buried inside the lipid layer. The two subunits of the 67,000 dalton chlorophyll-protein complex were isolated and characterized by a number of different methods. The chemical structure of the two polypeptides of 23,000 and 21,500 daltons is very similar. The possible role of these polypeptides for the assembly and organization of the chloroplast membrane is discussed. The results of the localization of the different components within the membrane structure provide the basis for a proposed model of the chloroplast membrane.

INTRODUCTION

In our previous work with the green alga *Acetabularia mediterranea*, we described a complex interaction between the

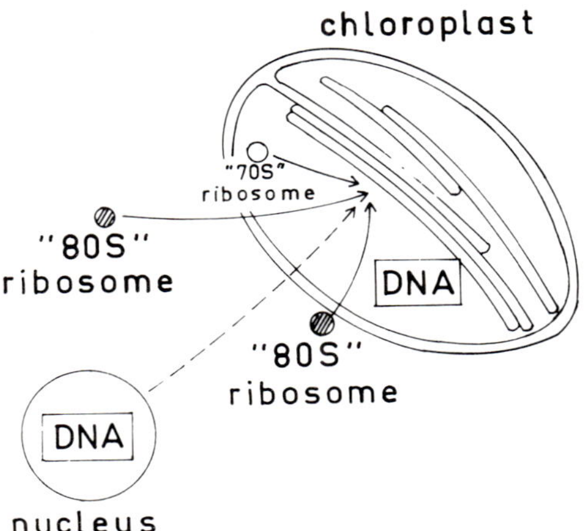

Figure 1. Schematic illustration of the nucleus-organelle interrelationships during the formation of chloroplast membranes.

nuclear and chloroplast genomes during the formation of the chloroplast membrane[1,2], which is summarized in Fig. 1. Some of the chloroplast membrane proteins are coded for by the nuclear DNA[1]. The chloroplast membrane proteins are either synthesized inside the organelle on chloroplast-specific 70S ribosomes or outside the organelle on two different groups of 80S ribosomes, one of which seems to be attached to the outer surface of the chloroplast while the second one is found in the cytosol[2] (Fig. 1). As an approach to an understanding of the biological meaning of this interrelationship, we are investigating the organization of the chloroplast membrane. It was the aim of this work, first to fractionate the chloroplast membrane into submembrane fragments; second, to purify the most prominent membrane proteins, the chlorophyll-protein complexes, from the isolated submembrane fragments and to characterize the chemical structure of these proteins; and third, to determine the localization of the chlorophyll-protein complexes within the membrane.

MATERIALS AND METHODS

The cultivation of *A. mediterranea*, the isolation of chloroplast membranes, the fractionation of the membranes, the electrophoretic separation and molecular weight estimation of the chloroplast membrane proteins, the pronase treatment and the iodination of the membrane were performed as described elsewhere[3,4]. The determination of the amino acid composition of the isolated polypeptides, the preparation of antibodies and the conditions for the trypsin and cyanogen bromide treatments will be described elsewhere[5].

RESULTS AND DISCUSSION

A. Fractionation of the chloroplast membrane

For the fractionation of the chloroplast membrane, the washed membrane preparation[3] was incubated with the detergent Triton X-100. The resulting membrane suspension could be resolved by sucrose gradient centrifugation into three different chlorophyll-containing bands A, B and C[3]. Fraction A contained only free chlorophyll. Fraction B of the washed chloroplast membrane (B_W) was identified as photosystem II while fraction C of the washed chloroplast membrane (C_W) was related to photosystem I[3].

The washed chloroplast membrane was solubilized in the presence of 0.2% SDS and was separated electrophoretically into 4 chlorophyll-containing bands (Fig. 2F). The fastest migrating chlorophyll band contained protein-free chlorophyll while the three other bands contained chlorophyll bound to proteins. The apparent molecular weights of these proteins were 125,000, 67,000 and 21,500 daltons[3]. In the fraction B_W only the 67,000 and 21,500 dalton chlorophyll-protein complexes were found (Fig. 2E) while in fraction C_W the 125,000 dalton chlorophyll-protein appeared (Fig. 2D). After staining the gel with Coomassie blue, additional protein bands appeared. Most of the polypeptides of fraction B_W did not appear in fraction C_W (Fig. 2A, B). This indicates an almost complete separation of the fraction B_W from fraction C_W. Since both submembrane fragments, B_W and C_W, contained a large number of polypeptides, it was not possible to isolate the chlorophyll-protein complexes directly from these fractions. Therefore, we fractionated the washed chloroplast membrane by a different procedure which involved two different steps.

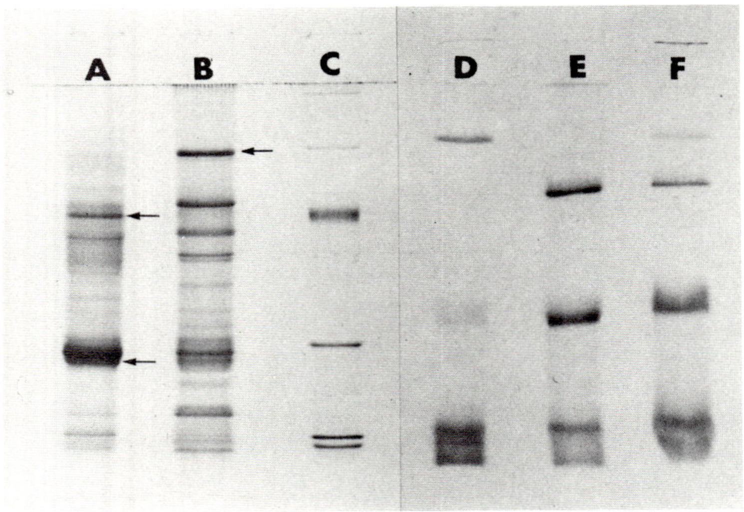

Figure 2. Chlorophyll and protein pattern after electrophoresis of the solubilized washed chloroplast membranes (F) and its subfractions B_W (A, E) and C_W (B, D) on polyacrylamide gels before (D - F) and after (A, B) Coomassie blue staining. The arrows indicate the position of chlorophyll-binding proteins. (C) Marker proteins[3].

First, the washed chloroplast membranes were treated with a solution containing EDTA and 2-mercaptoethanol. Under our experimental conditions, approximately 40% of the originally membrane-bound polypeptide species were solubilized and could be removed quantitatively from the remaining EDTA-insoluble chloroplast membrane (Fig. 3A, B)[4]. All the chlorophyll remained in the EDTA-insoluble membrane fraction and was at least partially bound to the three chlorophyll-protein complexes of 125,000, 67,000 and 21,500 daltons (Fig. 3B)[5].

In a second step, the EDTA-insoluble chloroplast membrane was incubated with the detergent Triton X-100. The resulting membrane suspension could be resolved by sucrose gradient centrifugation into three chlorophyll-containing bands A, B and C at approximately the same positions in the gradient as the three fractions of Triton X-100-treated washed chloroplast membranes. The fractions B and C of the EDTA-insoluble membranes (B_{EDTA} and C_{EDTA}) had similar chlorophyll a/b ratios and fluorescence properties and contained the same chlorophyll-protein complexes as the corresponding fractions B_W and C_W. However, fraction B_{EDTA} was photochemically inactive and both fractions, B_{EDTA} and C_{EDTA}, contained significantly fewer polypeptides than the fractions of the washed chloroplast membrane (Fig. 3C, D). Because of the smaller number of polypeptides, the chlorophyll-binding proteins of the two fragments B_{EDTA} and C_{EDTA} were isolated easily by the third fractionation step, preparative gel electrophoresis[4].

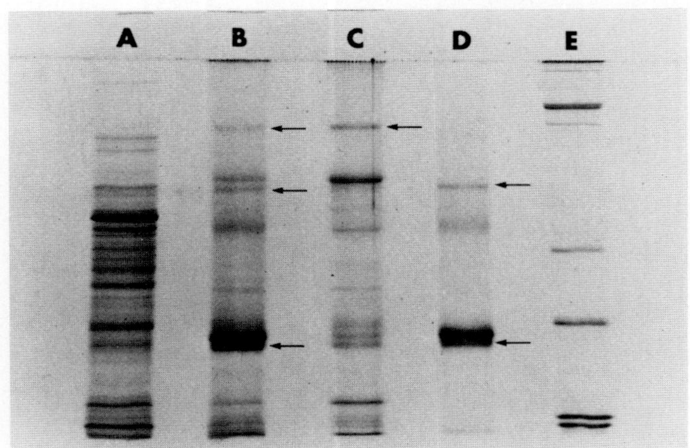

Figure 3. Electrophoresis of various membrane protein fractions after EDTA treatment of the chloroplast membranes of A. mediterranea. The gel was stained with Coomassie blue and shows the protein pattern of the EDTA-soluble protein fraction (A), the EDTA-insoluble membrane (B), and the fractions C_{EDTA} (C) and B_{EDTA} (D). Arrows indicate the position of chlorophyll-binding proteins. (E) Marker proteins[3].

B. Isolation of the chlorophyll-protein complexes

After preparative gel electrophoresis of the solubilized membrane proteins of fractions B_{EDTA} and C_{EDTA}, gel sections containing the three chlorophyll-protein complexes were cut out. The chlorophyll-binding proteins were eluted and reapplied to polyacrylamide gels.

Two chlorophyll-containing bands appeared upon re-electrophoresis of the 125,000 dalton chlorophyll-protein complex of fraction C_{EDTA}. Besides the 125,000 dalton chlorophyll-protein band, a band of free chlorophyll appeared. After Coomassie blue staining of the gel, two major protein bands were detected. In addition to the 125,000 dalton chlorophyll-binding protein, a major polypeptide of approximately 79,000 daltons appeared. Apparently, the 125,000 dalton chlorophyll-protein complex was unstable under our experimental conditions and was dissociated partially into free chlorophyll and one protein component of 79,000 daltons.

During re-electrophoresis of the 67,000 dalton chlorophyll-protein complex of fraction B_{EDTA}, the sample was resolved into three chlorophyll-containing bands. Apart from a 67,000 dalton chlorophyll-protein band there appeared a band of free chlorophyll and a 21,500 dalton chlorophyll-protein band. After Coomassie blue staining of the gel three protein bands were detected. In addition to the 67,000 dalton chlorophyll-binding protein, a second chlorophyll-binding polypeptide of 21,500 daltons, and a polypeptide of 23,000 daltons appeared (Fig. 4D). The 67,000 dalton chlorophyll-protein complex is apparently unstable under the conditions employed and was dissociated into two subunits of 23,000 and 21,500 daltons. The 21,500 dalton chlorophyll-binding polypeptide seems to be identical with the chlorophyll-protein complex of photosystem II in higher plants and other algae[6], which has been previously identified as the light-harvesting chlorophyll-protein complex of photosystem II[7].

Fraction B_{EDTA} contained only the 67,000 and 21,500 dalton chlorophyll-proteins, a 23,000 dalton polypeptide, and a minor component of 47,000 daltons (Fig. 3D). Since both the 23,000 and 21,500 dalton polypeptides are part of the 67,000 dalton chlorophyll-protein complex, there are actually only two proteins in fraction B_{EDTA}: the protein of 47,000 daltons, whose function is not known, and the 67,000 dalton chlorophyll-protein complex, which comprises approximately 80-90% of the total protein of fraction B_{EDTA}. This 67,000 dalton chlorophyll-protein probably represents the light-harvesting chlorophyll-protein complex of photosystem II in *Acetabularia*.

One may argue that the two subunits of the 67,000 dalton chlorophyll-protein complex are only two different electrophoretic forms of the same polypeptide and that the difference in electrophoretic mobility of these two protein bands is caused by their binding or non-binding to chlorophyll. We could exclude this possibility in several ways. Even after complete dissociation of chlorophyll from the 21,500 dalton polypeptide, both the 23,000 and 21,500 dalton polypeptides

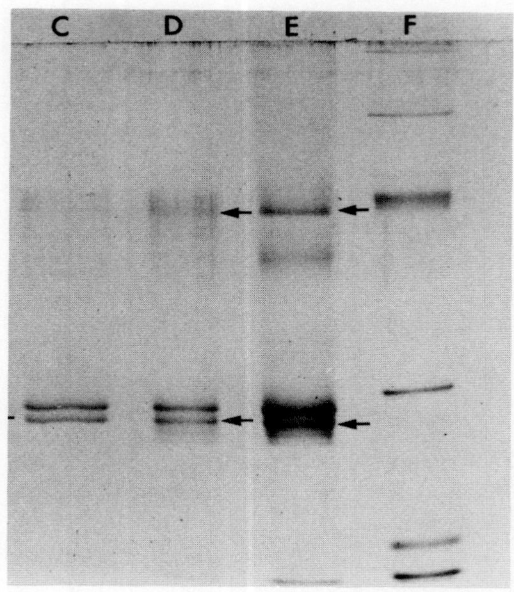

Figure 4. Re-electrophoresis of the 67,000 dalton chlorophyll-protein complex of A. mediterranea isolated in 1% (C) or 0.2% (D) SDS. (E) Electrophoresis of fraction B_{EDTA}. (F) Marker proteins[3]. The arrows indicate the positions of chlorophyll-binding proteins.

were still present in approximately the same amounts (Fig. 4C). Also, it was possible to separate the two subunits by preparative gel electrophoresis (Fig. 5A, B)[5].

The two isolated subunits were further characterized by comparison of their amino acid composition, by their immunochemical properties and by separating the peptide fragments obtained by trypsin and cyanogen bromide treatment.

The amino acid composition of the two subunits and the undissociated chlorophyll-protein complex of 67,000 daltons were determined and compared with that of the 125,000 dalton chlorophyll-protein complex (Fig. 6). The 125,000 and 67,000 chlorophyll-proteins are significantly different in their amino acid composition and thus seem to be different proteins. In contrast, the amino acid compositions of the two subunits

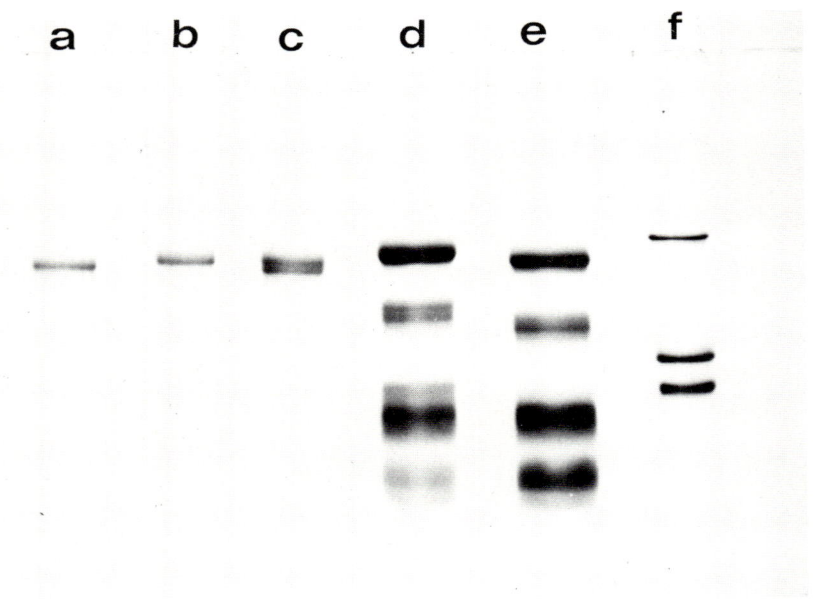

Figure 5. Electrophoresis of the cyanogen bromide fragments of the 23,000 (D) and the 21,500 (E) dalton subunits of the 67,000 dalton chlorophyll-protein complex of A. mediterranea. (A - C) Separation of the untreated subunits: (A) The isolated polypeptide of 21,500 daltons, (B) the isolated polypeptide of 23,000 daltons and (C) coelectrophoresis of the two isolated polypeptides. The BrCN-treatment was performed for 24 hours at 3°C in 70% formic acid.

of the 67,000 dalton chlorophyll-protein were so similar that any differences which may exist between the two polypeptides can only be revealed by other methods.

Antisera, which were prepared against the 67,000 dalton chlorophyll-protein gave precipitation lines on Ouchterlony double diffusion plates with the two isolated subunits, the undissociated 67,000 dalton chlorophyll-protein and fraction B_{EDTA}. The precipitation lines observed in all cases indicated immunochemical identity. The antisera did not react with the isolated 125,000 dalton chlorophyll-protein complex.

The different mobilities of the two subunits of the 67,000 dalton chlorophyll-protein during SDS polyacrylamide

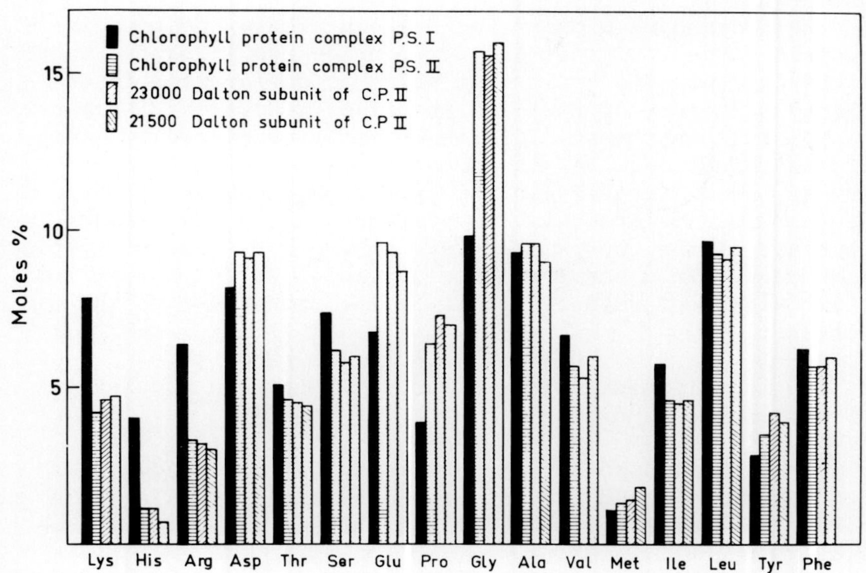

Figure 6. The amino acid composition of the 125,000 and 67,000 dalton chlorophyll-protein complexes and the 23,000 and 21,500 dalton subunits of the 67,000 dalton complex of A. mediterranea.

gel electrophoresis should reflect differences in the structure of the two polypeptides. The amino acid composition as well as the immunochemical properties did not indicate any significant differences between these two polypeptides. However, cyanogen bromide treatment as well as digestion with trypsin did reveal structural differences which could explain the difference in electrophoretic mobility of the two polypeptides.

Tryptic peptide maps of the isolated 23,000 and 21,500 dalton polypeptides showed approximately 17 detectable ninhydrin-positive spots, which were almost identical for both proteins. However, the 23,000 dalton subunit contained at least one tryptic peptide which was not found in the tryptic peptide pattern of the 21,500 dalton subunit, while the 21,500 dalton subunit differed in at least two tryptic peptides from the 23,000 dalton polypeptide.

The two isolated subunits were further characterized by comparison of their BrCN fragments. The cyanogen bromide fragments still exhibited at least partially the differences in molecular weight of the two polypeptides before the treatment (Fig. 5).

Both cyanogen bromide and trypsin cleave the proteins at specific sites. Differences between the resulting fragments of the two subunits could thus point to differences in the primary structure of these polypeptides. However, it cannot be excluded that these differences might be caused by secondary modifications. At the present time we cannot tell whether the differences in the apparent molecular weights of the two subunits are caused by differences in the primary structure of the two polypeptides or whether these polypeptides derive from one precursor molecule, which is modified in two different ways before it is incorporated into the membrane.

C. The localization of the chlorophyll-protein complexes within the membrane

The localization of the chlorophyll-protein complexes inside the thylakoid membrane was determined by using EDTA and pronase treatment and by labelling the surface-exposed proteins with ^{125}I.

Following the EDTA and pronase treatment of the washed chloroplast membrane, approximately 60% of the originally membrane-bound protein was removed from the membrane structure[4]. Electrophoretical analysis of the pronase-resistant membrane proteins shows that only the three chlorophyll-binding proteins of 125,000, 67,000 and 21,500 daltons are undegraded (Fig. $7B_1$). There is evidence that in addition to the three chlorophyll-binding proteins other smaller fragments are embedded in the pronase-treated membrane. The Coomassie blue-stained protein material in the unresolved front band increased significantly after pronase treatment[4] (Fig. 7B). This band contains fragments of molecular weights lower than approximately 9000. These fragments seemed to be part of originally larger membrane-bound proteins. A large portion of these proteins was degraded by pronase and removed from the membrane. However, some parts of these proteins seemed to be inaccessible to the enzyme and remained membrane-bound. Even though most of the membrane-bound proteins had been affected by the combined EDTA and pronase treatments, these treatments did not destroy the membrane structure as visualized in the electron microscope by thin-sectioning and freeze-fracturing techniques[4].

It cannot be expected that with the methods of EDTA and pronase treatment alone it would be possible to describe the surface topography of the chloroplast membranes. Thus, we used an additional procedure, enzymatic iodination according to Hubbard and Cohn[8], to label the chloroplast membrane. With this procedure we intended to clarify the following problem. The EDTA-soluble proteins comprise approximately 40% of the total protein of the washed chloroplast membranes. If these proteins were surface-bound as one might assume, their removal could influence the accessibility of the remaining proteins in the EDTA-insoluble membranes. This possibility was tested in the following two experiments.

In the first experiment the washed membranes were first iodinated. Then, the labeled membranes were treated with EDTA and 2-mercaptoethanol and the EDTA-soluble proteins were removed. The remaining EDTA-insoluble membranes were dissolved in the presence of SDS and the proteins separated electrophoretically. The distribution pattern of radioactivity in the gel indicates that in the washed membranes none of the EDTA-insoluble proteins were preferentially labeled (Fig. 7A). The large peak in the unresolved front band coincides with the zone of free chlorophyll and probably contains ^{125}I bound to lipids. This peak disappears in samples which had been extracted with acetone prior to electrophoresis.

In the second experiment, the chloroplast membrane was iodinated only after the EDTA-soluble proteins had been removed. If these latter proteins are at the surface, their removal could lead to a change in the accessibility of the remaining proteins in the EDTA-insoluble membrane. Indeed, the pattern of radioactivity of the EDTA-insoluble membrane proteins shows significant changes (Fig. 7C). In the EDTA-insoluble chloroplast membrane three main polypeptides became preferentially labeled with ^{125}I: Two peaks of 48,000 and 45,000 daltons and a major peak, which comigrated with the two polypeptides of 23,000 and 21,500 daltons. Although on this gel it was not possible to relate the radioactivity of the main peak to either one of these two polypeptides, it became evident after pronase treatment of the membrane that the radioactivity in this peak was bound only to the 23,000 dalton polypeptide. Parallel to the disappearance of radioactivity in this peak (Fig. 7C), the 23,000 dalton polypeptide was degraded and disappeared (Fig. $7B_1$). On the other hand, the 21,500 dalton chlorophyll-binding polypeptide was not affected by the pronase treatment.

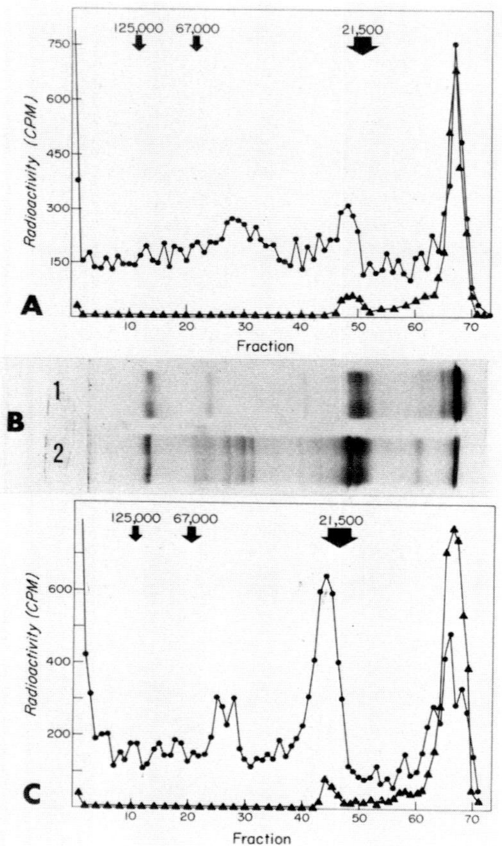

Figure 7. Electrophoresis of (^{125}I) lactoperoxidase-treated chloroplast membranes of A. mediterranea.

A) Washed chloroplast membranes were first iodinated and then extracted with EDTA. The EDTA-insoluble membranes were either solubilized and separated electrophoretically (●—●) or treated with pronase prior to solubilization of the membrane components (▲–▲). The arrows indicate the positions of the chlorophyll-binding proteins in the gel.

C) The washed chloroplast membranes were first extracted with EDTA and the EDTA-insoluble membranes were then iodinated as described[4]. The other experimental conditions were as described under Fig. 7A.

B) The polypeptide composition of the EDTA-insoluble chloroplast membrane before (2) and after (1) pronase treatment as revealed by Coomassie blue staining of the separated proteins in the gel.

These results indicate that the EDTA-soluble proteins were indeed on the surface and that they blocked, at least partially, the iodination of other membrane proteins. Only after the removal of the EDTA-soluble proteins, did the three proteins of 48,000, 45,000 and 23,000 daltons become accessible to ^{125}I and were preferentially labeled.

Based on our results, we were able to distinguish three groups of membrane proteins (Fig. 8). The first group of EDTA-soluble proteins was solubilized in the presence of EDTA and could be removed quantitatively from the remaining EDTA-insoluble chloroplast membrane. The second group of proteins seemed to consist of hydrophobic proteins, which are buried within the lipid layer of the membrane and which could not be reached by the surface probes. In the case of the chloroplast membranes of Acetabularia, only the chlorophyll-protein complex of 125,000 daltons and the 21,500 dalton subunit of the 67,000 dalton chlorophyll-protein complex seem to belong to the group of buried proteins. The third group of intermediary proteins seems to be linked with one part to the lipid layer probably by hydrophobic interaction, while the rest of the molecules remain outside the lipid layer where they can be reached by the surface probes. The intermediary proteins could link certain EDTA-soluble proteins to a buried protein, thus forming a functional unit.

For instance, one of the buried chlorophyll-binding polypeptides of 21,500 daltons together with the intermediary polypeptide of 23,000 daltons forms the chlorophyll-protein complex of 67,000 daltons. This complex, together with an additional minor component, can be isolated from the EDTA-insoluble membrane as a structural unit. In the washed chloroplast membranes, this unit forms together with several EDTA-soluble proteins the more complex, functional unit of photosystem II which can be isolated from the washed membranes by detergent treatment[3].

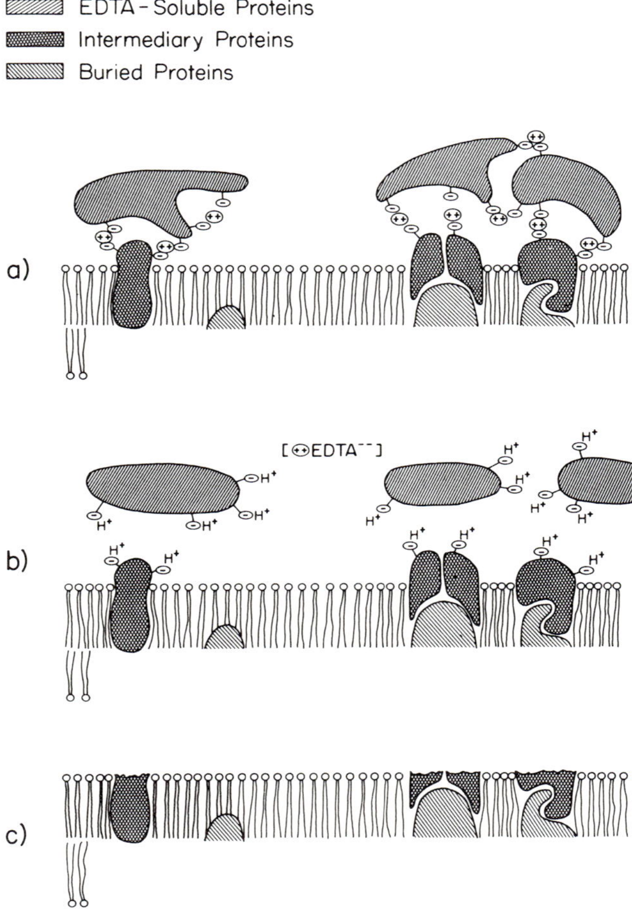

Figure 8. Schematic description of the effects of EDTA and pronase treatment on the chloroplast membrane of A. mediterranea. The washed chloroplast membrane before (A) and after the treatment with EDTA (B) and pronase (C).

As one of the major components of the chloroplast membrane, the 67,000 dalton chlorophyll-protein seems to play a crucial role in the assembly of the photosystem II particle as well as in the organization of the total membrane. It is possible that the two subunits of this complex as well as the other constituents of the photosystem II unit are synthesized on more than one of the different ribosome groups described previously for *Acetabularia*[2]. The spatial arrangement of these polypeptides within the membrane could be linked to the localization of the ribosome group on which they are synthesized. This possibility remains to be investigated in the future.

ACKNOWLEDGEMENTS

The author is grateful to Drs. J. M. Anderson, L. Bogorad, H. Chen, G. Miller, K. Miller, G. Richter, H. G. Schweiger, K. Steinback and C. L. F. Woodcock for cooperation, valuable suggestions and support.

Most of the experiments were done in the laboratory of L. Bogorad to whom the author is particularly grateful for his interest and encouragement throughout this work.

This investigation was supported by NATO, Deutsche Forschungsgemeinschaft and the Maria Moors Cabot Foundation.

REFERENCES

1. Apel, K. and Schweiger, H. G. (1972) Eur. J. Biochem. 25, 229.
2. Apel, K. and Schweiger, H. G. (1973) Eur. J. Biochem. 38, 373.
3. Apel, K., Bogorad, L. and Woodcock, C. L. F. (1975) Biochim. Biophys. Acta 387, 568.
4. Apel, K., Miller, K. R., Bogorad, L. and Miller, G. (1976) J. Cell Biol. 71, 876.
5. Apel, K., manuscript in preparation.
6. Thornber, J. P. (1975) Ann. Rev. Plant Physiol. 26, 127.
7. Thornber, J. P. and Highkin, H. R. (1974) Eur. J. Biochem. 41, 109.
8. Hubbard, A. L. and Cohn, Z. A. (1972) J. Cell Biol. 55, 390.

TEMPERATURE AND PHASE DEPENDENT EFFECT OF CYCLOHEXIMIDE ON THE INCORPORATION OF AMINO ACIDS INTO CHLOROPLAST MEMBRANE PROTEINS OF *ACETABULARIA*

T.-Y. Leong, D. O. Woodward and H. G. Schweiger

Max-Planck-Institut für Zellbiologie
Wilhelmshaven, Germany

SUMMARY

The incorporation of labeled amino acids into EDTA-insoluble proteins of the chloroplasts of *Acetabularia mediterranea* was studied in the presence and absence of cycloheximide during light and dark phases and at 20° and 25°. SDS polyacrylamide gel electrophoresis of these proteins, and subsequent measurement of the radioactive label incorporated into the different polypeptides revealed a peculiar temperature and phase dependent effect of cycloheximide on the incorporation into some polypeptides. There is at least one polypeptide, whose synthesis is strongly inhibited by cycloheximide at 20° in the light phase and at 25° in the dark phase, but is stimulated by cycloheximide at 20° in the dark phase and at 25° in the light phase. The molecular weight of this polypeptide is estimated to be approximately 39,000 daltons.

INTRODUCTION

The ultrastructure of chloroplasts from *Acetabularia* is subject to diurnal changes. The molecular mechanisms underlying these changes is unknown. More recently a two step model has been suggested[1] which might explain the biochemical basis of the circadian rhythm of photosynthesis rate. The two steps under consideration are the synthesis of "essential proteins" on 80S cytosol ribosomes and their integration into membranes, the two steps being interconnected by a feed back mechanism. The model implies that the peptide composition of membranes is subjected to diurnal changes. Moreover, the model predicts that the time of the day at which the changes occur depends on temperature. Here we want to report some preliminary results on the incorporation of amino acids into chloroplast membranes. These results are in agreement with the two step model.

MATERIALS AND METHODS

Cells of Acetabularia mediterranea were cultured as described[2,3] and were entrained (L:D 12:12) to a 24 hour cycle at 20° and 25°. For routine assays, 100 cells (2-2.5 cm in length) were incubated in 5 ml Erd-Schreiber medium[2,3] with an illumination of approximately 2500 lux. Preincubation began at 4.0 and 16.0 hours circadian time in the presence of cycloheximide (2µg/ml). After 30 minutes of preincubation, 100 µl (100 µCi) of ^{3}H-amino-acid mixture (Amersham Buchler) were added and the incubation allowed to proceed for 3 hours. The cells were then transfered to the chase medium[4] and incubated for 1 hour in the absence of cycloheximide. After this, chloroplasts were isolated and EDTA (disodium EDTA)-insoluble fractions were obtained as described[4]. These fractions were digested in SDS (sodium dodecyl sulfate) "Final Sample Buffer"[5] and separated on a slab polyacrylamide gel[6] employing a separation gel of 15% and 12.5% gel in the buffer system described[5]. Radioactivity in the 1mm gel slices was estimated by digesting the gel slices with 0.5 ml of tissue solubilizer (Soluene 300, Packard) at 60°C for 4 hours before being counted in 10 ml of toluene containing 0.4% Permablend III (Packard). Molecular weights were estimated from standard proteins[7].

RESULTS

In the present investigation, experiments were designed to analyze incorporation of amino acids into the EDTA-insoluble chloroplast membrane fraction of Acetabularia. Two different phases of the light dark cycles (circadian times 0400-0730 and 1600-1930) each at two different temperatures (20° and 25°C) were employed. The EDTA-insoluble chloroplast membrane fraction has been resolved by SDS polyacrylamide gel electrophoresis into at least 40 polypeptide bands[8]. The effects of cycloheximide on the incorporation of radioactivity into some of these polypeptides are summarized in Table 1 and Table 2. As shown in Table 1, at 20° and in the light phase, cycloheximide inhibits incorporation into polypeptide X (approximate molecular weight of 39,000 daltons), but stimulates incorporation during the dark phase. At 25°C, exactly the opposite is observed in the presence of the drug. This peculiar effect of cycloheximide is significantly observed in

TABLE 1

Appearance of labelled polypeptide X (39,000 daltons M.W.) in the EDTA-insoluble chloroplast membrane fraction

Temperature	Addition	Incorporation into polypeptide X	
		Light Phase	Dark Phase
20°	-CX	++	-
20°	+CX (2μg/ml)	-	++
25°	-CX	-	+
25°	+CX (2μg/ml)	++	-

TABLE 2

Incorporation of radioactive amino acids into EDTA-insoluble chloroplast membrane proteins (24,000 and 22,500 M. W.)

Temperature	Addition	Incorporation into polypeptide	
		Light Phase	Dark Phase
20°	-CX	++	+
20°	+CX (2μg/ml)	-	-
25°	-CX	++	+
25°	+CX (2μg/ml)	-	-

a few polypeptides, but particularly in polypeptide X. In contrast to this observation, as shown in Table 2 for two polypeptides of approximately 24,000 and 22,500 daltons molecular weight, cycloheximide inhibits the incorporation under all the experimental conditions. Most of the polypeptides in the EDTA-insoluble chloroplast membrane fraction behave similarly, i.e. the incorporation into most of the polypeptides in the EDTA-insoluble fraction is inhibited by cycloheximide in both the light and dark phases and at both 20° and 25°C.

DISCUSSION

The present study reveals that the incorporation of amino acids into most of the polypeptides in the EDTA-insoluble chloroplast membrane fraction is inhibited by cycloheximide under all the experimental conditions. This type of behavior is represented by the polypeptides which have molecular weights of 24,000 and 22,500. The incorporation into these components which are supposed to be subunits of the photosystem II complex[9], is inhibited by cycloheximide under all conditions. The two polypeptides are preferentially synthesized in the light phase (Table 2). However, there is at least one polypeptide (polypeptide X), whose synthesis is inhibited by the drug only under certain specific conditions (temperature and phase) and is even stimulated by cycloheximide under other conditions.

The "asymmetric" temperature dependent effect of cycloheximide exhibits a striking similarity with the effect of the same inhibitor on the circadian rhythm of O_2-evolution in *Acetabularia*. Cycloheximide has been shown[10,11] to shift the phase of the circadian rhythm of photosynthetic rate at 20° in the middle of the dark phase and at 25° in the middle of the light phase.

ACKNOWLEDGEMENTS

The technical assistance of Mrs. Tatjana Grimminger is gratefully acknowledged. We thank Dr. B. Cairns for critically reading the manuscript.

The experiments described in this paper are submitted by T.-Y. Leong to the Freie Universität Berlin in partial fulfillment of the requirements for a doctor's degree.

REFERENCES

1. Schweiger, H. G. and Schweiger, M. (1977) Intern. Rev. Cytol. in press.
2. Hämmerling, J. (1963) Ann. Rev. Pl. Physiol. 14, 65-92.
3. Schweiger, H. G. (1969) Curr. Top. Microbiol. Immunol. 50, 1-36.
4. Apel, K. and Schweiger, H. G. (1973) Eur. J. Biochem. 38, 373-383.

5. Laemmli, U. K. (1970) Nature 227, 680-685.
6. Studier, F. M. (1973) J. Mol. Biol. 79, 237-248.
7. Weber, K. and Osborn, M. (1969) J. Biol. Chem. 244, 4406-4412.
8. Leong, T.-Y., Woodward, D. O. and Schweiger, H. G. in preparation.
9. Apel, K., Bogorad, L. and Woodcock, C. L. F. (1975) Biochem. Biophys. Acta 387, 568-579.
10. Karakashian, M. W. and Schweiger, H. G. (1976) Proc. Natl. Acad. Sci. USA 73, 3216-3219.
11. Karakashian, M. W. and Schweiger, H. G. (1976) Exp. Cell Res. 98, 303-312.

BIOSYNTHESIS IN ISOLATED *ACETABULARIA* CHLOROPLASTS. III. COMPLEX LIPIDS

Fenton D. Moore and Irene Tschismadia

Biology Department
John Carroll University
Cleveland, Ohio
and
Ohio State University
Columbus, Ohio

ABSTRACT

Biosynthesis of complex lipids has been examined in isolated chloroplasts of *Acetabularia mediterranea* employing $NaH^{14}CO_3$, 1-^{14}C-acetate and {U}-^{14}C-glycerol. The major phospholipids were phosphatidylcholine and phosphatidylglycerol with lesser amounts of phosphatidylserine, phosphatidylinositol and diphosphatidylglycerol present. Monogalactosyldiglyceride and digalactosyldiglyceride were the major galactolipids with a minor component of polygalactosyldiglyceride. Sulfolipid, plastoquinone, glycerol, sterol glycoside and pigments were identified as products. Over 80% of the labeled lipoidal material exclusive of pigments and neutral lipids was accounted for.

In comparing the utilization of substrates, acetate was 4% as efficient as CO_2 in labeling lipids and glycerol 16%. Total phospholipid incorporation was 14.5% for CO_2, 24.6% for acetate and 32.4% for glycerol. Total galactolipid incorporation was 37.6% for CO_2, 31.7% for acetate and 19.9% for glycerol. The phosphatidylglycerol:phosphatidylcholine ratio was 3.2:1 and the monogalactosyldiglyceride:digalactosyldiglyceride ratio was 1.7:1.

Based upon acetate incorporation in light and dark it is proposed that the synthetic pathways of phosphatidylglycerol, phosphatidylserine and diphosphatidylglycerol are intraplastidal while those of phosphatidylcholine and the precursors of galactolipids are extraplastidal.

INTRODUCTION

In a continuing investigation of the synthetic potential of isolated *Acetabularia mediterranea* chloroplasts and the identification of their components, the biosynthesis of the complex lipids has been examined. *Acetabularia* chloroplasts are useful for studying biosyntheses for a number of reasons. First, they have been shown to be photosynthetically normal for long periods *in vitro*[1-3]. Secondly, isolated *Acetabularia* chloroplasts have already been shown to be capable of a variety of complex syntheses including protein amino acids[4], pigments[5,6], plastoquinones[7,8] and RNA[9]. With regard to lipid synthesis, their major advantage is that they multiply continuously throughout the log phase of growth[10]. Dubacq and Puiseux-Dao[11] have taken advantage of this log growth to study the relationship between lipid synthesis and chloroplast structure. Most studies of lipid synthesis are limited to greening of etiolated tissues[12], etioplasts[13] or periods of leaf expansion[14,15].

Studies of the relative efficiency of various carbon substrates in lipid synthesis is currently contradictory. Sherratt and Givan[16] claimed that CO_2 was not incorporated into the lipids of isolated pea chloroplasts while acetate was readily incorporated but other investigators have noted CO_2 incorporation into lipids of isolated chloroplasts[15,17]. We have therefore undertaken a study of the relative incorporation of CO_2, acetate and glycerol into the chloroplast lipids.

Although the synthesis of the chloroplast-limited galactolipids has been extensively studied, little is known of the site of synthesis of the major membrane phospholipids (see 18-20 for reviews). Studies of galactlipid synthesis which have been performed indicate that galactolipids which may have a structural function in the thylakoid related to Photosystem I [21] require translocation of precursors from the cytoplasm to the chloroplast[22-24].

MATERIALS AND METHODS

Acetabularia mediterranea (Lamouroux) completely free of contaminating algal species was cultured employing the methods and media described by Shephard[25]. Cells used in the experiments were 1-2 cm in length and in the log phase of growth.

Chloroplasts were isolated and incubated in mannitol-based media. Both the media and isolation techniques have been previously described and evaluated in detail[4]. All chloroplast preparations were completely free of contaminating bacteria. Chlorophyll was determined spectrophotometrically according to the method of Arnon[26] and ranged from 40-190 μg chlorophyll per incubation. Isolated chloroplasts were incubated with ^{14}C-sodium bicarbonate (Sp. Act. 55.3 mC/mM), 1-^{14}C-sodium acetate (Sp. Act. 59.9 mC/mM), {U}-^{14}C-glycerol (Sp. Act. 9.1 mC/mM), ^{35}S-sodium sulfate (Sp. Act. 25 mC/mM) or ^{32}P-disodium orthophosphate (Sp. Act. 951 mC/mM) for 1.5-3 hr at 1400 fc and 19-21 C. All labels except glycerol were employed in both light and dark incubations. To compare the relative efficiency of the carbon substrates, a single chloroplast preparation was divided into equal aliquots and incubated with different radioactive labels. All subsequent procedures were identical. Sodium bicarbonate served as the control and was sampled to determine fixation rate.

At the end of the incubation period, chloroplasts were collected by centrifugation, washed with 10% NaCl to remove the incubation medium and repelleted. To prevent lipolytic activity 2 ml of boiling isopropanol were added to each pellet and maintained at boiling temperature for 2 min[27]. Lipids were extracted according to the procedure of Bligh and Dyer[28]. All solvents were of spectral or reagent grade and deoxygenated with N_2 prior to use. The extract was dried under a N_2 stream, redissolved in a few drops of chloroform and spotted on a Silica Gel G thin layer plate. The chromatogram was developed in two dimensions using the solvent system of Lepage[29]. The procedure of Henninger and Crane[30] was used in four experiments to selectively extract plastoquinones. This extract was treated as above. After development, lipids were visualized employing specific spray reagents[31] and their pattern traced on plastic sheets. All chromatograms were contact radioautographed. The traces were overlaid on the resultant radioautographs. For comparative purposes exposure periods and development were identical. Radioautographs were scanned with a Photovolt Densitometer to quantitate relative incorporation into different lipids.

The following abbreviations are used: PGDG = polygalactosyldiglyceride, PS = phosphatidylserine, PI = phosphatidylinositol, GLY = glycerol, PC = phosphatidylcholine, SL = sulfolipid, PG = phosphatidylglycerol, PL = uncharacterized phospholipids, PGP = diphosphatidylglycerol, DGDG = digalactosyldiglyceride, MGDG = monogalactosyldiglyceride, PQ = plastoquinone, SG = sterol glycoside, UNK = unknown and PE = phosphatidylethanolamine.

RESULTS

Nineteen experiments were performed to establish the chromatographic fingerprint and identify individual spots. Phospholipids were located by selective incorporation of ^{32}P and identified by specific spray reagents and published Rf values[29]. The major membrane phospholipids were PG and PC. Minor components included PS, PI and PGP. In addition two other spots (#10 and #12, Fig. 1 B and C) incorporated ^{32}P in both light and dark. They were not labeled with CO_2 (Fig. 1 A) but incorporated both acetate and glycerol. They accounted for less than 3% of total carbon incorporation with either label but more than 15% of total phosphorus incorporation. Although unidentified, these compounds do not appear to be breakdown products as phosphatidic acid which is indicative of lipase activity[20] was never observed. Neither spot was PE. Sulfolipid was identified as the only spot incorporating ^{35}S. Galactolipids were identified by specific spray reagents and their Rf's as MGDG, DGDG and PGDG. Two spots were determined to be PQ's by chromatographing the heptane extract of the CO_2 labeled chloroplasts. Spot #17 (Fig. 1 A, B and C) was tentatively identified as SG based upon its response to specific spray reagents but was not further characterized. Glycerol was identified by chromatographing a standard. Pigments were identified by visual inspection of the chromatograms.

In order to compare the relative efficiency of various substrates in lipid synthesis, a single chloroplast preparation was divided into equal aliquots in 21 experiments. Preliminary experiments indicated that acetate and glycerol were not utilized at rates high enough to permit equal exposure times of the chromatograms. Therefore, subsequent experiments were performed with a differential in specific activities of CO_2:acetate:glycerol = 2.01:59.9:9.1. With the exception of the label, all other parameters and manipulations were identical. Resultant radioautographs were scanned densitometrically. Ratios of the areas under the curves for acetate and glycerol with respect to CO_2 were determined for each spot (Table 1). The cofactors, ATP, NADPH and acetyl CoA, were not employed as they should not be limiting in isolated chloroplasts undergoing normal photosynthesis[1-3]. Non-ionic detergents were omitted as they disrupt chloroplast integrity and virtually eliminate CO_2 fixation.

Figure 1 (opposite page). Contact radioautograph of the chromatograms of the complex lipids labeled in vitro. A = $NaH^{14}CO_3$ (Sp. Act. 2.01 mC/mM), B = 1-^{14}C-acetate (Sp. Act. 59.9 mC/mM), C = [U]-^{14}C-glycerol (Sp. Act. 9.1 mC/mM). 1 = PGDG, 2 = PS, 3 = UNK, 4 = PI, 5 = GLY, 6 = PC, 7 = SL, 8 = UNK, 9 = PG, 10 = PL, 11 = PGP, 12 = PL, 13 = UNK, 14 = DGDG, 15 = MGDG, 16 = PQ, 17 = SG, 18 = PQ, 19 = UNK, 20 = pigments and neutral lipids. Dashed circles = spots which are too light to copy well photographically. Unlabeled spots are degradation products variably present.

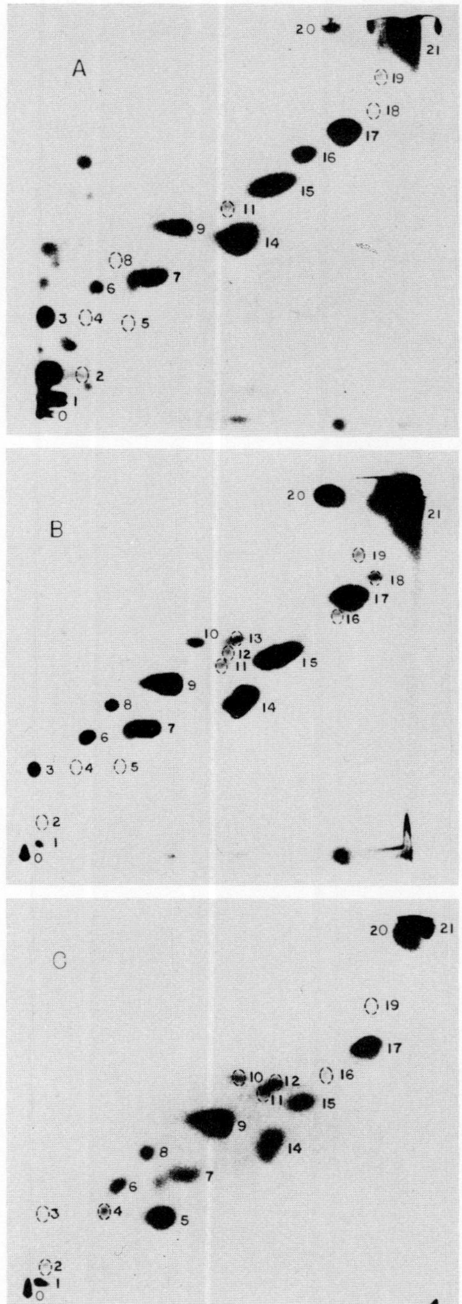
A
0
1
2
3
4
5
6
7
8
9
11
14
15
16
17
18
19
20
21
B
0
1
2
3
4
5
6
7
8
9
10
11
12
13
14
15
16
17
18
19
20
21
C
0
1
2
3
4
5
6
7
8
9
10
11
12
14
15
16
17
19
20
21

TABLE 1

Ratio of incorporation into specific compounds of 1-^{14}C-acetate and {U}-^{14}C-glycerol with respect to $NaH^{14}CO_3$

Spot number [a]	Compound	Ratios of Areas under Curves: 1-^{14}C-acetate / $NaH^{14}CO_3$		Ratios of Areas under Curves: {U}-^{14}C-glycerol / $NaH^{14}CO_3$
1	PGDG	(0.28)*	0.07[b]	0.06[b]
2	PS	(0.04)	0.01	0.03
3	UNK	(0.97)	0.24	0.32
4	PI	(0.20)	0.05	0.51
5	GLY	(0.12)	0.03	5.65[b]
6	PC	(0.24)	0.06	0.19
7	SL	(0.16)	0.04	0.13
8	UNK	(2.35)	0.58	3.35
9	PG	(0.28)	0.07	0.41

10	PL		c	c
11	PGP	(0.16)	0.04	0.39
12	PL		c	c
13	UNK		d	d
14	DGDG	(0.12)	0.03[a]	0.10[b]
15	MGDG	(0.20)	0.05[a]	0.08[b]
16	PQ	(0.01)	0.003	0.03
17	SG[e]	(0.12)	0.03	0.15
18	PQ	(0.49)	0.12	f
19	UNK	(0.08)	0.02	0.04
20	Pigments	(0.41)	0.10	0.06

**bracketed figures show acetate normalized relative to glycerol.*

a) numbers correspond to Figure 1.

b) figures are meaningless; see text.

c) absent in $NaH^{14}CO_3$ *labeled lipids.*

d) absent in $NaH^{14}CO_3$ *and* $1\text{-}^{14}C$*-acetate labeled lipids.*

e) tentative identification.

f) absent in [U]-^{14}C*-glycerol labeled compounds.*

Sodium bicarbonate was the most efficiently utilized substrate for lipid synthesis. Total acetate incorporation was 4% of total CO_2 incorporation while glycerol was 16%. The relative efficiency of acetate and glycerol can be ascertained (Table 1) when the ratio of incorporation of acetate to CO_2 is normalized with respect to the ratio of glycerol to CO_2. Acetate was a significantly less efficient label only for PI but was more efficient than glycerol for labeling PQ and pigments. The efficienty of acetate relative to glycerol for GLY, PG and PGP cannot be determined as the labeled glycerol biased the data.

In spite of the different levels of incorporation in absolute terms (Table 1) the distribution of the label into the phospholipids was remarkably constant with respect to PG and within experimental error when compared as percent of phosphorus labeled compounds (Table 2). PC was poorly labeled with glycerol while PS was disproportionately high. Acetate labeled PI and PGP to approximately 50-60% of the other two substrates. The most striking difference was the total absence of CO_2 incorporation into the two PLs. When expressed as a percent of total incorporation (Table 2) the substrates differed significantly with respect to the phospholipids, galactolipids and plastoquinones. Fourteen and one half percent of the CO_2, 24.6% of the acetate and 32.4% of the glycerol was incorporated into phospholipids. Glycerol was incorporated into galactolipids to a level 40-60% that of CO_2 and acetate. Neither acetate nor glycerol was an efficient label for the plastoquinones. Incorporation of {U}-^{14}C-glycerol in GLY was meaningless and made the total incorporation spuriously high.

In comparing light and dark incubations, ^{32}P and ^{35}S behaved differently. Sulfur in the dark was incorporated to a level approximately 1/3 of the incorporation in light while phosphorus was incorporated equally in both light and dark. Dark incorporation of CO_2 was nearly zero which is indicative of photosynthetic fixation into the lipoidal material. Glycerol was not incubated in the dark. Results of the dark incubation with acetate are particularly interesting (Fig. 2). MGDG was labeled in the dark to only 1% that in light. DGDG, PI and PC were labeled in the dark to less than 0.05% that in light. PGDG, PQs and pigments were unlabeled in dark. This would indicate that ^{32}P labeling in the dark may be due to substitution rather than synthesis as all phospholipids were labeled to equal levels in both light and dark. SL, SG and the PLs were labeled in the dark with acetate to a level equal to that of SL incubated in the dark with ^{35}S. This may indicate that ^{35}S label was incorporated rather than

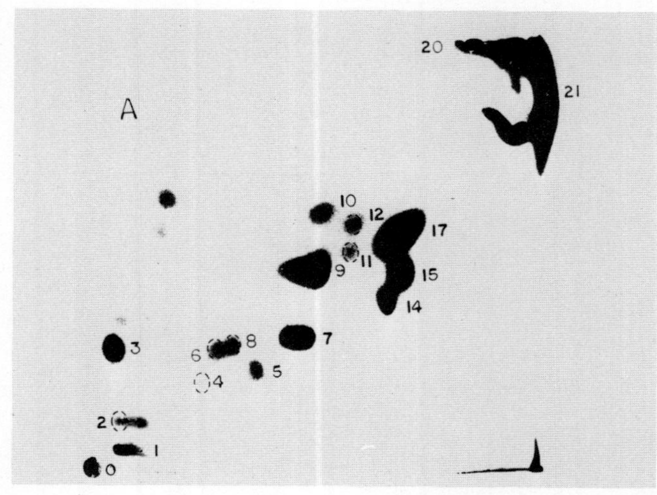

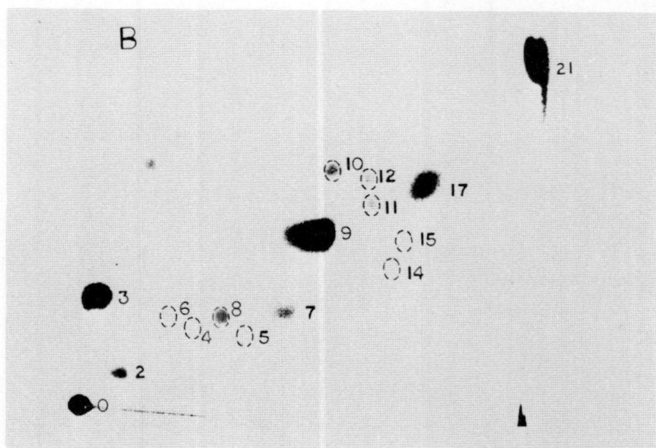

Figure 2. Contact radioautograph of the chromatograms of the complex lipid labeled in vitro with 1-^{14}C-acetate. A = incubation in light, B = incubation in dark. See Figure 1 for spot identification.

TABLE 2

Percent of total incorporation of $NaH^{14}CO_3$, 1-^{14}C-acetate and {U}-^{14}C-glycerol into specific compounds and distribution of the labels into the phospholipids as a percentage of total phosphorus labeled compounds

Compound	$NaH^{14}CO_3$		1-^{14}C-Acetate		{U}-^{14}C-Glycerol	
	% of Total Incorporation	% of P-Labeled Compounds	% of Total Incorporation	% of P-Labeled Compounds	% of Total Incorporation	% of P-Labeled Compounds
PG	9.3	64.1	15.0	61.0	21.4	66.0
PC	3.3	22.1	4.3	17.5	3.4	10.5
PI	0.7	4.8	0.8	3.3	2.0	6.2
PGP	0.8	5.5	0.7	2.8	1.8	5.6
PS	0.5	3.5	0.9	3.7	2.5	7.7
PL	0	0	2.9	11.7	1.3	4.0
MGDG	12.9		17.5		6.2	

DGDG	16.2		12.7		10.5	
PGDG	8.5		1.5		3.2	
SL	9.5		10.6		8.0	
SG	13.9		12.3		13.9	
PQ	4.8		1.3		0.7	
GLY	0.4		0.4		14.5	
% of total incorporation accounted for	80.7		80.9		89.4	

substituted. PS, UNKs (#3 and #8, Fig. 2 B), PG and PGP incorporated at approximately 2/3 of the light rate.

DISCUSSION

The lipids of *Acetabularia mediterranea* chloroplasts have been identified. Major phospholipids were PC and PG with PS, PI and PGP as minor components. Two other phospholipids were noted but not characterized. They may be lysophospholipids which are poorly extracted with chloroform and methanol[32]. PE could not be demonstrated as a chloroplast component which agrees with findings in spinach[33] and bean[34] chloroplasts. Major galactolipids were MGDG and DGDG with a minor component of PGDG. Other lipoidal components identified were SL, PQs, pigments and a sterol, tentatively identified as SG. A variety of sterols have been identified and characterized as components of spinach chloroplast envelope membranes[35]. Other sterols may be present but the amount of material employed in this study was too low to detect them. Of the lipid extract, excluding pigments and neutral lipids, approximately 80% of the total label incorporated was accounted for (Table 2).

CO_2 was a 25-fold better substrate than acetate for lipid synthesis and better than glycerol by 6-fold. This would imply either that the isolated chloroplasts have a decided preference for recently fixed CO_2 rather than exogenous substrates or that acetate and glycerol cannot freely cross the chloroplast membrane. Previous experiments with isolated *Acetabularia mediterranea* chloroplasts have shown the former to be true[4]. Acetate was the only useful label in dark incubation and incorporated to 34% of the light rate. Although no attempt was made to quantitate the complex lipids directly, their relative ratios can be estimated based upon incorporation. One must, however, assume that the incorporation represented *de novo* synthesis and that degradation was minimal. Based upon incorporation the ratio of PG to PC varied from 3.2:1 for CO_2 and acetate to 6:1 for glycerol. Since the glycerol label biased the data, the ratio of 3.2:1 is more realistic. This value is of the same order as reported for spinach[22] and bean[34] chloroplasts. The ratio of MGDG to DGDG varied with both substrate and length of incubation as previously noted[15]. With an increase in incubation periods, the label incorporation appears first in MGDG and then in DGDG and PGDG. This corresponds with kinetic studies of acetate and CO_2 incorporation into the galactolipids[14]. The ratio of incorporation into MGDG to DGDG leveled at 1:1.7. This is slightly low relative to the frequently reported value of 1:2 in chloroplasts of spinach[22,33,36], beans[34] and maize and sorghum[37] but is considerably higher than the 1:1 ratio reported in Euglena[38,39]. In discussing MGDG:DGDG ratios, the integrity of the chloroplasts must be evaluated as the chloroplast envelope is the site of incorporation of uridine diphosphate galactose into galactolipids[22-24]. Loss of plastid integrity would reduce the percentage of total incoration into galactolipids. This does not however appear to be the case as CO_2 incorporation was linear during the incubation and the 4% incorporation level of acetate was similar to that previously reported[40]. The ratio of total galactolipids to total phospholipids ranged from 1:0.6 with glycerol, 1.3:1 with acetate and 2.6:1 with CO_2. This disparity appears to be due to the disproportionate incorporation of glycerol and acetate into the phospholipids.

The above data are related to the efficiency of substrate utilization and do not directly deal with the localization of the required enzymes. However, the distribution of acetate into specific galactolipids and phospholipids in light and dark incubation suggests enzymatic compartmentalization. In the dark, the only significantly labeled galactolipid was MGDG but to a level less than 1% of the light rate. The light-dependent galactolipid synthesis has been previously reported but the limiting factor(s) in the dark has not been determined[13]. The phospholipid labeling pattern in the dark indicated that PS, PG and PGP were labeled to over 60% of the light rate while PC and PI were labeled to less than 0.05%. The requirement for light in the synthesis of PC is particularly puzzling. Based upon the proposed biosynthetic pathways for glycerolipids[20], it would appear that PG, PS and PGP are synthesized in a cellular compartment which has an adequate supply of triphosphate nucleotides and reducing compounds. It is proposed that this compartment is the chloroplast. On the other hand, the synthetic pathway leading to PC and the precursors for the galactolipids exist in another compartment, probably microsomal, and are limited by the lack of the necessary cofactors in the dark. This contention would seem to be supported by the studies of the intracellular localization of the enzymes involved in both galactolipid and phospholipid syntheses. Aldose reductase, uridine diphosphate-glucose pyrophosphorylase and uridine diphosphoglucose 4-epimerase required for uridine diphosphate galactose synthesis have been claimed to be microsomal[41]. Our results of light and dark incubation with acetate appear to confirm that at least a portion of the galactolipid synthetic pathway is extraplastidal and part intraplastidal. Similarly, it has been proposed that the rapidly labeling PC is associated with the microsomal fraction while the rapidly labeling PG is associated with the chloroplast[14,42]. Location for the synthetic pathways for other phospholipids is unresolved but our results would indicate that PG, PS and PGP are synthesized in the plastid.

This work was supported in part by NIH grant HD-00020-10 to F. D. M. and by the Biology Department of John Carroll University.

REFERENCES

1. Shephard, D. C., Levin, W. B. and Bidwell, R. G. S. (1968) Biochem. Biophys. Res. Comm. 32, 413-420.
2. Bidwell, R. G. S., Levin, W. B. and Shephard, D. C. (1970) Plant Physiol. 45, 70-75.
3. Shephard, D. C. and Bidwell, R. G. S. (1973) Protoplasma 76, 289-307.
4. Shephard, D. C. and Levin, W. B. (1972) J. Cell Biol. 54, 279-294.
5. Moore, F. D. (1971) Abstracts of papers, 11th annual meeting of the American Society for Cell Biology.
6. Moore, F. D. and Shephard, D. C. (1976) Protoplasma, in press.
7. Tschismadia, I. (1975) J. Cell Biol. 67, 435 a.
8. Tschismadia, I. and Moore, F. D. in preparation.
9. Berger, S. (1967) Protoplasma 64, 13-25.
10. Shephard, D. C. (1965) Exptl. Cell Res. 37, 93-110.
11. Dubacq, J. P. and Puiseux-Dao, S. (1974) Plant Science Letters 3, 241-250.
12. Trémolières, A. and Lepage, M. (1971) Plant Physiol. 47, 329-344.
13. Panter, R. A. and Boardman, R. K. (1973) J. Lipid Res. 14, 664-671.
14. Slack, C. R. and Roughan, P. G. (1975) Biochem. J. 152, 217-228.
15. Williams, J. P., Watson, G. R., Kahn, M-U. and Leung, S. (1975) Plant Physiol. 55, 1038-1042.
16. Sherratt, D. and Givan, C. V. (1973) Planta 113, 47-52.
17. Bishop, R. S., Perry, M. J. and Schreiber, R. W. (1969) Can. J. Bot. 47, 667-673.
18. Kates, M. (1970) Advan. Lipid Res. 8, 225-265.
19. Kates, M. and Wassef, M. K. (1970) Ann. Rev. Biochem. 39, 323-358.
20. Mazliak, P. (1973) Ann. Rev. Plant Physiol. 24, 287-310.
21. Krupa, Z. and Baszynski, T. (1975) Biochim. Biophys. Acta 408, 26-34.
22. Douce, R., Holtz, R. B. and Benson, A. A. (1973) J. Biol. Chem. 248, 7215-7222.
23. Douce, R. (1974) Sci. 852-853.
24. Van Hummel, H. C., Hulsebos, Th. J. M. and Wintermans, J. F. G. M. (1975) Biochim. Biophys. Acta 380, 219-226.
25. Shephard, D. C. (1970) in Methods in Cell Physiology (Prescott, D., ed) Vol. IV, pp 49-69, Academic Press, New York.

26. Arnon, D. I. (1949) Plant Physiol. 24, 1-15.
27. Kates, M. and Eberhardt, F. M. (1957) Can. J. Bot. 35, 895-902.
28. Bligh, E. G. and Dyer, W. J. (1959) Can. J. Biochem. 39, 323-358.
29. Lepage, M. (1964) J. Chromatog. 13, 99-103.
30. Henninger, M. D. and Crane, F. L. (1966) J. Biol. Chem. 241, 5190-5196.
31. Stahl, E. (1969) Thin Layer Chromatography, Springer-Verlag, New York.
32. Bjerve, K. S., Daae, L. N. W. and Bremer, J. (1974) Anal. Biochem. 58, 238-245.
33. Poincelot, R. P. (1971) Biochem. Biophys. Acta 239, 57-60.
34. Mackender, R. O. and Leech, R. M. (1974) Plant Physiol. 53, 496-502.
35. Poincelot, R. P. (1973) Arch. Biochem. Biophys. 153, 134-142.
36. Webster, D. E. and Chang, S. B. (1969) Plant Physiol. 44, 1523-1527.
37. Bishop, D. G., Anderson, K. S. and Smillie, R. M. (1971) Biochim. Biophys. Acta 231, 412-414.
38. Matson, R. S., Fei, M. and Chang, S. B. (1970) Plant Physiol. 45, 531-532.
39. Lin, M. F. and Chang, S. B. (1971) Phytochem. 10, 1543-1549.
40. Hawke, J. C., Rumsby, M. G. and Leech, R. M. (1974) Phytochem. 13, 403-413.
41. Konigs, B. and Heinz, E. (1974) Planta 118, 159-169.
42. Marshall, M. O. and Kates, M. (1974) Can. J. Biochem. 52, 469-482.

HETEROGENEITY OF THE PLASTID POPULATION AND CHLOROPLAST DIFFERENTIATION IN *ACETABULARIA MEDITERRANEA*

D. Hoursiangou-Neubrun, J. P. Dubacq and S. Puiseux-Dao

Laboratoire de Biologie cellulaire végétale
Université Paris VII
and
Laboratoire de Physiologie cellulaire
Université Paris VI
Paris, France

ABSTRACT

The unicellular alga *Acetabularia mediterranea* contains numerous small chloroplasts which are not all similar and are distributed along a morphological apicobasal gradient in the cylindrical cell. In this article additional information is given on the gradient itself, the thylacoid morphology and the pigment and lipid content at the different levels of the alga. All the data are consistent with the previously proposed hypothesis that plastids in the apices behave similarly to proplastids in higher plants and that mature organelles found in the stalk age towards the base. These results are discussed in relation to a film which shows that chloroplast morphology is linked to intracellular streaming activity.

INTRODUCTION

Acetabularia cells show a morphological and physiological apicobasal gradient. The nucleus is found in the basal part which is differentiated into rhizoids; growth and morphogenesis take place in the apical part[1]. Several physiological parameters such as cytoplasmic RNA content[2] and synthesis[3], protein synthesis[4], and photosynthesis[5,6], vary according to their position in the stalk.

The gradient also involves the chloroplast population as has been observed with the light[7] and the electron microscope[8,9,10]. The plastid morphology statistically differs when the apical, median and basal regions are compared. The characteristics concerned are: the size and form, the storage content, the number, length and stacking of the thylacoids and the stroma density. Some physiological plastid capacities also vary along the same gradient: photosynthetic metabolism[5,6], fluorescence at low temperature[11,12], and multiplication[8]. The synthesis of 16 S and 23 S RNAs, mainly chloroplast RNAs, has been shown to take place along the apicobasal gradient[3].

The plastid gradient depends upon the culture conditions[10] but it can be concluded that in all cases the cells contain three main chloroplast categories the proportions of which are modulated in the different cell portions.

Some additional evidence is given here concerning the existence and the properties of the various chloroplast types; the data are discussed in relation to a film analyzing the cytoplasmic movements in the apical, mid and basal regions.

MATERIALS AND METHODS

Cultures

The algae were cultured by the usual procedures: sea-water enriched with NO_3^-, PO_4^{---} and soil extract; temperature 20° C; light: 1000-1200 lux, LD 12-12 [13]. *Acetabularia* selected for the experiments were 15-20 mm in length and had no reproductive cap.

Chloroplast isolation and electron microscope controls

Homogenates were prepared at 4° C with algae previously maintained at this temperature for 1 or several hours. The cells were sectioned into fragments in a buffered solution (pH 7.2 - phosphate buffer 0.15 M or pH 6.6 - tris maleate buffer 0.2 M) containing sucrose (0.4 M or 0.6 M). In some cases BSA (bovine serum albumin : 1%), EDTA (ethylene diamine tetracetate : 10^{-3} M), or, DTT (dithiothreitol : 10^{-3} M) were added, but none proved advantageous. After homogenizing in a Potter homogenizer (20 teflon plunger movements) and filtering the suspension through cheese cloth, the filtrates were layered on to sucrose solutions in centrifuge tubes. Centrifugations were carried out in a swinging bucket rotor (Sorvall centrifuge) at 1000 to 10,000 xg.

The green bands of chloroplasts and pellets were fixed (glutaraldehyde : 4%, 1 h; OsO_4 : 1%, 3/4 h) in the homogenization buffer and embedded into araldite. Sections stained with uranyl acetate and lead citrate were examined with Hitachi HU 12 and Philips EM 300 microscopes.

Chloroplast membrane preparation for electron microscope observation

Isolated chloroplasts were resuspended at 4° C in an ammonium acetate solution (10^{-3} M), containing bacitracin (50 µg/ml). The suspensions were centrifuged at 30,000 xg for 10 minutes. The pellets were diluted with the ammonium acetate solution and centrifuged once again. Then fractions of those latter pellets containing thylacoids were transferred to grids and treated for negative staining with fresh solutions of 1% uranyl formate[14]. Some of these pellets were also fixed and embedded according to the procedure given for isolated chloroplasts.

Pigment analyses

Photosynthetic pigments were extracted either in pure acetone or in an acetone-methanol mixture; both techniques were equivalent. The pigments were characterized by silica gel thin layer chromatography. Chlorophyll and carotenoid contents were estimated as usual[15,16].

Lipid analyses

The procedure for preparing the total lipid fraction was derived from that described by Bligh and Dyer[17]. The algae or the pellets were fixed with methanol, then ground and added to chloroform. The chloroform phase obtained by centrifugation contains the lipids. The lipids were separated from each other using thin layer chromatography according to Gardner's technique[18] as modified by Grenier et al.[19]. The fatty acid composition of the chloroformic extract was analyzed by gas chromatography after methylation[20,21].

RESULTS

Chloroplast isolation

A. Isolation of three plastid categories

When the homogenate (0.4 M) is deposited on a discontinuous sucrose gradient 1.6 M - 0.8 M - 0.6 M and centrifuged (1000 g, 20 minutes), three bands and a small pellet are obtained (Fig. 1). Each band and the pellet, resuspended and separately centrifuged (4000 g, 10 minutes) were examined under the electron microscope after fixation and embedding. The storage content and the thylacoid morphology show that the light band is enriched in apical type chloroplasts, the mid band in median type organelles and the heaviest one in basal

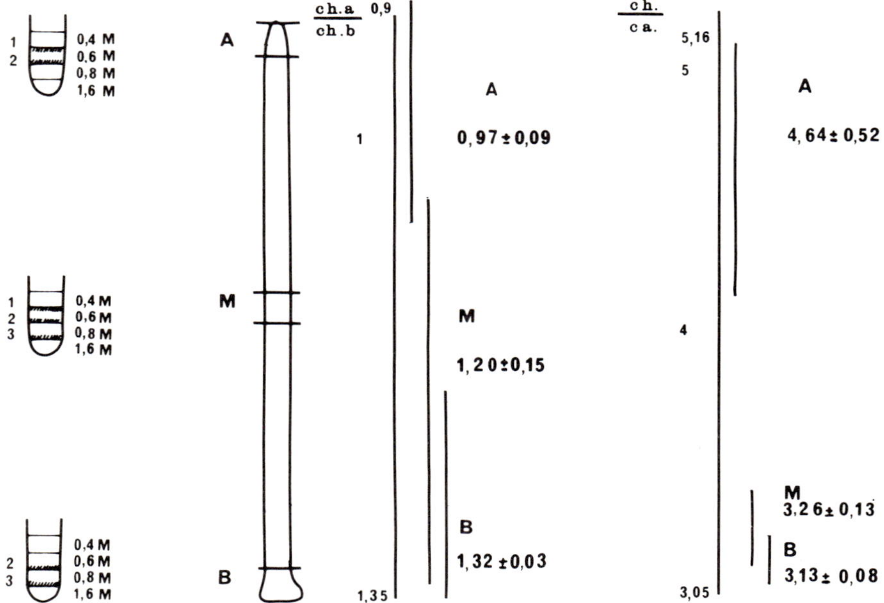

Figure 1. On the left, bands of chloroplasts after centrifugation of an homogenate (0.4 M) obtained from apical (A), median (M) and basal (B) fragments 2mm in length. Mid fragments as well as entire algae give 3 bands, apical parts only the 2 lightest ones, basal parts only the 2 heaviest ones. In the middle, chlorophyll a: chlorophyll b ratio values (chl a/chl b) in the 3 types of fragments; the ratios are very similar, however apical parts have a significantly lower ratio. On the right, chlorophyll: carotenoid ratios (chl/ca) from the same fragments; apical plastids clearly are different from the others.

Plate I (opposite page). a, b, c: Chloroplasts isolated from the lightest, the median and the heaviest band obtained as in Figure 1 d, e, f; Chloroplasts in the algae, in the apical, mid and basal regions respectively. (bar = 1 micron)

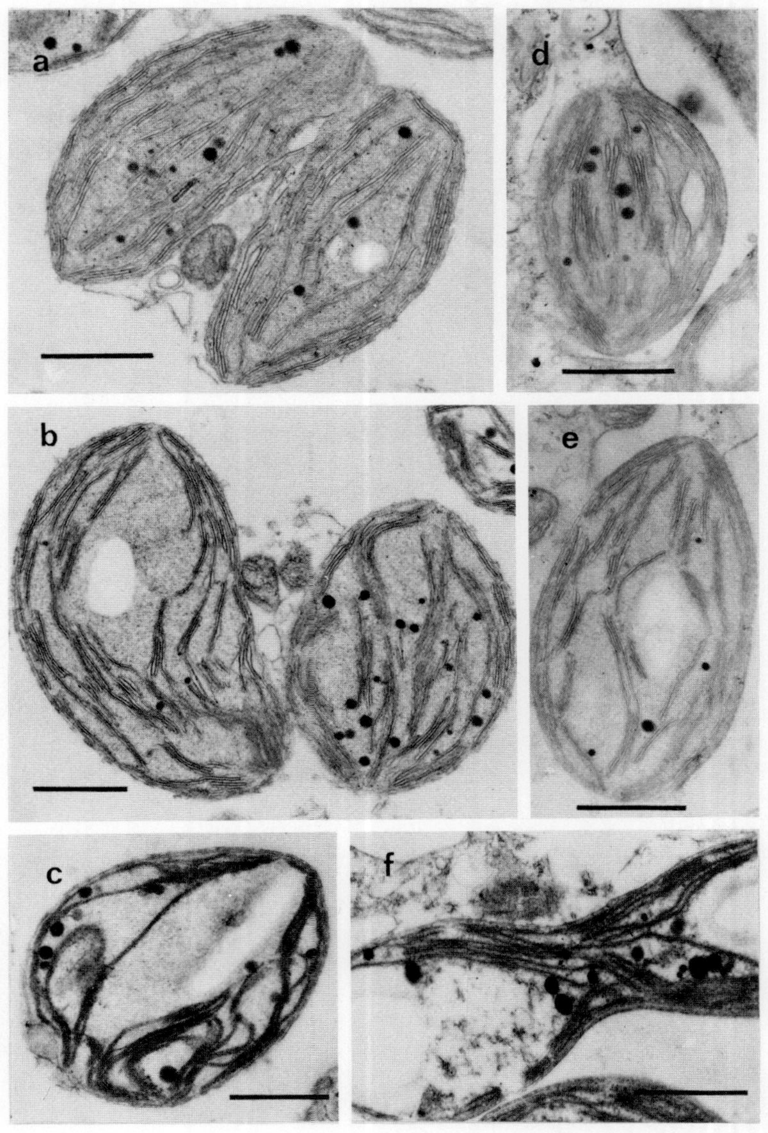
a
b
c
d
e
f

plastids (Pl. I); the small white pellet contains very large often broken chloroplasts with huge polysaccharide grains and isolated storage grains.

Such a technique allows the separation of three fractions of rather homogeneous organelles. When it is used to prepare plastids not from entire cells but from fragments, one can observe that the basal parts give the two heaviest bands, the median fragments give three bands and the apical parts only the two lightest ones (Fig. 1).

Chloroplasts prepared in such a way are more or less contaminated with mitochondria and some bacteria. Counting on micrographs shows that the lightest band is less pure. Moreover plastids are often enveloped with a thin cytoplasmic layer which isolates several chloroplasts and mitochondria (Pl. I, a and b).

B) Isolation of pure chloroplast fractions

The above results clearly indicate that the described technique is of interest to demonstrate the heterogeneity of the chloroplast population, but not for obtaining pure fractions. After studying the procedure given by Bidwell et al.[22], a new simple technique was developed. The homogenate (0.4 M) is deposited on a sucrose gradient made of only two solutions (0.8 M and 1.6 M). After centrifugation (1000 g, 20 minutes) the 0.8 M section contains most of the chloroplasts while mitochondria and bacteria remain in the 0.4 M section. The 0.8 M solution is then centrifuged (10,000 g, 10 minutes) and gives a pellet containing well preserved isolated plastids and only very few mitochondria and membrane fragments (Fig. 2; Pl. II a and b). Apical, median and basal portions of the cells were used and plastid membranes were prepared from the organelles as described above and in Figure 2.

The membrane of the different chloroplasts

Electron microscope observation of pellets after the osmotic shock in ammonium acetate (10^{-3} M) mainly shows two categories of thylacoids which are more or less inflated vesicles, large ones and small discs.

The apical organelles especially give rise to discs which can form short chains attached to medium sized thylacoids (Pl. III and IV). On the larger membranes one can observe thin furrows. Many particles are found all over and around the different membranes.

Very compactly assembled material is obtained from the plastids of the mid stalk. However, on some grids one can distinguish large thylacoids with particles and folds. Some

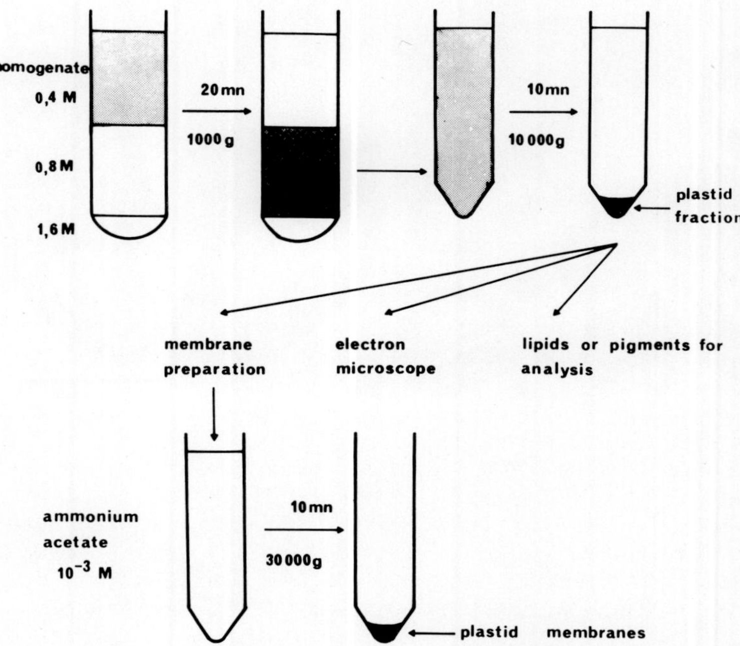

Figure 2. Top: isolation procedure for obtaining a pure chloroplast fraction. Bottom: preparation of a thylacoid fraction.

Plate II (overleaf).

a and b. Chloroplasts isolated by the procedure shown in Figure 2.

c and d. Sections of isolated thylacoids from apical plastids.

e. Sections of isolated membranes from basal chloroplasts.

(bar = 1 micron)

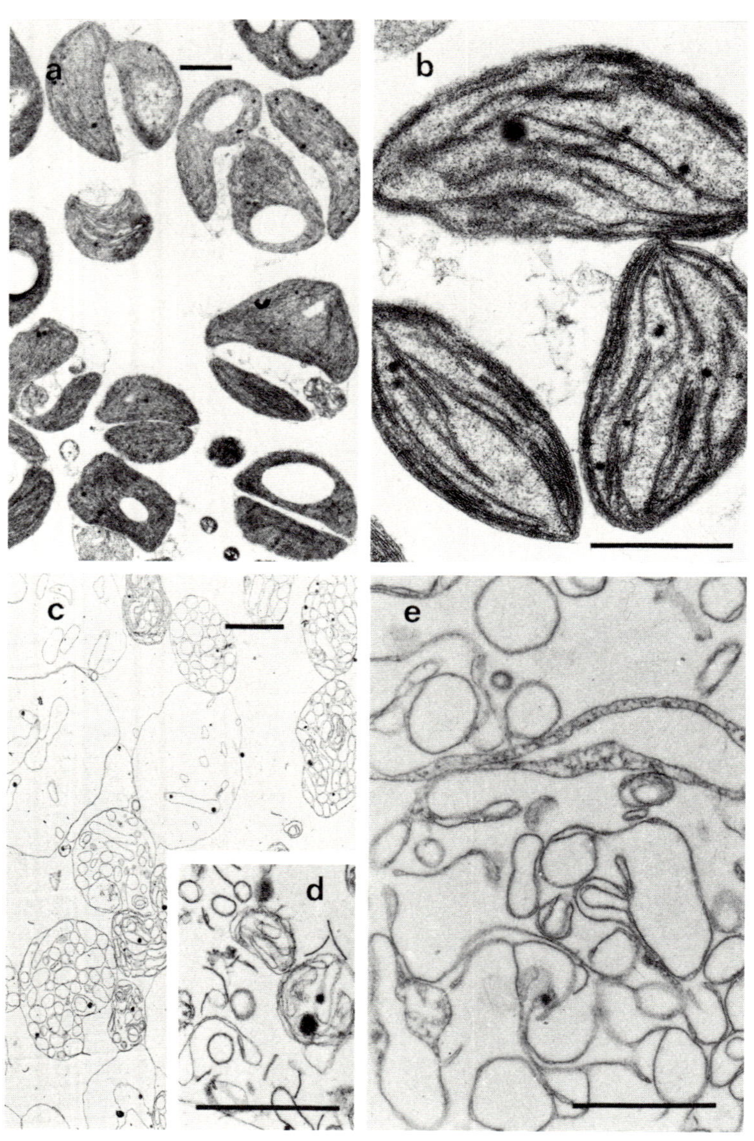
a
b
c
d
e

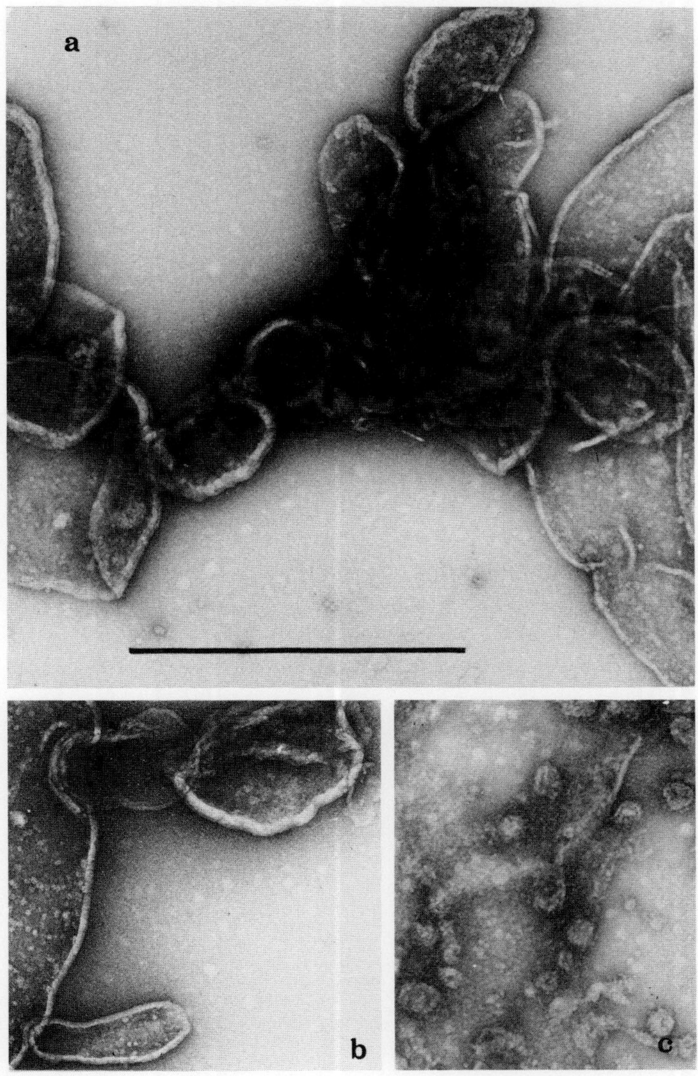

Plate III.

a and b. Isolated thylacoids from apical chloroplasts.

c. Associations of granules observed around the thylacoids.

(negative staining; bar = 1 micron)

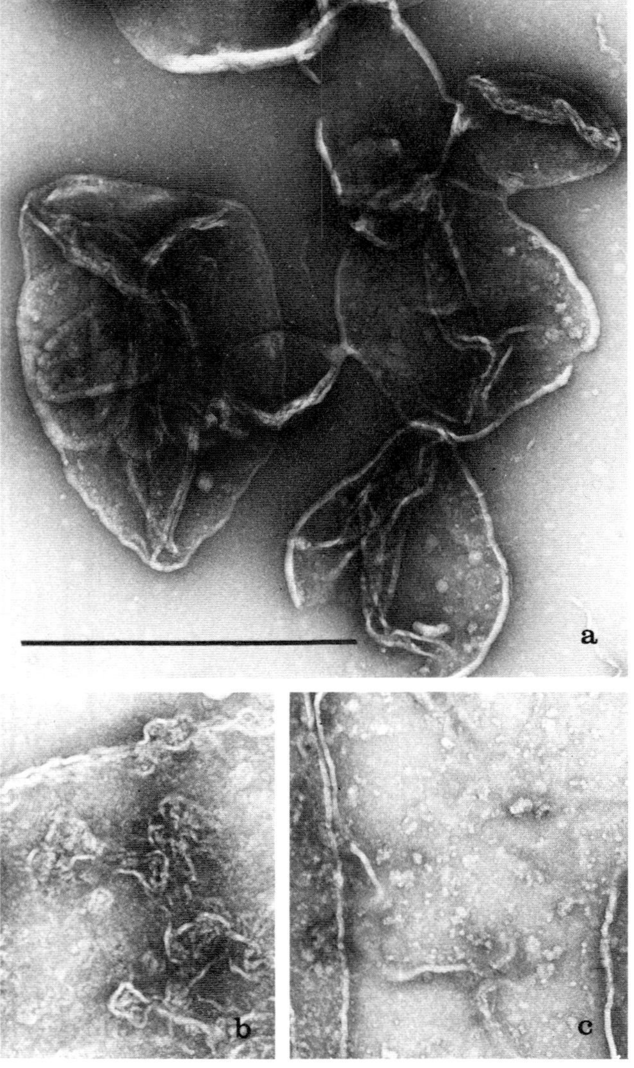

Plate IV.
a. Isolated thylacoids from apical plastids.
b and c. Granules associated with the membranes.
(negative staining; bar = 1 micron)

of these folds are due to the technical procedure; but others are clearly defined well-stacked double folds. Moreover, long chains of firmly attached discs are associated with the large thylacoids, frequently masking them.

The basal chloroplasts contain very large membranes with rare folds and discs, and only a few particles. On the thylacoid surface, holes are often visible; through these perforations, one sees a thin layer (Pl. VI and VII). Some of the thylacoids seem to consist only of one of these thin layers; they carry bundles of filaments and particles (Pl. VII).

When the membranes are embedded, the sections show large more or less inflated vesicles, apparently attached to each other and numerous discs or small vesicles, inside or outside the largest ones. Discs and vesicles often form chains. The thylacoids, discs as well as larger ones, are smaller and more frequently unattached in apical fractions; they often show a close flattened configuration when obtained from median or basal plastids.

Plates V, VI and VII on following pages:

Plate V. Thylacoids from median chloroplasts.
a. Groups of thylacoids with double folds.
b. Piles of stacked discs.
(negative staining; bar = 1 micron)

Plate VI. Thylacoids from basal plastids.
a. Large thylacoids with holes and rare associated discs.
b. Thylacoids with short folds.
(negative staining; bar = 1 micron)

Plate VII. Thylacoids from basal chloroplasts.
a. Large thylacoid with holes.
b. Clear membrane with bunches of filaments and granules which seems to correspond to a thylacoid reduced to one of its sides.
(negative staining; bar = 1 micron)

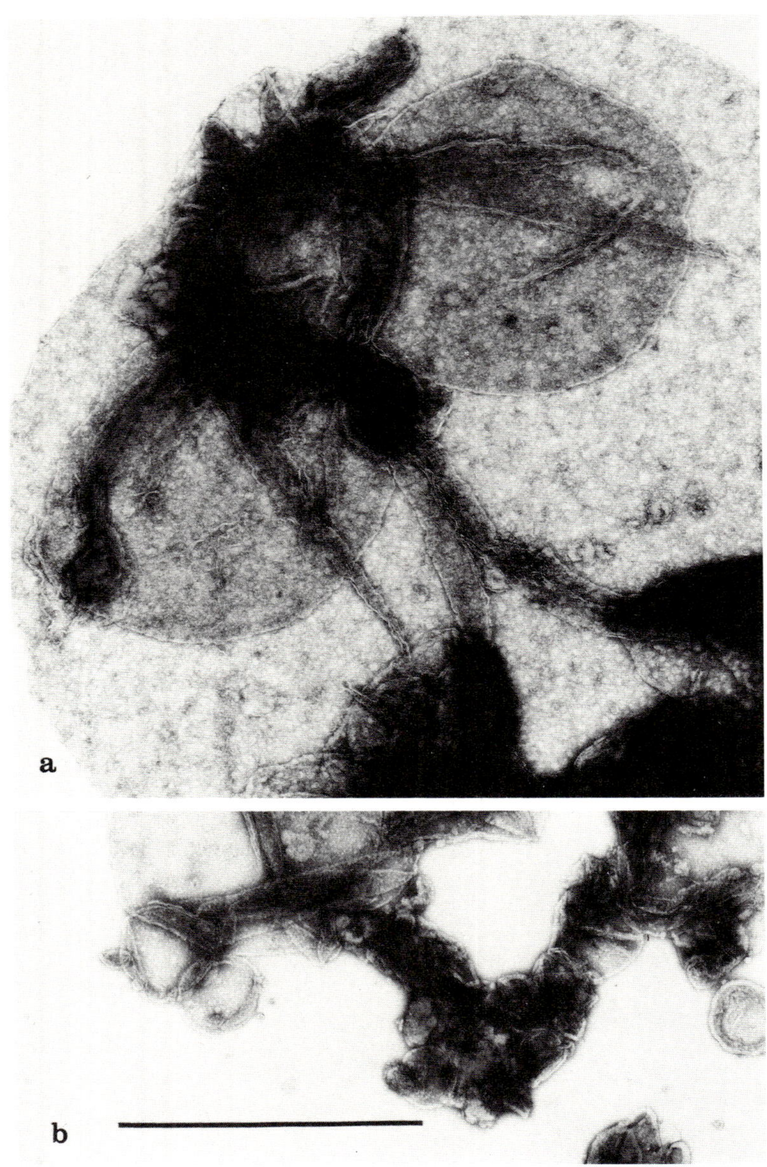
a
b

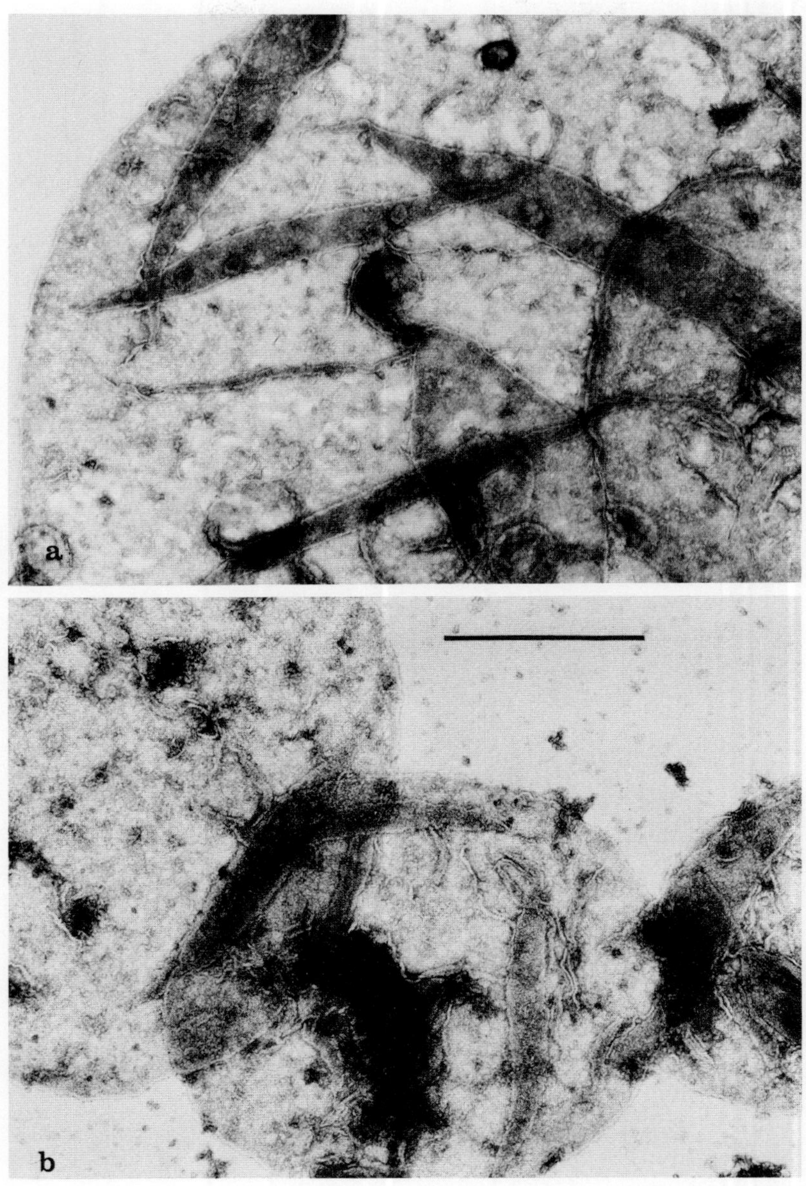
a
b

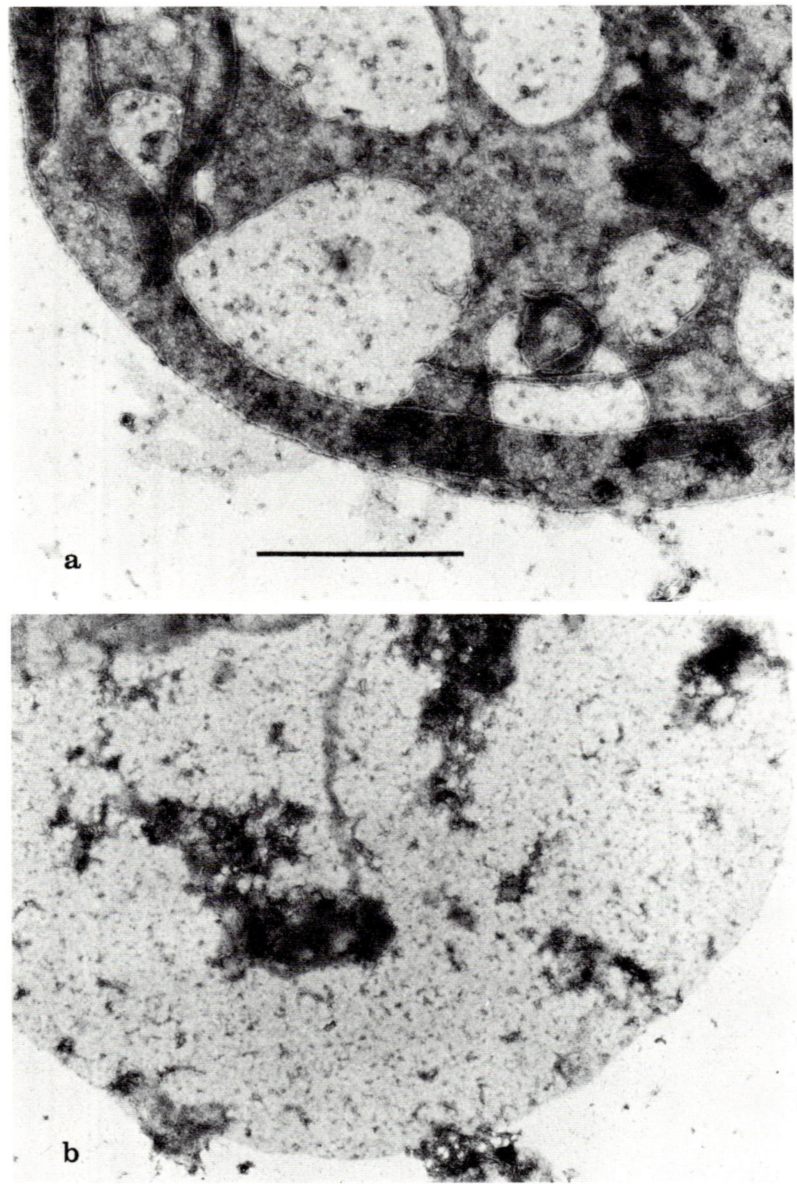
a
b

Analyses of pigments and lipids

Due to the low quantities of organelles isolated from the different cell fragments (2 mm long) and because most of the cytoplasmic mass in Acetabularia consists of the chloroplasts, assays were more frequently made directly on apical, median and basal parts. However the data obtained on plastids isolated from the fragments were similar, but they were at the limit of detection and for this reason not reported here.

A. Pigments

In our culture conditions, Acetabularia cells contain chlorophylls a and b and the following carotenoids: lutein, β-carotene, violaxanthin and neoxanthin, the latter two in traces. The chlorophyll content is about 45 μg/mg protein and the carotenoid content about 14 μg/mg protein. Apical plastids have less pigment than the others (Fig. 3).

An evaluation of the chl a/chl b ratio gives about 1.2. This ratio varies along the stalk, it increases from the apex towards the base (Fig. 1); the amplitude of this variation depends upon the experimental series and can be less than reported in Figure 1. The ratio chlorophylls/carotenoids decreases from the apical part towards the rhizoids and very clearly the apical chloroplasts differ from the others.

B. Lipids

We have paid attention to membrane lipids and especially galactolipids which are characteristic of plastids. In Figure 3 one observes that apices are poor in phospholipids and galactolipids. The content is higher in the mid region particularly for digalactosyldiglycerids (DGDG). DGDG is again less abundant in the bases while median and basal fragments have similar quantities of phospholipids and monogalactosyldiglycerids.

Unsaturated fatty acids are also mostly found in chloroplasts. In Figure 4 fatty acids are in larger proportions in the stalk (middle and basal regions). Moreover the unsaturated fatty acid content decreases from the mid portion towards the base. Besides a comparison of the length of fatty acid chains seem to indicate a growth from the apex towards the rest of the cell (Fig. 4)

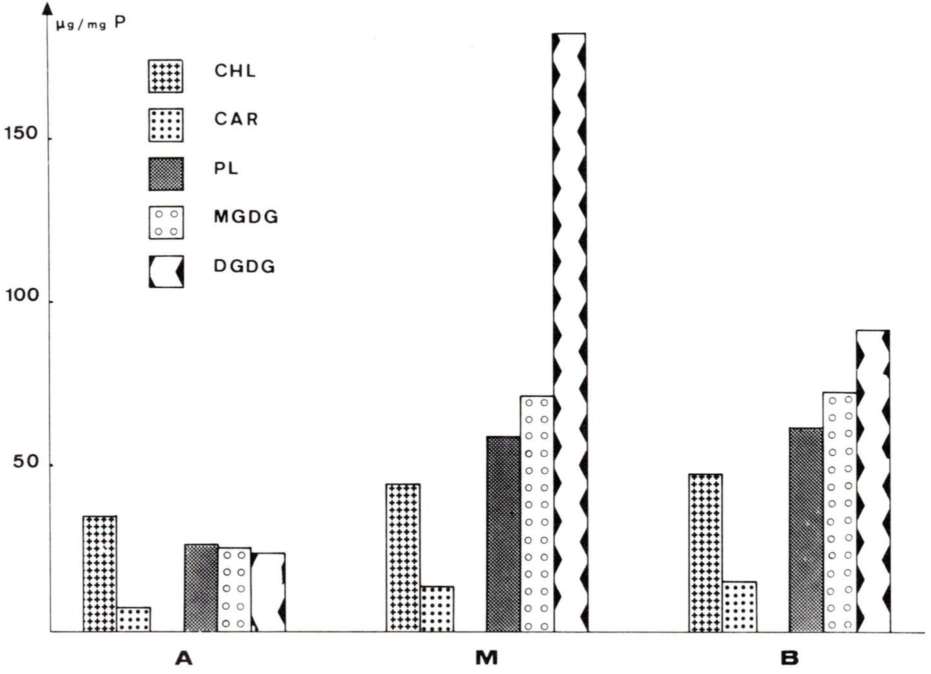

Figure 3. Pigment (chlorophylls: CHL; carotenoids: CAR) and lipid (phospholipids: PL; monogalactosyldiglycerids: MGDG; digalactosyldiglycerids: DGDG) content per mg protein in apical (A), median (M) and basal (B) fragments.

Pigments, particularly carotenoids, are less abundant in apices. The membrane lipid level is very much lower in the apical fragments; moreover the DGDG content decreases from the mid region towards the base.

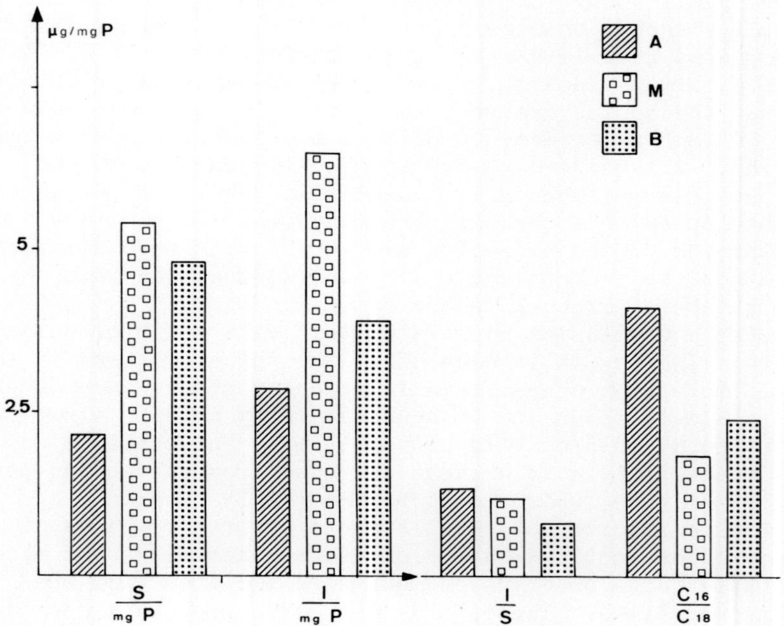

Figure 4. Fatty acids in apical (A), median (M) and basal (B) fragments. On the left are reported the saturated fatty acids (S/mg P) and the unsaturated fatty acids (I/mg P) content per mg protein. The values are higher in M and B fragments; unsaturated fatty acids decrease from the mid part towards the base. On the right are given ratios: I/S, unsaturated fatty acids over saturated fatty acid content; C_{16}/C_{18}, content of fatty acids with 16 carbon chains over content of fatty acids with 18 carbon chains.

DISCUSSION

The separation of three chloroplast bands on a sucrose gradient confirms the conclusions drawn from the cytological observations that have indicated the existence of three main plastid categories in Acetabularia stalks[7-10]. As one obtains only the two lightest bands with apical fragments and the two heaviest ones with the basal parts, it can be concluded that the reported heterogeneous distribution of the organelles along an apicobasal gradient is also true. Centrifugation data given by Lüttke et al. seem to prove that such a situation is found in other Acetabularia and siphonaceous green algae[23].

The thylacoids isolated from apical plastids are in general small; they form inflated vesicles or discs which are not well attached to each other. On the contrary, median chloroplasts give larger membranes as well as piles of discs, all very firmly stacked. From the basal plastids, most of the obtained thylacoids are very large and moreover they show holes or look as if made up of only one membrane having lost one side. All those data are in good agreement with the previous observations on sections[10] the conclusion of which was that apical chloroplasts are young, and forming new discs; the plastids of the midregion are mature with more numerous and larger, well organized and closely associated membranes, while the basal organelles are aging.

Such a conclusion correlates well with the biochemical results. Indeed, it is clear that the apical content is low for all molecules characteristic of chloroplasts such as pigments, galactolipids and unsaturated fatty acids. Also, the proportion of chlorophylls among pigments and the DGDG and unsaturated fatty acid content decrease from the median part towards the base, which could be the result of aging.

Some morphological details are noteworthy: pairs of thylacoids on sections can be due to stacked discs but also to the double folds observed on membranes isolated from the median organelles. These folds may correspond to a considerable increase in the photosynthetic surface. They probably arise at the level of the furrows described on apical thylacoids, and micrographs show in Plates III and IV suggest they are possibly formed by associating particles.

Several authors[5,6] have reported an apicobasal gradient for photosynthetic activities in Acetabularia with a decrease from the apex towards the base. This does not exactly fit with our observations indicating that apical plastids must show low photosynthetic capabilities. However the differences are very easy to explain. The authors have cut the algae in two or three parts of the same length. So the apices were linked to very large portions of stalk and thus were diluted. For this reason, we have used 2 mm long fragments to avoid the masking of apical plastid peculiarities.

The problem that arises is how in one single cell with one nucleus and one chloroplast strain[10], such a heterogeneous plastid population at various differentiation stages can be maintained in spite of an active cellular streaming. When filming the cytoplasmic movements, it became evident that a very clear correlation exists between the rate of movement of cytoplasmic strands and the appearance of the chloroplasts they transport. Fine strands moving at a high speed are found in the apical part, more rarely in the others; they always contain smaller organelles. On the contrary, large masses of cytoplasm are visible in the stalk, especially near the base; they move slowly and transport larger chloroplasts. In some rhizoids the cytoplasm does not move; huge round plastids full of storage material are found in them. In slowly growing cells, for example in algae transferred into pure seawater, the intracellular streaming decreases after some days; in these conditions, cytoplasmic masses moving very slowly are observed from the base up to the mid region; large chloroplasts are then visible in the whole basal halves[10]. So we can conclude that chloroplast differentiation is influenced by cytoplasmic streaming, perhaps at the level of intergenomic cooperation between the nucleus and the chloroplasts by modulating the transfer of molecules or the transport of organelles to a site where key molecules are synthesized.

REFERENCES

1. Hämmerling, J. (1953) Intern. Rev. Cytol. 2, 475.
2. De Vitry, F. (1965) Bull. Soc. Chim. Biol. 47, 1375.
3. Naumova, L. P., Pressman, E. K. and Sandakchiev, L. S. (1976) Plant Science Letters 6, 231.
4. Woodcock, C. L. F. and Dazy, A. C. unpublished data.
5. Issinger, O., Maas, I. and Clauss, H. (1971) Planta 101, 360.
6. Vanden Driessche, T. (1974) in M. Avron, Proceedings of the Third International Congress on Photosynthesis, Elsevier Scientific Publishing Company, Amsterdam, p. 745.
7. Puiseux-Dao, S. (1962) Rev. Gén. Bot. 819, 409.
8. Puiseux-Dao, S. and Dazy, A. C. (1970) in J. Brachet and S. Bonotto, Biology of Acetabularia, Academic Press, London, p. 111.
9. Boloukhere, M. (1972) J. Microscopie 13, 401.
10. Hoursiangou-Neubrun, D. and Puiseux-Dao, S. (1974) Plant Science Letters 2, 209.
11. Sironval, C., Bonotto, S. and Kirchmann, R. (1973) Plant Science Letters 1, 47.
12. Dujardin, E., Bonotto, S., Sironval, C. and Kirchmann, R. (1975) Plant Science Letters 5, 209.
13. Lateur, L. and Bonotto, S. (1973) Bull. Soc. Roy. Bot. Belg. 106, 17.
14. Leberman, R. (1965) J. Mol. Biol. 13, 606.

15. Strain, H. H. and Svec, W. A. (1966) in L. P. Vernon and G. R. Seely, The Chlorophylls, Academic Press, New York and London, p. 50.
16. Wintermans, J. F. and De Mots, A. (1965) Biochem. Biophys. Acta 109, 448.
17. Bligh, E. G. and Dyer, W. S. (1959) Canad. J. Biochem. Biophys. 37, 911.
18. Gardner, H. W. (1968) J. Lipid Res. 9, 139.
19. Grenier, G., Tremolieres, A., Therrien, M. P. and Willemot, C. (1973) Physiol. Vég. 11, 253.
20. Metcalfe, L. P., Schmitz, A. A. and Pelka, J. A. (1966) Anal. Chem. 38, 514.
21. Lechevallier, D. (1966) C. R. Acad. Sci. 263, 1849.
22. Bidwell, R. G. S., Levin, W. B. and Shephard, D. C. (1969) Plant Physiol. 44, 946.
23. Lüttke, A., Rahmsdorf, U. and Schmid R. (1976) Z. Naturforsch. 31 c, 108.

FLUORESCENCE EMISSION SPECTRA OF APICAL, MIDDLE AND BASAL CHLOROPLASTS OF *ACETABULARIA* AND *BATOPHORA* AT STAGE 4

S. Bonotto, E. Dujardin, R. Kirchmann and C. Sironval

Département de Radiobiologie
Centre d'Etude de l'Energie Nucléaire
Mol, Belgium
and
Laboratoire de Photobiologie
Université du Sart-Tilman
Liège, Belgium

SUMMARY

The 77° K fluorescence emission spectra (FES) is a good method for distinguishing chloroplasts extracted from the apical, middle and basal region of the stalk of *A. mediterranea*, *A. peniculus* and *B. oerstedii* at stage 4. Differences exist between the three species. In *A. peniculus*, the fluorescence emission at 700-720 nm is dominant even in basal extracted chloroplasts. Our results suggest the existence of a FES apico-basal gradient in the three species investigated.

INTRODUCTION.

It is well established that *Acetabularia mediterranea* contains an heterogeneous population of numerous plastids distributed along a morphological gradient[1,2,3]. The apical chloroplasts are small and poor in carbohydrate grains, contain numerous lamellae and divide. In the basal region of the cell, chloroplasts are bigger and are full of storage material; their lamellae are reduced and they divide relatively rarely compared to the apical plastids. The ultrastructural organization of the chloroplasts in *A. peniculus* and in *B. oerstedii* is similar to that observed in *A. mediterranea*. Moreover, as in *A. mediterranea*, the plastid population of *A. peniculus* and *B. oerstedii* is morphologically heterogeneous. However, using ultrastructure alone, it is rather difficult to distinguish the plastids of the three algae, though some small morphological differences seem to exist, for example, between the chloroplasts of A. mediterranea and A. peniculus[8].

In this paper we show that the fluorescence emission spectra technique, successfully used in previous work[4,5], permits chloroplasts of the apical, middle and basal region of the stalk of the three species investigated to be distinguished.

MATERIALS AND METHODS

The algae, Acetabularia mediterranea, Acetabularia peniculus and Batophora oerstedii, were cultivated following the methods reported previously[6,7,8]. These three algae possess, at maturity, well known species-specific morphological characters (Fig. 1). However, their cellular organization is very similar: They appear as cylindrical stalks fixed by their bases which are differentiated into rhizoids. Only cells at stage 4 [9] were used in this work (Fig. 2). The number of sterile whorls present on the stalk varied considerably from one species to another, as illustrated in Figure 2. In B. oerstedii, between 10 and 20 sterile whorls may be present on the stalk at stage 4. Chloroplasts were extracted,

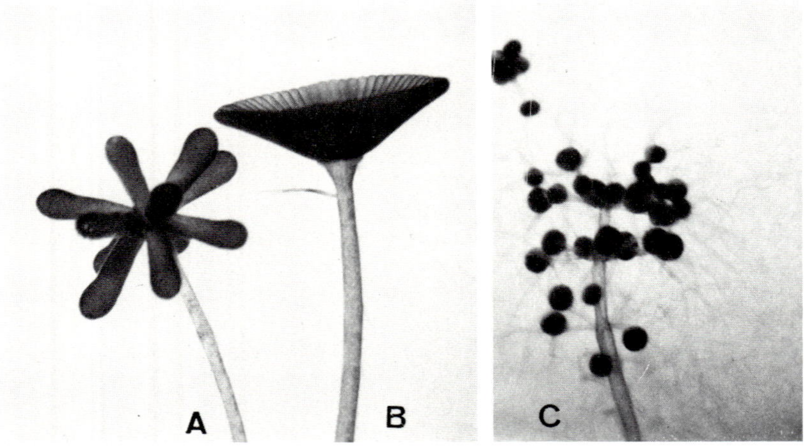

Figure 1. Species-specific morphological characters of Acetabularia peniculus (A), Acetabularia mediterranea (B) and Batophora oerstedii (C).

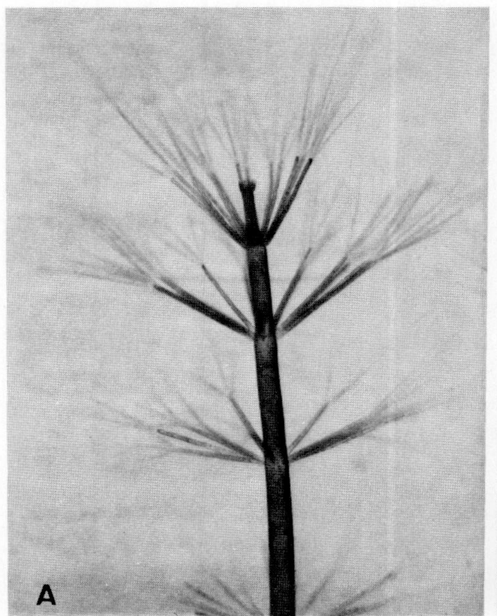

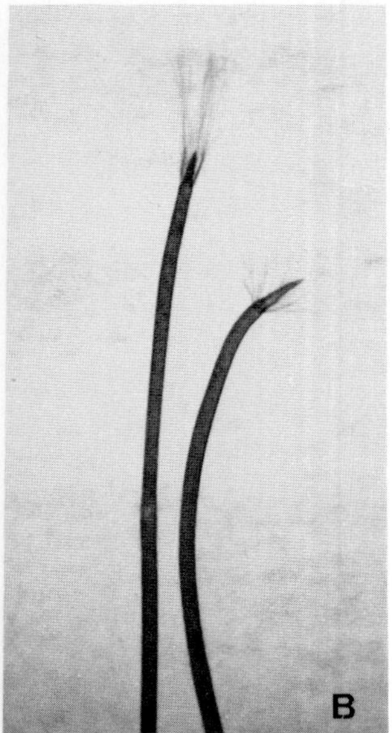

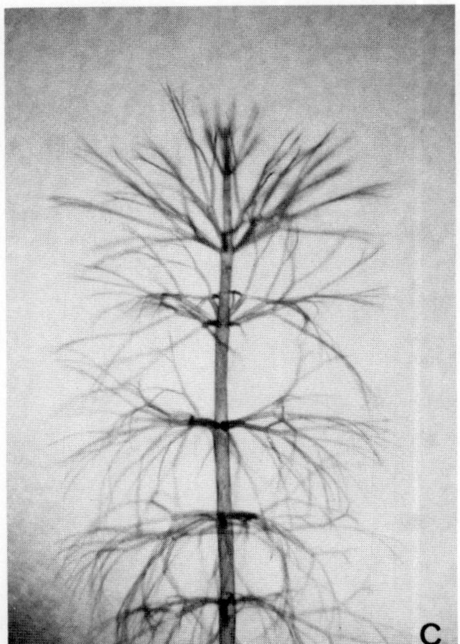

Figure 2. Acetabularia mediterranea (A), Acetabularia peniculus (B) and Batophora oerstedii (C) at stage 4. Note the number of sterile whorls. B. oerstedii may have 20 or more sterile whorls on the stalk.

in the afternoon, from 5 mm stalk segments in the buffered medium of Shephard and Levin[10] and filtered rapidly on small Millipore filters covered with a piece of bolting silk, which retain the cellular wall fragments. The filters were mounted into a holder, as illustrated in Figure 3, and analysed for their fluorescence at 77° K by the procedure described by Sironval et al.[11,12].

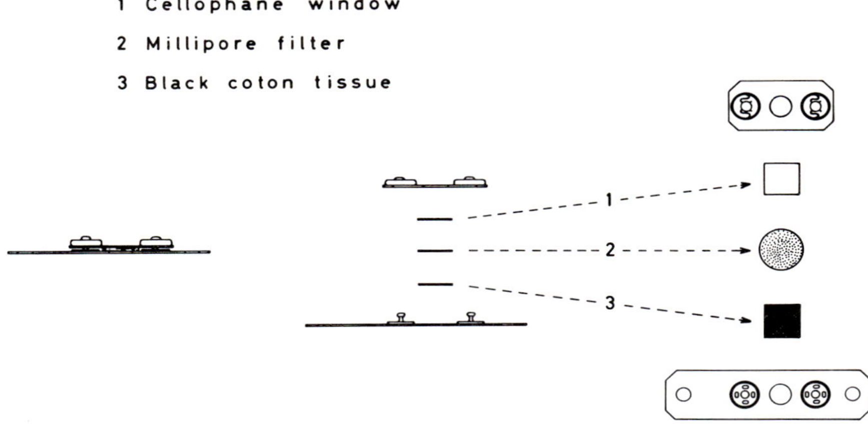

Figure 3. Schematic drawing showing how a Millipore filter with a deposit of extracted chloroplasts is mounted into a holder. The black cotton tissue is used to avoid reflection of incident light[11,12].

RESULTS

Acetabularia

The 77° K fluorescence emission spectra (FES) of chloroplasts extracted from the apical, middle and basal region of the stalk of A. mediterranea and of A. peniculus are reproduced respectively in Figures 4 and 5. Figure 4 shows that in A. mediterranea the three types of chloroplast are distinguishable: apical chloroplasts give maximal emission at 700-720 nm, whereas basal chloroplasts have their maximal

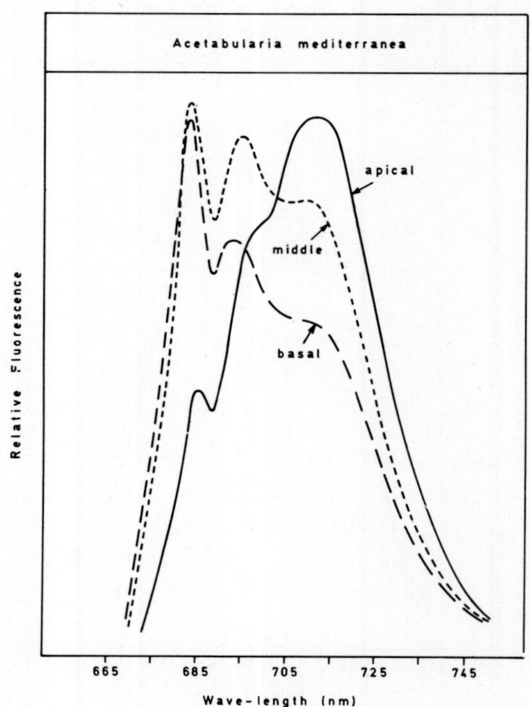

Figure 4. Acetabularia mediterranea: fluorescence emission spectra (FES) of apical, middle and basal chloroplasts.

emission at 685-690 nm. Middle chloroplasts give a FES which is intermediary between the two others.

In A. peniculus (Fig. 5) the apical chloroplast FES is rather similar to the apical chloroplast FES of A. mediterranea (maximal emission at 700-720 nm). In A. peniculus, the middle and basal chloroplast FES are undistinguishable one from the other, although they are

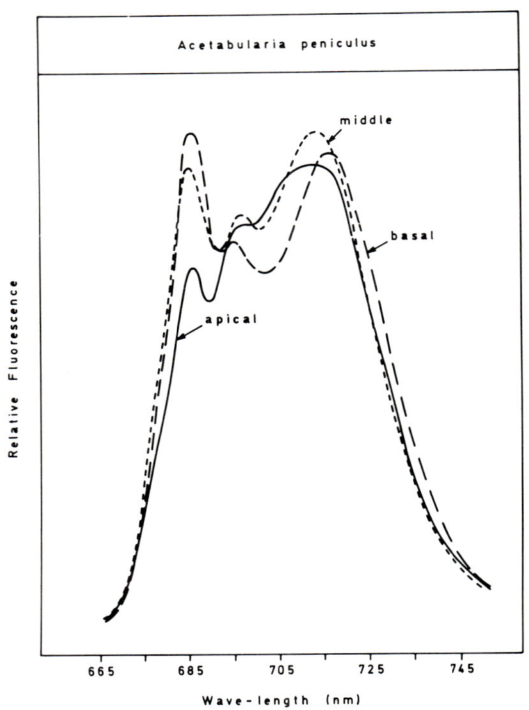

Figure 5. Acetabularia peniculus: fluorescence emission spectra (FES) of apical, middle and basal chloroplasts.

distinguishable from the FES of the apical chloroplasts.

Batophora

In this species, the FES of the apical chloroplasts is also clearly distinguishable from the FES of middle and basal chloroplasts (Fig. 6). The Batophora apical chloroplast FES

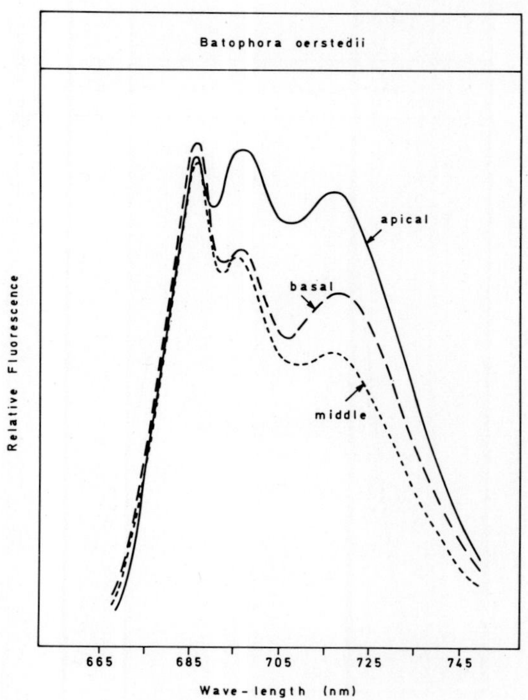

Figure 6. Batophora oerstedii: fluorescence emission spectra (FES) of apical, middle and basal chloroplasts.

is similar to the FES of A. mediterranea middle chloroplasts (compare Fig. 4 with Fig. 6). On the other hand, Batophora middle and basal chloroplasts have FES similar to the FES of A. mediterranea basal chloroplasts (see Figs. 4 and 6).

Comparison of basal chloroplasts FES in the three species

Figures 7 and 8 emphasize the differences existing between the basal chloroplast FES of A. mediterranea, B. peniculus and B. oerstidii. The figures show that by the fluorescence emission technique it is possible to distinguish

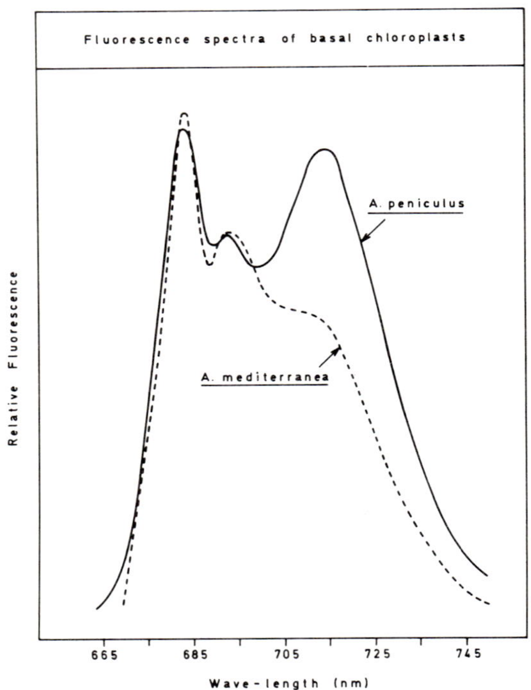

Figure 7. Comparison of fluorescence emission spectra (FES) of basal chloroplasts from A. mediterranea and A. peniculus.

basal chloroplasts of A. peniculus from those of A. mediterranea or of B. oerstedii. However, basal chloroplasts of A. mediterranea and of B. oerstedii can not be distinguished by this technique.

DISCUSSION

The FES profiles of apical, middle and basal chloroplasts of A. mediterranea, A. peniculus and B. oerstedii confirm the heterogeneity of these organelles. In the vegetative cells

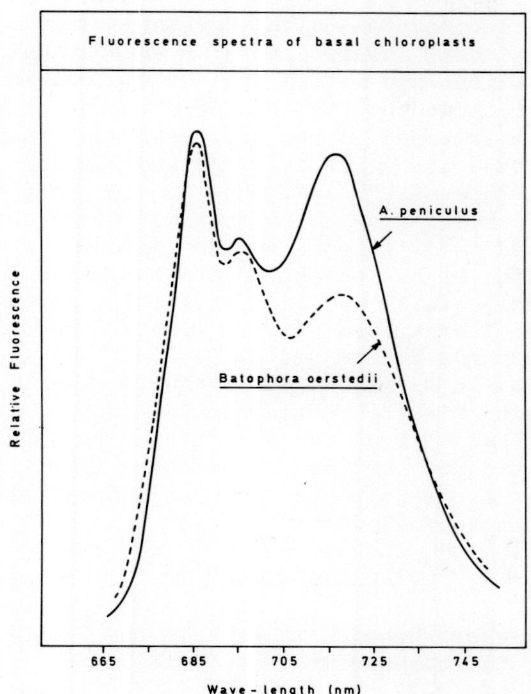

Figure 8. Comparison of fluorescence emission spectra (FES) of basal chloroplasts from A. peniculus and B. oerstedii.

(stage 4) of A. mediterranea, the chloroplasts are distributed according to an apico-basal morphological[1,2,3,8,13,14,15] and physiological[16] gradient. Moreover, in the same species, the organization of the chloroplast genome shows also an apico-basal gradient[17]. The results reported in this paper extend the concept of the apico-basal gradient (FES gradient) to two other species of the Dasycladaceae: A. peniculus and B. oerstedii. The existence of the chloroplast gradient in other species (A. cliftonii, A. major) is suggested by the recent work of Luttke et al.[18], who separated, by isopycnic gradient centrifugation, four subpopulations of chloroplasts, having different buoyant densities. It is quite likely that the chloroplast gradient occurs also in other not yet investigated *Acetabularia* species. Thus it may be a general feature.

It is to be noted that the FES apico-basal gradient of the chloroplasts is maintained in the cell in spite of protoplasmic streaming[19,20,21,22], which is sensitive to cytochalasin B[23]. Information on chloroplast movement in *Acetabularia* is still insufficient for understanding how chloroplast gradient and motion are correlated. We do not know the path followed by the chloroplasts into the stalk. How great is their speed in the different regions of the cell (quantitative data are still lacking) and how does it vary at the different times of the day? How do the cytoplasmic hydrodynamic forces influence chloroplast size? Are chloroplasts subjected to a 'to and fro' motion only, restricted to a limited portion of the stalk, or are they able to migrate through the whole stalk? At first sight it seems that the first of these alternatives is more likely. See also the paper of Hoursiangou-Neubrun et al.[3].

Our results on extracted chloroplasts clearly show that the FES gradient reflects the intrinsic state of the chloroplasts rather than that of the surrounding cytoplasm. The differences found for the FES of the three investigated species may perhaps permit the fate of chloroplasts in grafted cells to be followed[24].

ACKNOWLEDGEMENTS

This work was supported in part by the "Fonds de la Recherche Scientifique Fondamentale Collective" and by NATO Research Grant n° 1027. We thank Mr. G. Nuyts and Mrs. Madeleine Meurice for their technical assistance, Mr. G. Bas for the photos, Mr. A. Geusens for the graphs and Mrs. Jeannine Romeyer-Luyten for typewriting the text. We are indebted to Professor Simone Puisseux-Dao, who kindly provided *Acetabularia peniculus* and *Batophora oerstedii* plants.

REFERENCES

1. Puiseux-Dao, S. and Dazy, A. C. (1970) In "Biology of *Acetabularia*" (J. Brachet and S. Bonotto, eds.) pp. 111-122, Academic Press, New York and London.
2. Puiseux-Dao, S., Dazy, A. C., Hoursiangou-Neubrun, D. and Matthys, E. (1972) In "Biology and Radiobiology of Anucleate Systems" (S. Bonotto, R. Goutier, R. Kirchmann and J. R. Maisin, eds.), Vol. 2, pp. 101-125, Academic Press, New York and London.

3. Hoursiangou-Neubrun, D., Dubacq, J. P. and Puiseux-Dao, S. (1977) These Proceedings, p.175, Academic Press, New York and London.
4. Sironval, C., Bonotto, S. and Kirchmann, R. (1973) Plant Science Letters 1, 47.
5. Dujardin, E., Bonotto, S., Sironval, C. and Kirchmann, R. (1975) Plant Science Letters 5, 209.
6. Lateur, L. (1963) Rev. Algol. n. s. 1, 26.
7. Lateur, L. and Bonotto, S. (1973) Bull. Soc. Roy. Bot. Belgique 106, 17.
8. Puiseux-Dao, S. (1970) Acetabularia and cell biology, 162 p., Logos Press, London.
9. Bonotto, S. and Kirchmann, R. (1970) Bull. Soc. Roy. Bot. Belgique 103, 255.
10. Shephard, D. and Levin, W. B. (1972) J. Cell. Biol. 54, 279.
11. Sironval, C., Brouers, M., Michel, J. M. and Kuiper, Y. (1968) Photosynthetica 2, 268.
12. Sironval, C., Kirchmann, R., Bronchart, R. and Michel, J. M. (1968) Photosynthetica 2, 57.
13. Boloukhère, M. (1972) J. Microscopie 13, 401.
14. Hoursiangou-Neubrun, D. and Puiseux-Dao, S. (1974) Plant Sicence Letters 2, 209.
15. Hoursiangou-Neubrun, D. and Puiseux-Dao, S. (1975) XII Int. Bot. Congress, Leningrad, Abstracts 2, 293.
16. Issinger, O., Maas, I. and Clauss, H. (1971) Planta 101, 360.
17. Mazza, A., Bonotto, S. and Felluga, B. (1977) These Proceedings, p.123, Academic Press, New York and London.
18. Lüttke, A., Rahmsdorf, U. and Schmid, R. (1976) Z. Naturforsch. 31 c, 108.
19. Kamiya, N. (1960) Ann. Rev. Plant Physiol., 11, 323.
20. Bouck, G. B. (1964) In "Primitive Motile Systems in Cell Biology" (R. D. Allen and N. Kamiya, eds.), pp. 7-18, Academic Press, New York and London.
21. Williams, N. S. and Terborgh, J. (1970) Plant Physiology 46, 1.
22. Puiseux-Dao, S. (1972) Bull. Soc. Bot. France, Mémoires (Coll. Morphologie), pp. 71-88.
23. Brachet, J. and Tencer, R. (1973) Acta Embryologiae Experimentalis 83-104.
24. Puiseux-Dao, S., Valet, G. and Bonotto, S. (1970) C. R. Acad. Sci. Paris 271, 1354.

TEMPORARY PERIODIC LOCALIZATION OF THE CHLOROPLASTS IN THE FORM OF TRANSVERSE BANDS, IN THE STALK OF *ACETABULARIA MEDITERRANEA*

C. Sironval, S. Bonotto, M. Paques and E. Dujardin

Laboratoire de Photobiologie
Département de Botanique
Université de Liège
Liège, Belgium
and
Département de Radiobiologie
Centre d'Etude de l'Energie Nucléaire, C.E.N.-S.C.K.
Mol, Belgium

ABSTRACT

Whole and anucleate *Acetabularia* cells show transverse bands in the stalk as well as in the sterile whorls. Band formation is induced by stirring the cells at day-break. Newly formed bands persist for several hours in the dark, but disappear in the light after some tens of minutes. Band formation is due to chloroplast accumulation and can be detected by scanning frozen cells at 77° K with a pencil of blue light (436 nm). No explicit mention of band formation in *Acetabularia* has been previously made, although bands are clearly visible in many pictures published in the literature. The biological significance of the bands remains unknown.

INTRODUCTION

Our attention has been called to a phenomenon which we were subsequently able to find by examining closely the illustrated papers in the literature, and of which no explicit mention seems to have been made before. It consists of the observation that giant *Acetabularia* cells, cultivated in the laboratory, sometimes exhibit more or less transverse bands, which can be seen by the naked eye. Figure 1 is a photograph of these bands magnified four times. Figure 2 gives details of the bands, at 4 different magnifications. The ring-shaped

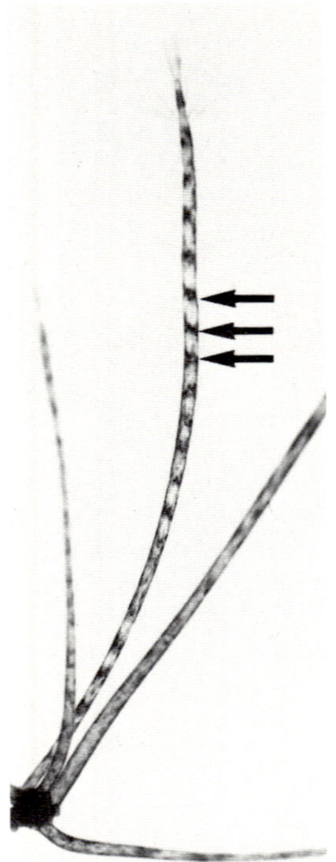

Figure 1. Whole *__Acetabularia__* *cell (stage 4) showing distinct bands (arrows) along the entire stalk. (x 4).*

image originates from the alternation of green and much less green transverse zones roughly perpendicular to the stalk axis. In Figure 1, about twenty green bands are visible. The distance between successive bands is rather constant (λ = 0.7 - 1 mm), from the base of the apex. Band frequency in 0.25 - 0.30 mm wide stalks is about 10 per cm. We tried to find out the conditions of allowing band formation and to

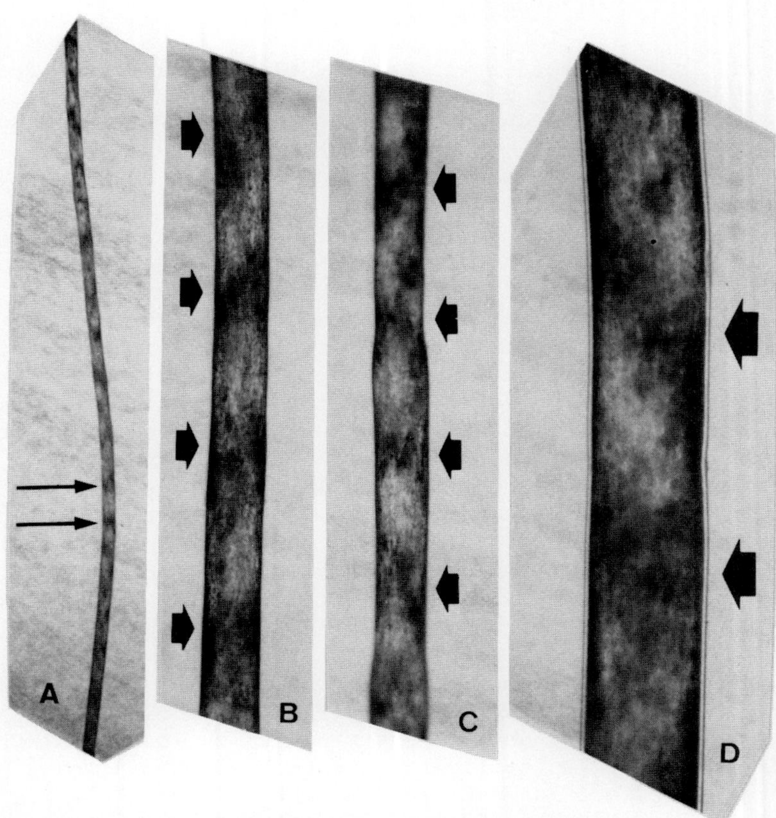

Figure 2. Bands in the stalk of whole cells, at four different magnifications: A (x 6), B (x 30), C (x 25), D (x 50). The arrows indicate the green bands, where chloroplast accumulation occurred.

and to investigate their nature. We summarize here our present knowledge of this matter.

MATERIALS AND METHODS

Acetabularia mediterranea were cultivated following the methods reported previously[1,2]. The plants were given artificial light as reported in these proceedings[3]. The device used for scanning the cell fluorescence at 77° K will be described elsewhere. The photographs of *Acetabularia* were taken with a fixed ordinary camera or with an automatic Polaroid camera mounted on a Reichert microscope.

RESULTS AND DISCUSSION

Band formation occurs in healthy plants during the growth phase (Stages 3 to 7; rarely at stage 8 [4]. Bands appear suddenly in a stalk, which was previously entirely devoid of bands. The transition to the ring-shaped image occurs mostly at day-break (from night to day); it is promoted by gently stirring the culture medium. The action of taking an *Acetabularia* cell from its culture vessel may be sufficient to induce the bands. A typical experiment is described below.

During the night, a few hours before day-break, whole and anucleate algae are gently stirred for 60-120 min: there is not band formation in darkness. The algae are then allowed to remain stationary for 60 min in the dark. At day-break, the algae are gently stirred: when withdrawn from the culture vessels they look as in Figure 3 A. This figure shows 4 whole cells (at the left) and 4 cells which have been enucleated for 5 days (at the right), from the same culture: band formation is clearly visible in all the stalks, although it does not appear so clearly as in Figure 1. After further stirring of the algae for 1 min in the light, they look as in Figure 3 B. If the algae are left in the light without stirring for 35 min., the bands disappear (Fig. 3 C). Stirring the algae once more in the light, produces only a few bands which appear rather faintly (Fig. 3 D). The above experiment demonstrates that stirring has by itself no effect (in the dark; or in the light: compare Figures 3 A and 3 B) or that its effect is weak (in the light: compare the Figures 3 C and 3 D). However, if stirring coincides with day-break, it generally induces band formation. Band disappearance in the light is concomitant with relatively rapid movements, as shown in Figure 4. This figure shows the same cell photographed shortly after stirring at day-break (Fig. 4 A) and 1 minute later (Fig. 4 B). The two bands visible in Figure 4 A between whorls 2 and 3 (arrows) are shifted, becoming a little

Figure 3. Band formation in whole and in anucleate cells.
A. Cells stirred at day-break.
B. The same cells as in A, but again stirred in the light for 1 min.
C. The same cells as in B, after 35 min. resting in the light.
D. The same cells as in C, but once more stirred in the light (x 3.5).

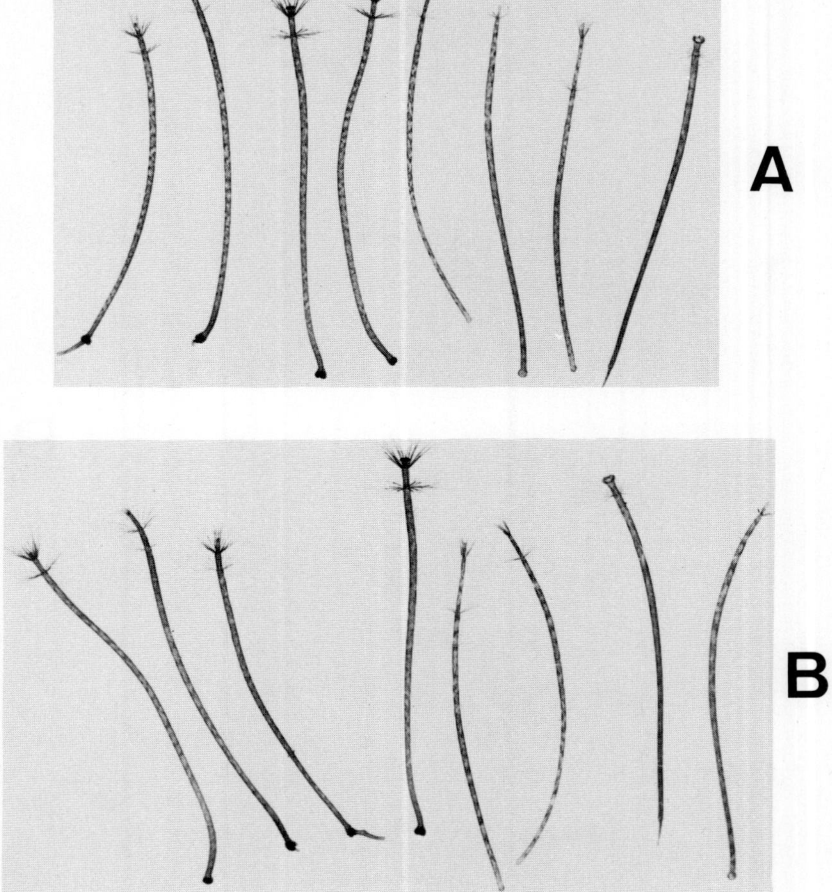

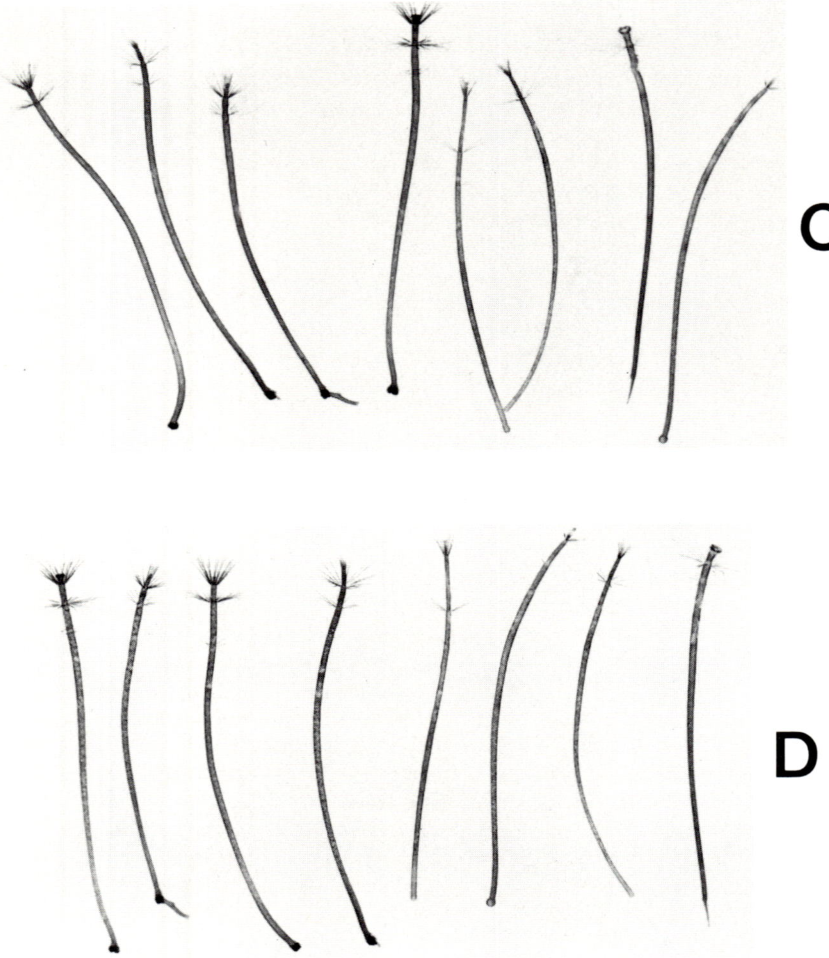

Figure 3 C, D. See previous page for legend.

diffuse 1 minute later (Fig. 4 B). Figure 4 B shows also a band midway between whorls 3 and 4 (arrow), which was absent 1 minute before (compare with Fig. 4 A), when a band was adjacent to whorl 4.

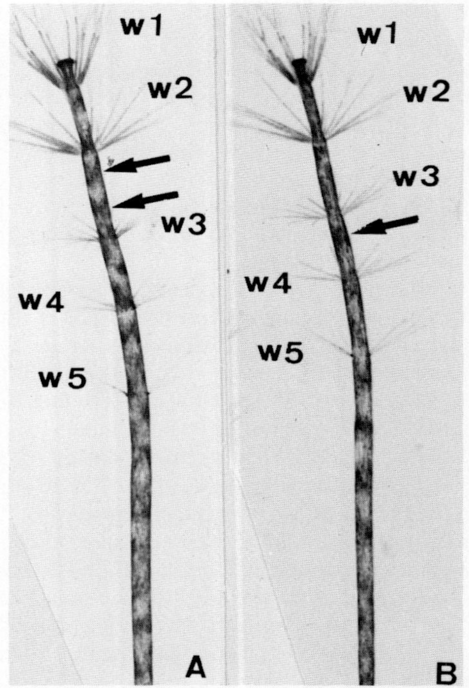

Figure 4. Rapid movements in the stalk by band disappearance in the light.

A. Whole cell showing two distinct bands (arrows) between whorl 2 (W2) and whorl 3 (W3) and another band adjacent to whorl 4 (W4).

B. The same cell, photographed 1 min. later: note that only a band is now visible between W2 and W3.

The two pictures of the same cells have been taken after focussing, with a fixed camera. For this reason the magnification is different (A: x 10; B: x 8.5).

If after stirring in the light at day-break, the banded algae are brought back to darkness, the bands persist for several hours; returning to the non-banded state is thus promoted by light.

The alternation of green and clear bands in the stalk is due to the accumulation of chloroplasts in the green bands. Chloroplast movements are thus involved in band formation.

It has been possible to show, by scanning frozen algae with a pencil blue light (436 nm), that the amount of fluorescence emitted at 77° K by the chlorophylls _in situ_ is lower in banded than in non-banded cells. This could be due to fluorescence quenching in the green bands, which are overcrowded with chloroplasts. Consequently, the difference in the fluorescence emitted by green and clear bands is reduced, although green bands are unambiguously revealed by a series of fluorescence peaks in the recordings (Fig. 5). In non-banded cells (having lost, or not having acquired the bands), the amount of fluorescence emitted by the chlorophylls varies from one region to another along the stalk, but without any clear periodicity.

Chloroplast movements at a transition from darkness to more or less bright light, or vice versa, have been widely studied and described in the literature (see for example the experiments by Zurzycki on _Lemna trisulca_ and on _Funaria hygrometrica_[5-9] and the film produced by the same author; see also the recent review paper of Seitz[10]. In the case of the _Acetabularia_ stalk, one is surprised by the rapidity of band formation and by the periodicity of the bands, suggesting a concerted structural organization along the whole stalk. The bands seem to move like waves along the stalk (Fig. 4 A and B). The observed ring shaped-images are also reminiscent of the bands found in the (chemical) Zhabotinski reaction[11,12], as illustrated in the book published by Glansdorff and Prigogine[13] (pages 147 and 148). Stirring at day-break may certainly be considered as a perturbation and one can postulate that the banded state is the result of a process deriving from an instability induced by the transition from darkness to light. In any case, the movements involved are independent of the presence of the nucleus, since band formation occurs in whole as well as in anucleate cells (Fig. 3). It is to be noted that band formation is sometimes visible only or mainly in the whorls (Fig. 6). The whorls reproduced in Fig. 5 B, page 9, of the review paper by Brachet[14] show the presence of distinct bands. Some cells in the papers by Schweiger et al.[15] and by Vanden Driessche[16] also show bands. In the work of Vanden Driessche[16], bands are clearly seen in whole as well as in anucleate cells, treated or not by morphactins. Her results suggest that

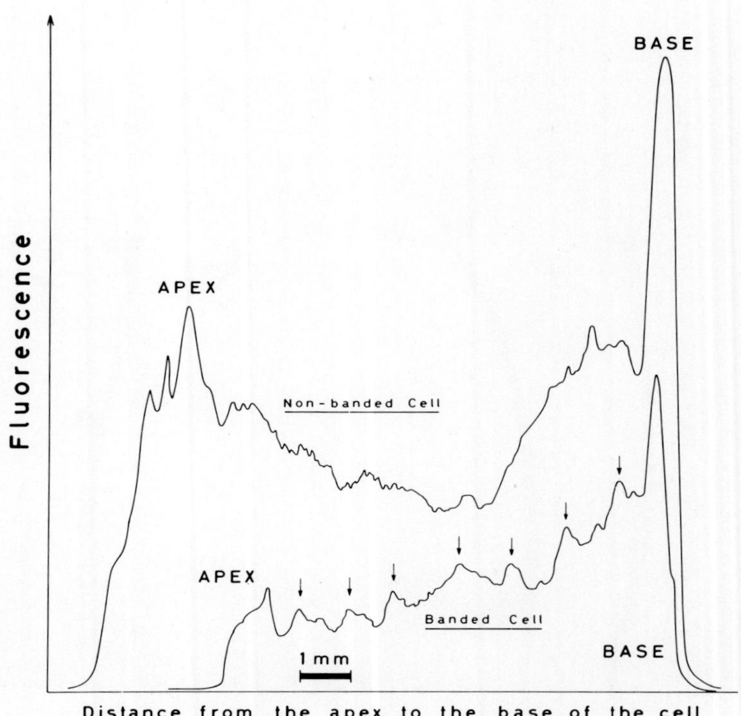

Figure 5. Fluorescence at 77° K of a whole non-banded and of a whole banded cell, scanned by a pencil of blue light (436 nm). The arrows show fluorescence peaks, which correspond to the bands.

morphactins have no action on band formation in whole and in anucleate cells.

Some other cases of band formation are found in the literature, in the stalks of Acetabularia crenulata[4], or in the sterile whorls of Bornetella oligospora, Neomeris, Acetabularia kilneri and Acetabularia dentata (see G. Valet, doctoral thesis[17]). These observations show that band

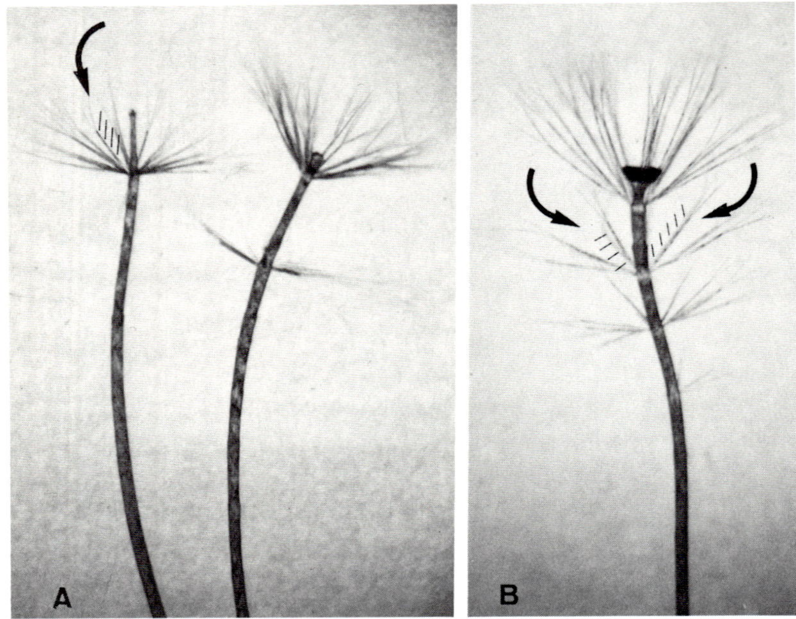

Figure 6. Two examples (A, B) of cells with bands in the sterile whorls (arrows). The fine bands are indicated by small lines (x 6).

formation is a phenomenon common to several species of the Dasycladaceae.

ACKNOWLEDGEMENTS

This work has been supported in part by the "Fonds de la Recherche Scientifique Fondamentale Collective" and by NATO Research Grant n°1027. We thank Mr. G. Nuyts for the technical assistance, Mr. R. Sauveur and Mr. G. Bas for the photographic work, Mr. A. Geusens for the graph and Mrs.

Jeannine Romeyer-Luyten for typewriting the text. We are indebted to Mr. L. Lateur, who kindly provided young cultures of Acetabularia.

REFERENCES

1. Lateur, L. (1963) Rev. Algol. n. s. 1, 26.
2. Lateur, L. and Bonotto, S. (1973) Bull. Soc. Roy. Bot. Belgique 106, 17.
3. Bonotto, S. and Sironval, C. (1977) These Proceedings, p. 241. Academic Press, New York and London.
4. Bonotto, S. and Kirchmann, R. (1970) Bull. Soc. Roy. Bot. Belgique 103, 255.
5. Zurzychi, J. (1962) Acta Soc. Bot. Pol. 31, 489.
6. Zurzychi, J. (1965) Acta Soc. Bot. Pol. 34, 637.
7. Zurzychi, J. (1967a) Acta Soc. Bot. Pol. 36, 133.
8. Zurzychi, J. (1967b) Acta Soc. Bot. Pol. 36, 143.
9. Zurzychi, J. (1972) Acta Protozool. 11, 189.
10. Seitz, K. (1975) In "Marine Ecology" (Otto Kinne, ed.), Vol. 2 pp. 451-497. John Wiley & Sons, London, New York, Sydney, Toronto.
11. Zhabotinsky, A. M. (1964) Biofizika 2, 306.
12. Zhabotinsky, A. M. (1968) Russ. J. Phys. Chem. 42, 1649.
13. Glansdorff, P. and Prigogine, I. (1971) Structure, stabilité et fluctuations, 288 p. Masson et Cie Editeurs, Paris.
14. Brachet, J. (1968) In "Current Topics in Developmental Biology" (A. Monroy and A. Moscona, eds.), Vol. 3, pp. 1-36. Academic Press, New York and London.
15. Schweiger, H. G., Werz, G. and Reuter, W. (1969) Protoplasma 68, 354.
16. Vanden Driessche, T. (1974) Protoplasma 81, 323.
17. Valet, G. (1968) Contribution à l'étude des Dasycladales, pp. 1-216. Doctoral Thesis, University of Paris.

PLASTIDIAL HETEROGENEITY DURING THE DEVELOPMENTAL CYCLE OF *ACETABULARIA MEDITERRANEA*

Esther Dujardin, Silvano Bonotto and Cyrille Sironval

Laboratoire de Photobiologie
Université de Liège
Liège, Belgium
and
Département de Radiogiologie
Centre d'Etude de l'Energie Nucléaire, C.E.N.-S.C.K.
Mol, Belgium

ABSTRACT

The authors have investigated, using the 77° K fluorescence emission method, how chloroplasts change during the developmental cycle of *Acetabularia mediterranea*. The experiments were performed using whole and anucleate cells. The facts suggest that, in *Acetabularia*, plastidial heterogeneity not only depends on the position in the cell (spatial differentiation), but is also closely related to cell ontogenesis (temporal differentiation).

INTRODUCTION

We have previously shown that the characteristics of the 77° K fluorescence emission spectra prove the heterogeneity of the chloroplasts in *Acetabularia mediterranea*[1,2]. Chloroplast heterogeneity in *Acetabularia* has been demonstrated also using light and electron microscopy[3-6]. On the other hand, we show elsewhere in this volume, that the 77° K fluorescence of chloroplasts of *Acetabularia peniculus* differs from that of chloroplasts of *Acetabularia mediterranea* and of *Batophora oerstedii*[7].

The 77° K fluorescence emission spectrum is a useful tool, because it relates to the structural organization of the plastid lamellae. The study of this emission provides a sensitive and reproducible method which requires a small amount of plant material, for investigating the relationships between the pigment-protein complexes collecting and utilizing the absorbed light energy inside the chloroplast lamellae.

The spectra have three emission bands: the first, at 685 nm, originates from light collecting pigments; the second and the third, at 695-700 and 710-720 nm, arise respectively from the photoactive centers II and I of photosynthesis. When the intensity of the emission at 695-720 nm decreases with respect to the emission at 685 nm, one can infer a change in the structural organization of the lamellae, the transfer of energy towards the photoactive centers being reduced. Also, the emission of center I sometimes increases at the expense of that of center II, and inversely, because the energy becomes transferred preferentially towards one or another type of center, or for some other reason[3]. Thus, in the studies involving an analysis of the fluorescence emission spectra, the chlorophylls behave as internal markers reflecting structural (organizational) features of the chloroplast lamellae.

In our first investigations[1], we repeatedly submitted the algae to large temperature transitions, from 293° K to 77° K and vice versa, in order to test the stability of the *in situ* molecular organization of the lamellae, and we compared in this respect chloroplasts of the apical to those of the basal region of the *Acetabularia* stalk. The changes induced by these thermic transitions in the relative intensities of the emission bands suggested that the chloroplasts of the base were intrinsically different from those of the apex. In subsequent investigations[2], we extracted the chloroplasts, which were then rapidly collected on Millipore filters covered with a piece of bolting silk (see ref. 7), and we improved the quality of the fluorescence spectra. We found that extraction increased the differences between spectra of apical and basal chloroplast. We defined for both apical and basal, extracted chloroplasts a typical spectrum: the "apical type" spectrum and the "basal type" spectrum. We were able to demonstrate that basal chloroplasts could arise from apical ones, and inversely, by experimenting on anucleate cells and on regenerating basal nucleate fragments. Of particular interest was the finding that, in the absence of the nucleus, chloroplasts exhibiting initially a spectrum of the basal type and acquired, in a few days, a spectrum of the apical type. The fluorescence emission spectra at 77° K were also used to show that the lamellar structure of middle stalk chloroplasts undergoes circadian changes[8].

In the present paper we use the 77° K fluorescence emission method for describing how chloroplasts change during the developmental cycle of *Acetabularia mediterranea*.

MATERIAL AND METHODS

The procedure used has been reported by Dujardin et al.[2]. A 5 mm portion of the apical or of the basal region of the stalk is homogenized in the buffer of Shephard and Levin[9]. The homogenate is filtered as described in this volume[7]. In some experiments, the fluorescence of whole cells or of parts of cells is examined: in this case the material is deposited on a buffered Millipore filter, which is mounted into a holder (see Fig. 3 of ref. 7). The holder is frozen at 77° K and the fluorescence emission is registered[10,11].

RESULTS AND DISCUSSION

Figure 1 A reproduces two, randomly chosen fluorescence emission spectra of 1 mm young plantlets (stage 3,S_1 [12]). These spectra are similar to the spectrum of the apical region of 2.5 cm plants at stage 4: one easily recognizes three bands (at 685, 695 and 715 nm) having about the same intensity. In Figure 1 B and 1 C, a series of spectra of chloroplasts extracted from the apex (B) or from the base (C; with the rhizoids) of the stalk are superposed. They belong to plastids extracted at day 0 from 2.5 cm long whole cells (stage 4,S_{25},W_3) and then 20, 40 and 55 days later. The profiles of the spectra of basal chloroplasts undergo only small changes (Fig. 1 C). In contrast, the profiles of apical chloroplasts spectra (Fig. 1 B) change markedly: the intensity of the emissions at 695 and at 710-720 nm first increases considerably in comparison to the intensity of the emission at 685 nm, which becomes very low between day 10 and day 20. However, later on, especially after day 40, the spectrum of the apical chloroplasts approaches that of basal chloroplasts. This change seems to be independent of direct control of the nucleus, as shown by the spectra in Figure 1 D, which are derived from apical chloroplasts from anucleate algae, of the same age as the algae of Figure 1 B and 1 C.

Figure 2 shows specta pertaining to full grown cells when caps contain secondary nuclei (stage 9) and then cysts (stage 10). Figure 2 A gives the spectrum of the stalk at these stages: the same type of spectrum is consistently found from the time when the stalk becomes "empty," after migration of secondary nuclei. In this spectrum, the emission at 685 nm is predominant over the other two emissions at 695 and 710 nm, which appear as satellites of the major peak. On the contrary, in the reproductive caps with secondary nuclei (Fig. 2 B), or cysts (Fig. 2 C), chloroplasts emit fairly well at 695 and at 715 nm. The chloroplasts extracted from these caps have a spectrum intermediate between the apical and the basal type. The spectrum of whole cysts from ripe caps is shown in Figure

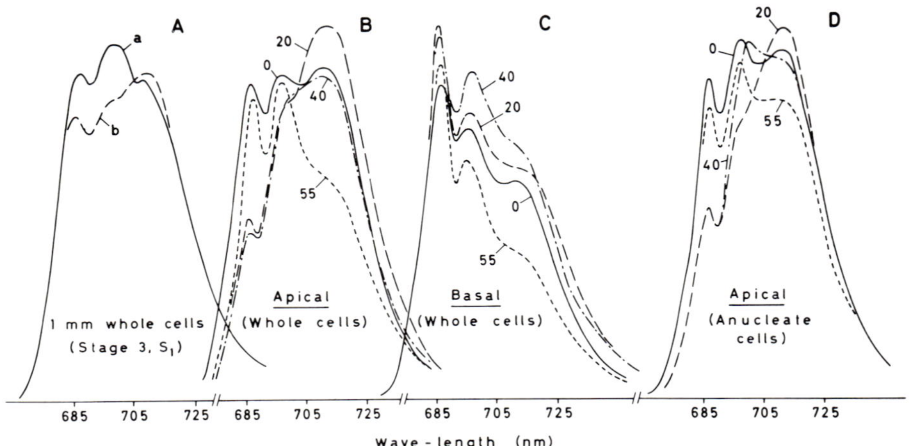

Figure 1. 77° K fluorescence emission spectra.

A. Young 1 mm long plantlets (a) and total chloroplasts extracted from these plantlets (b).

B. Chloroplasts extracted from the apex (5 mm) of 2.5 cm long whole cells at stage 4 (time 0) and 20, 40 and 55 days later respectively.

C. Chloroplasts extracted from the base (5 mm with the rhizoids) of 2.5 cm long whole cells at stage 4 (time 0) and 20, 40 and 55 days later respectively.

D. Chloroplasts extracted from the apex (5 mm) of 2.3 cm long anucleate cells at stage 4 (time 0) and 20, 40 and 55 days later respectively.

2 D: it looks similar to the spectrum emitted by 1 mm young plantlets (compare with Fig. 1 A).

Figure 3 gives spectra of chloroplasts of sterile whorls. The sensitivity of the method permits the examination, one by one, of the whorls separated from one single cell. Figure 3 A compares the spectra of the whorls 1, 3 and 4 ordered by

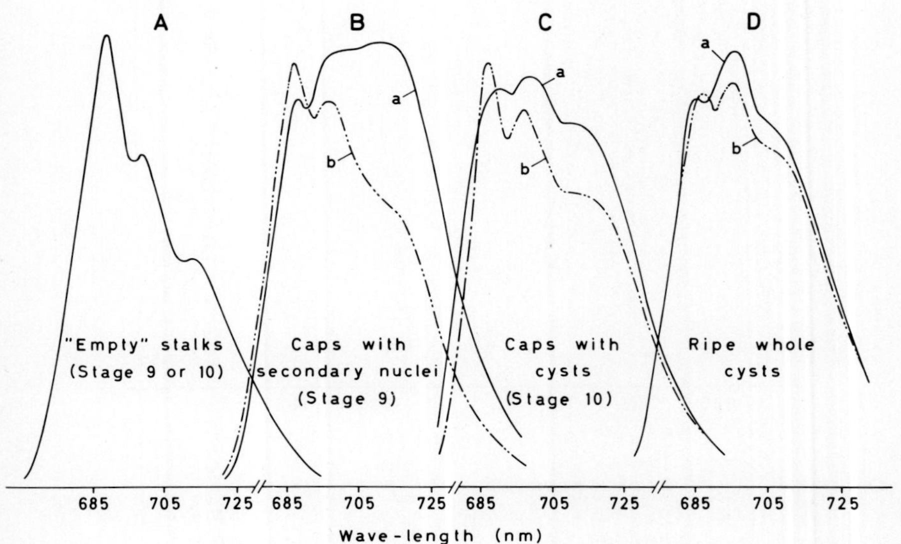

Figure 2. 77° K fluorescence emission spectra.

A. Typical spectrum of an "empty" stalk at stage 9 or 10.

B. Chloroplasts extracted from caps with secondary nuclei (stage 9). Two examples (a, b) of extreme spectra are shown.

C. Chloroplasts extracted from caps with cysts (stage 10). Two examples (a, b) of extreme spectra are shown.

D. Spectra of two (a, b) preparations of ripe whole cysts, repeatedly purified by sedimentation in filtered sea-water.

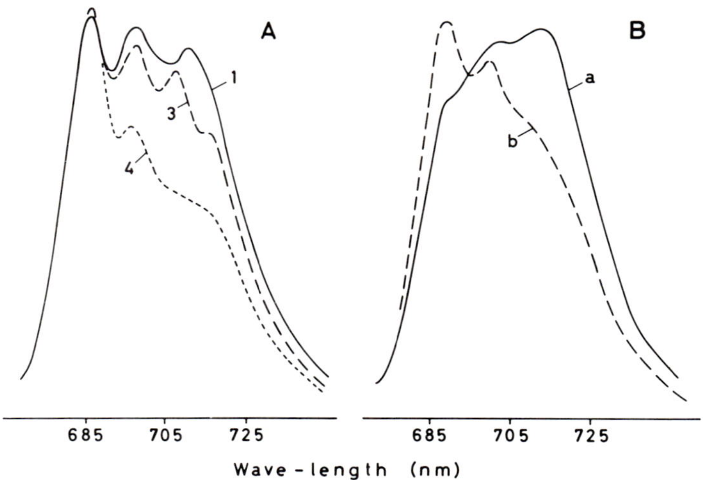

Figure 3. 77° K fluorescence emission spectra.

A. Sterile whorl of order 1, 3 and 4. Whorl 1 is the youngest one, whereas whorl 4 is the oldest one.

B. Chloroplasts extracted from a young cap of a cell at stage 7 (a) and from the whorl of order 1, still present on the stalk, but already "aged" (b).

starting from the apex of one cell. The chloroplasts of whorl 1 and 3 clearly have a spectrum type intermediate between the apical and the basal type. Whorl 4 has a spectrum of the basal type, although it belongs to a region of the stalk whose chloroplasts exhibit a spectrum of the apical type. This indicates that:

1. chloroplasts of two neighboring parts of one single cell may be very different;
2. the whorls are distinguished from the stalk by having chloroplasts with differing spectra.

These conclusions are also supported by observations on cells with a young cap and a whorl nearby: the spectrum of the cap approaches the apical type, whereas that of the whorl looks like the basal type (Fig. 3 B).

Figure 4 summarizes the facts showing that in the giant Acetabularia cell plastidial heterogeneity is closely connected to cellular ontogenesis. Chloroplast heterogeneity is not a static phenomenon. It becomes more and more accentuated during plant development and it is particularly clear when stalk growth is maximal (stage 4). This suggests that the photosynthetic activity of the chloroplasts should also vary according to their localization and to ontogenetic stage. Moreover, chloroplast evolution seems to be in some way specific in the Dasycladaceae since, using the fluorescence emission, it is possible to distinguish chloroplasts of Acetabularia peniculus from those of Acetabularia mediterranea and of Batophora oerstedii, when the plants are at stage 4, as shown in ref. 7.

On the other hand, the situation in the whorls implies that the change from the apical to the basal chloroplast type may reflect chloroplast aging. In Acetabularia mediterranea the whorls are deciduous structures which fall off at a certain age, i.e. at a certain stage of morphological differentiation[13-19]. If this idea, namely that a spectrum of the basal type corresponds to aged chloroplasts, is extended to the whole cell, one is led to qualify as "young" the chloroplasts of the apex, and as "older" or "aged" those of the base of the stalk (stage 4), or those which remain in the "empty" stalk. The latter are apparently degenerating.

ACKNOWLEDGEMENTS

This work was supported in part by the "Fonds de la Recherche Scientifique Fondomentale Collective" and by NATO Research Grant n° 1027. We thank Mrs. Madeleine Meurice and Mr. G. Nuyts for their technical assistance, Mr. G. Bas for the photos, Mr. A. Geusens for the graphs and Mrs. Jeannine Romeyer-Luyten for typewriting the text.

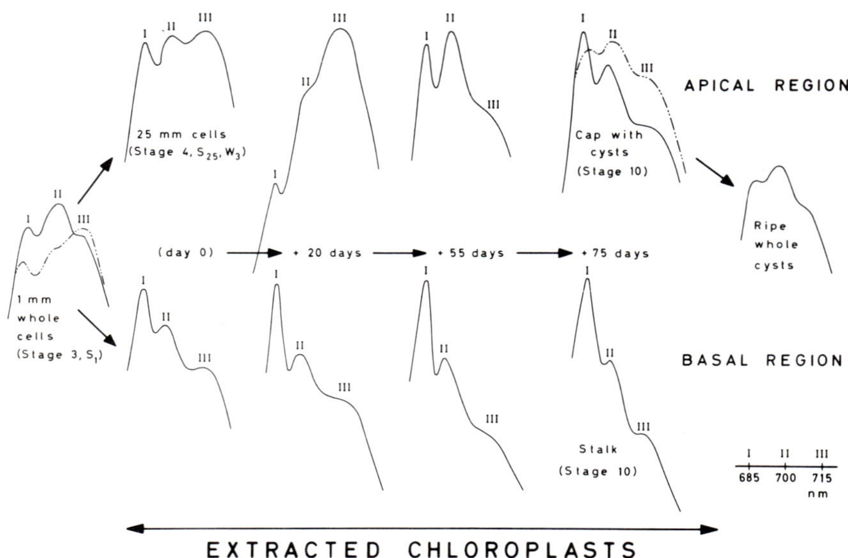

Figure 4. Schematic representation of the changes in 77° K fluorescence emission spectra of Acetabularia chloroplasts, during the developmental cycle of the plant.

REFERENCES

1. Sironval, C., Bonotto, S. and Kirchmann, R. (1973) Plant Science Letters 1, 47.
2. Dujardin, E., Bonotto, S., Sironval, C. and Kirchmann, R. (1975) Plant Science Letters 5, 209.
3. Shephard, D. (1965) Exp. Cell Research 37, 93.
4. Puiseux-Dao, S. and Dazy, A. C. (1970) In "Biology of Acetabularia" (J. Brachet and S. Bonotto, eds.), pp. 111-122, Academic Press, New York and London.

5. Puiseux-Dao, S., Dazy, A. C., Hoursiangou-Neubrun, D. and Matthys, E. (1972) In "Biology and Radiobiology of Anucleate Systems" (S. Bonotto, R. Goutier, R. Kirchmann and J. R. Maisin, eds.), Vol. 2, pp. 101-125. Academic Press, New York and London.
6. Hoursiangou-Neubrun, D. and Puiseux-Dao, S. (1974) Plant Science Letters 2, 209.
7. Bonotto, S., Dujardin, E., Kirchmann, R. and Sironval, C. (1977) These Proceedings, p. 195, Academic Press, New York and London.
8. Vanden Driessche, T., Dujardin, E., Magnusson, A. and Sironval, C. (1976) Int. J. Chronobiology 4, 111.
9. Shephard, D. and Levin, W. B. (1972) J. Cell Biol. 54, 279.
10. Sironval, C., Brouers, M., Michel, J. M. and Kuiper, Y. (1968) Photosynthetica 2, 268.
11. Sironval, C., Kirchmann, R., Bronchart, R. and Michel, J. M. (1968) Photosynthetica 2, 57.
12. Bonotto, S. and Kirchmann, R. (1970) Bull. Soc. Roy. Bot. Belgique 103, 255.
13. Puiseux-Dao, S. (1962) Rev. Gen. Bot. 319, 409.
14. Bonotto, S. (1969) Bull. Soc. Roy. Bot. Belgique 102, 165.
15. Declève, A., Van Gorp, U., Bouloukhère, M. and Bonotto, S. (1972) In "Biology and Radiobiology of Anucleate Systems" (S. Bonotto, R. Goutier, R. Kirchmann and J. R. Maisin, eds.), Vol. 2, pp. 259-293. Academic Press, New York, London.
16. Gibor, A. (1973a) Protoplasma 78, 195.
17. Gibor, A. (1973b) Protoplasma 78, 461.
18. Gibor, A. (1974) Portugaliae Acta Biologica 14, 295.
19. Adamich, M., Gibor, A. and Sweeney, B. M. (1975) J. Phycol. 11, 364.

IV GROWTH AND MORPHOGENESIS

CELL ELONGATION IN *ACETABULARIA*

A. Gibor

University of California
Santa Barbara, California

The appearance of an *Acetabularia* cell, as that of all other living organisms, is a resultant of the interaction of the genetic potential and environmental factors. The classic work of Hammerling established the role of the nucleus and its genome in the appearance of *Acetabularia* cells[1]. In the following I want to describe observations on the effects of some environmental factors on the development of these cells; I will consider primarily the elongation of the cells.

Usually elongation is symmetrical, resulting in a straight cell axis with equally spaced sterile or fertile whorls. Asymmetrical cell elongation results in the appearance of curved cells. A number of experimental conditions were found which can cause curving of *Acetabularia* cells. As yet I have no physiological explanation for the observed asymmetrical growth.

A. Apical elongation

Elongation of *Acetabularia* cells occurs typically at the apex. This was shown clearly by time lapse photography[2]. Also from electron-microscopical observations on the distribution of golgi vesicles Werz[3] concluded that the cells grow by apical elongation.

In recent studies I demonstrated that illumination of the apical region of the cell is essential for elongation[4]. Cells which were grown with only their apical portions exposed to light were found to elongate as much or even more than cells which were totally illuminated. On the other hand cells with only their apical portions kept in dark stopped elongating (Table 1). Is the light effect due to localized photosynthesis or to a photomorphogenic effect on the cell apex? I demonstrated that DCMU, a photosynthesis inhibitor, if applied only to the apical region of the cells caused the stopping of

TABLE 1

Cell Elongation of A. major

Days	Culture Conditions	# cells	Original length (mm)	Change in length (mm)	% change
10	Total in light	19	399	+106	26.6
10	Total in dark	18	394	+ 16	4.1
10	Apex in light	19	451	+186	41.2
16	Total in light	10	272	+135	49.6
16	Apex in light	9	261	+107	41

The elongation of cells cultured in dark, light or with only the apical few millimeters exposed to light was measured after the indicated number of days. Growing cells with only their apices in light were pulled into the dark chamber every second day.

elongation (Table 2). Thus photosynthesis in the apical region of the cell is essential for elongation. However other morphogenetic effects of light on the apical regions can not be excluded. Another interesting and important conclusion from these observations is that intracellular translocation of photosynthesis products and of DCMU is lacking or is very slow.

Unique physiological properties of the cell apex of Acetabularia are suggested from the reported electrical properties of the growing cell apex. It is claimed that endogenous electric currents flowing between the growing cell apex and its base are essential for growth. Electric isolation of the cell apex from the base was found to block cell growth[5]. We do not know yet whether light exposure of the apex is required to induce the electric current flow.

TABLE 2

Effect of DCMU on Cell Elongation in the Light

Days	Culture Conditions	# cells	Original length (mm)	Change in length (mm)	% change
14	No DCMU	9	147	85	57.8
14	+ DCMU	5	80	1	1.2
14	Apex in DCMU	9	192	3	1.6
14	Base in DCMU	9	187	30	16.0

DCMU solution to a final concentration of 10^{-6} M was added to one of the chambers of a culture vessel. The effect on cell elongation was measured after the indicated number of days.

B. Asymmetric growth

1. Curving due to sterile hair removal

After surgical removal or irradiation of the sterile hair from one side of A. mediteranea, the cell is seen to curve towards the side from which the hair was removed or irradiated (Fig. 1)[6]. Obviously unequal lengths of the cell result from the operation. The rapid curving (it is seen within two days), and the region of the cell which curves indicate that the curving zone is not at the elongating apex. Curving occurs near the region where the mature whorls are. This region of the cell is normally not elongating since the distances between mature whorls or between scars of whorls which were shed is quite constant.

However, for curving to occur, the difference in length between the sides of the cell will be only a fraction of the cell diameter, and this will not be readily measurable.

Although we reported that the curving occurs only if the cells are maintained under conditions which promote active cell elongation we can not state whether the curving is due to the preferential elongation of one side or whether it results from shortening of the side of the cell from which the hair was removed.

We found recently that mature Acetabularia cells can shorten. Cells which were kept in light in the presence of DCMU (10^{-6} M) and carefully measured were found to have shortened after several days[7]. Curving could thus result from either unequal elongation or shortening of the sides of the cell.

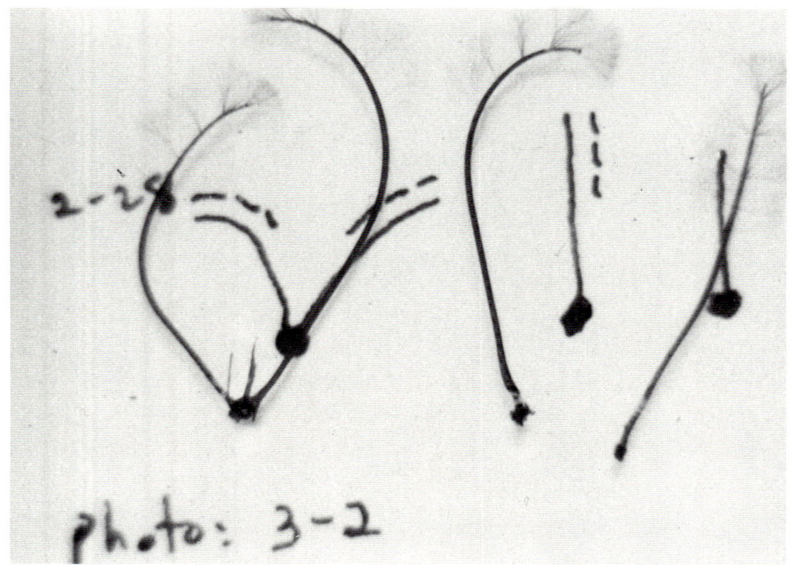

Figure 1. Photograph of cells 3 days after shaving hair of one side of the cell. The line drawn in the background indicates the appearance of the cells before the operation, the broken lines indicate the shaven side. The cell on the right was not shaven.

2. Curving due to unequal illumination

Phototropism, the directed growth of organisms in relation to a light source, was reported for Acetabularia cells growing in nature[8]. The appearance of undisturbed cultures of A. major, growing under illumination from one side clearly indicates that the cells are growing towards the light. (Fig. 2).

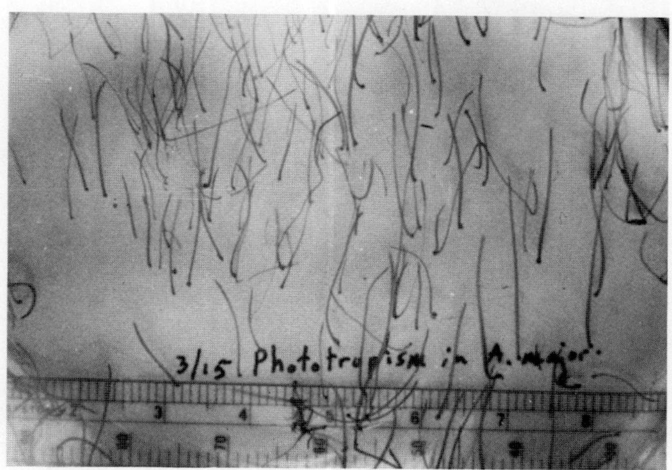

Figure 2. A culture dish of undisturbed A. major cells-- growing oriented towards the light source.

We experimented further with the phototropic responses of A. major. The availability of the relatively non toxic contact-glue, cyanoacrylate, enabled us to glue Acetabularia cells in a definite orientation towards the light source. A minute droplet of the glue was placed on the dry bottom of a petri-dish. A cell was blotted carefully and then placed with the desired segment coming into contact with the glue-droplet. Adhesion occurs instantly, and the dish can then be carefully filled with culture medium and oriented as desired. Such glued cells were found to grow towards the light source.

Cells which were glued in their middle were found to be able to curve both at the apical and basal ends (Fig. 3). It is thus evident that changes in length of the cells, sufficient to cause curving, can occur throughout the entire cell length.

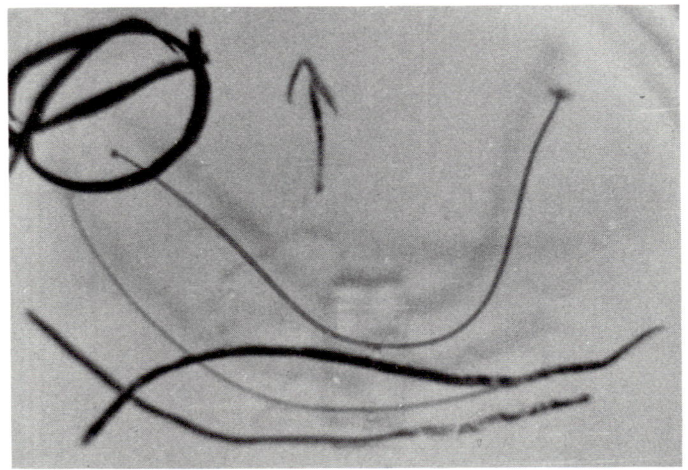

Figure 3. Two A. major cells, glued in their middle and growing towards the light source (Arrow). The black lines drawn in the background represent the appearance of the cells when glued down.

In a further attempt to demonstrate the region of the cell which elongates I marked the length of cells with carbon particles and then glued them down for cultivation. The growing cells were photographed daily. The images of the photographs of the cell were projected onto ruled paper and their outlines traced by hand. Fig. 4 is an example of such a composite figure. The daily changes in the cell and its zone of curving are readily seen from the series of tracings. It is clear that curving occurred well below the apical region of the growing cell.

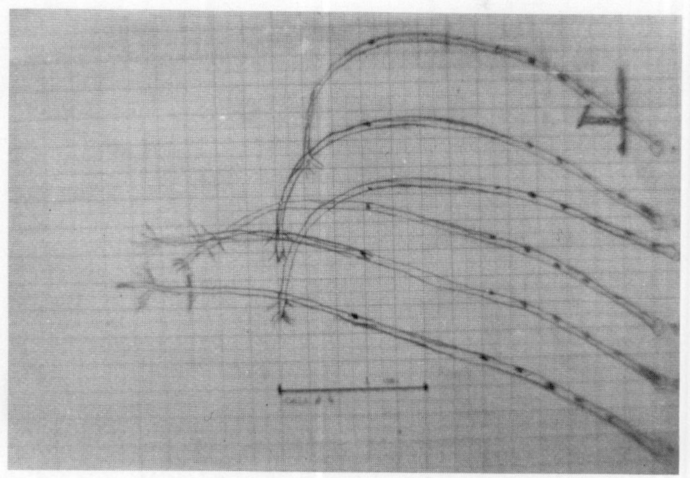

Figure 4. Hand tracing of the daily changes in appearance of a glued cell. Day-1 is the top tracing. Day-6, bottom drawing.

3. Curving in response to gravity

In some experiments which were conducted for other purposes I planted A. mediteranea cells in an inverted position, i.e. with their apical portions pointing downward. After several weeks of growth under such conditions the cells were found to have curved upward. Fig. 5 is an example of such an experiment in which nucleated and enucleated cells were grown inverted to the gravity vector. These observations suggest that the cells respond to gravity and tend to grow in a negative geotropic sense. The curved growth in response to gravity is very slow. It required at least a week of active growth before a noticeable curvature was observed.

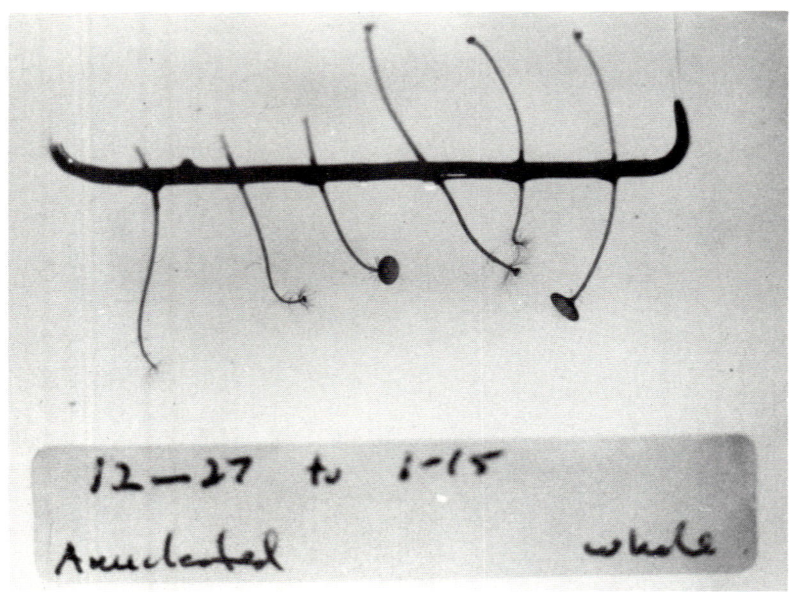

Figure 5. A. mediteranea cells growing inverted, attached to a glass rod.

The nature of the physiological factors which are responsible for changes in length in different sectors of the cell are not known. It is interesting, however, to note that the two *Acetabularia* species which we used, *A. mediteranea* and *A. major*, differ in their responses to the environmental factors which we examined. *A. mediteranea* responded to gravity while *A. major* did not. On the other hand, *A. major* readily curved in response to unilateral illumination while *A. mediteranea* did not. Similarly the effect of removal of sterile hair on bending of the cells is readily demonstrable with *A. mediteranea* but not with *A. major*. By nuclear transplantation it should be possible to determine whether phototropism for example is genetically controlled.

REFERENCES

1. Hammerling, J. (1963) Ann. Rev. Plant Physiol. 14, 65-92.
2. Martynov, L. A. et al. (1972) Second Symposium on Acetabularia.
3. Werz, G. (1970) Current Topics in Microbiology and Immunol. 51, 27-62.
4. Gibor, A. (1976) (abstract) Cell Biol. 70, (part 2), 219a (paper submitted to Plant Physiol.).
5. Novak, B. (1975) Protoplasma 83, 178-182.
6. Gibor, A. (1973) Protoplasma 78, 461-465.
7. Gibor, A. (unpublished results).
8. Nasr, A. H. (1939) Revue Algology 11, 347-350.

EXPERIMENTAL STUDIES ON THE PHOTOTROPISM OF *ACETABULARIA MEDITERRANEA* AND *ACETABULARIA CRENULATA*

Silvano Bonotto and Cyrille Sironval

Département de Radiobiologie
Centre d'Etude de l'Energie Nucléaire
Mol, Belgium
and
Laboratoire de Photobiologie
Université du Sart-Tilman
Liège, Belgium

SUMMARY

Experiments performed under controlled conditions have shown that in *Acetabularia mediterranea* as well as in *Acetabularia crenulata*, the growing stalk displays a positive phototropism. Moreover, *Acetabularia* cells are capable of reorienting their stalk when light direction changes. The rhizoids of both species exhibit a negative phototropism.

INTRODUCTION

In nature, *Acetabularia* cells are fixed to the rocks or other substrata by their rhizoids, the stalk growing towards the light. The length of the stalk and the size of the reproductive cap clearly depend on light intensity. The plants living in shallow waters have short stalks and large caps, those living in deep waters possess long stalks and small caps. Very long (10 cm) *Acetabularia mediterranea* having a small cap were observed by Brachet on a Greek amphora found at a depth of 20 m[1]. The vertical standing of a natural population of *Acetabularia* cells shows that the plant is subjected to the orienting action of the force of gravity. The geotropism of *Acetabularia* is evident also in laboratory cultures, when the plants are fixed to the bottom of the bottles or to pebbles. The first observations on the phototropism of *Acetabularia* were made in 1937 on the species *Acetabularia calyculus* growing in the Red Sea[2]. By placing the collected plants in a glass basin next to a window (as

Professor J. Feldmann had done before for the alga *Derbesia Lamourouxii*[3]), Nasr observed that the old plants exposed their caps towards light direction; young plants without cap showed also a clear positive phototropism. However, the same author was unable to observe any phototropism in *Acetabularia möbii* and *Acetabularia mediterranea*[2]. In contrast with this early report, a clear positive phototropism of the stalk has been occasionally observed in *Acetabularia mediterranea* cultivated in the laboratory by S. Puiseux-Dao[4], by S. Bonotto and by L. Lateur (unpublished observations). New interesting observations on *Acetabularia* phototropism were reported by Aharon Gibor at the fourth IRGA Symposium (see these proceedings).

In this paper, we report some observations on the phototropism of *Acetabularia mediterranea* and of *Acetabularia crenulata*, indicating that these unicellular algae may be useful for research in this field.

MATERIALS AND METHODS

The cultures of *Acetabularia mediterranea* and *Acetabularia crenulata* were obtained following the methods reported previously[5,6]. The experiments were started with zygotes (stage 2) or with young plants being at stage 3 [7]. At this stage the algae stick to the bottom of the glass vessels[6] and become more and more attached as the growth of the rhizoids continues. The plants were submitted to light-dark cycles of 12:12 h, the light period being given from 9 a.m. to 9 p.m. The fluorescent tubes (Phytor LF-40 W, ACEC) gave an illuminance of 600 lux at the level of the vessels. The wavelengths emitted by these daylight tubes range from 400 to 700 nm[8]. The culture vessels were illuminated at an angle $\alpha = 55^{\circ}$ (see Fig. 4) and maintained in the laboratory at 23-24° C. The culture medium was renewed every week. The photographs of the *Acetabularia* cells were taken after overturning the vessels.

RESULTS

Acetabularia mediterranea

Young plants at stage $3,S_1$ [7] were cultivated for 70 days. A positive phototropism of the stalk was already observed after 3 weeks. After 70 days, most of the plants were at stage $4,S_7,W_1$ [7] and had their stalk oriented in the light direction. In a few plants, the rhizoids grew in the opposite direction, suggesting a negative phototropic reaction. In order to confirm this reaction of the rhizoids, young plants at this stage $3,S_2$ [7] were cultivated for 42 days. Figure 1 shows that in most plants, stalk growth occurred towards the

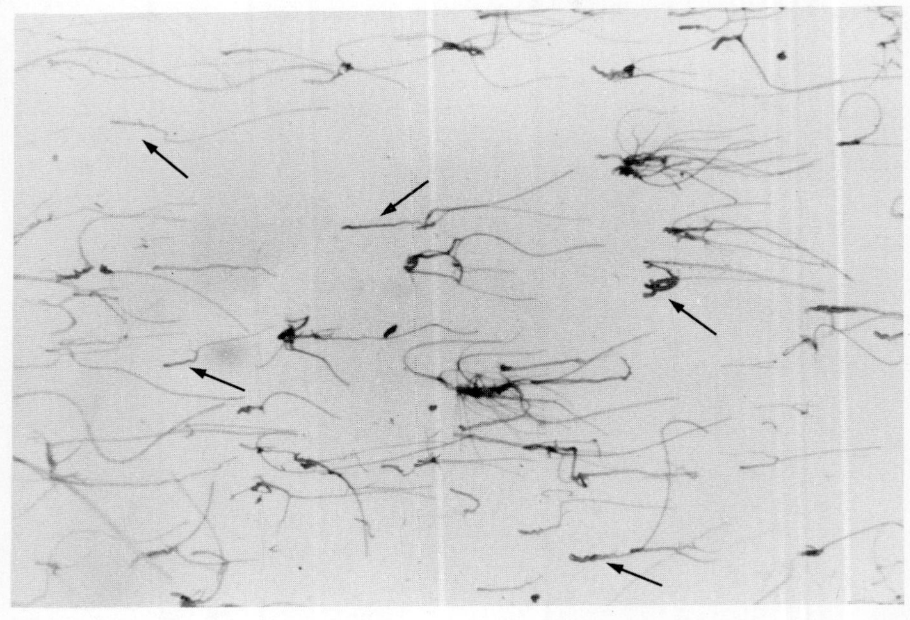

Figure 1. Acetabularia mediterranea. Young plants cultivated for 42 days with light at an angle of 55°; the stalk and the rhizoids show a positive and a negative (arrows) phototropism respectively.

light. On the contrary, the rhizoids grew in the opposite direction (arrows), showing clearly a negative photropism, and they became abnormally long.

Acetabularia crenulata

Young plants at stage 3,S_3 [7] were cultivated for 78 days. The phototropic reaction was more pronounced than in A. mediterranea, practically all the plants having their stalk in a straight line with the light direction (Fig. 2). Figure 3 also shows that in A. crenulata the rhizoids display a negative phototropism (arrows) and that their length increases

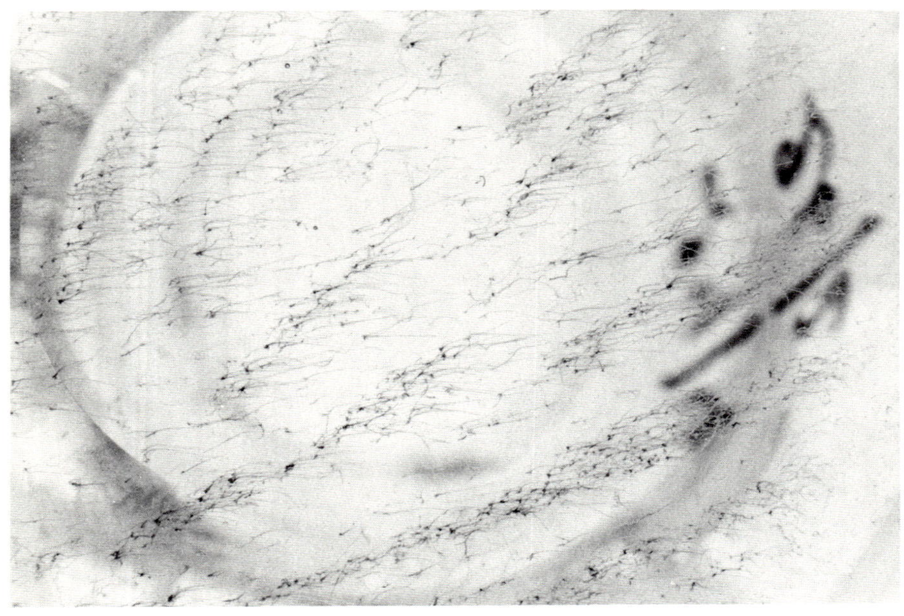

Figure 2. Acetabularia crenulata. Positive phototropism of the stalk.

abnormally. In another culture, zygotes (stage 2) were used. The plants were cultivated for 86 days, when they reached stage 4,S_7,W_1 7. At that time they had the stalk directed towards light (positive phototropism) and the rhizoids oriented in the opposite direction (negative phototropism). The plants were then subjected to a perpendicular illumination (α = 90°) and cultivated for further 25 days. At the end of this period (stage 4,S_{10},W_2) most of the plants had turned towards light, the region of curvature of the stalk being some millimeters above the rhizoids. No apparent changes were observed in the rhizoids. This experiment, schematically represented in Figure 4, shows the capability of A. crenulata of reorienting when the direction of the light changes.

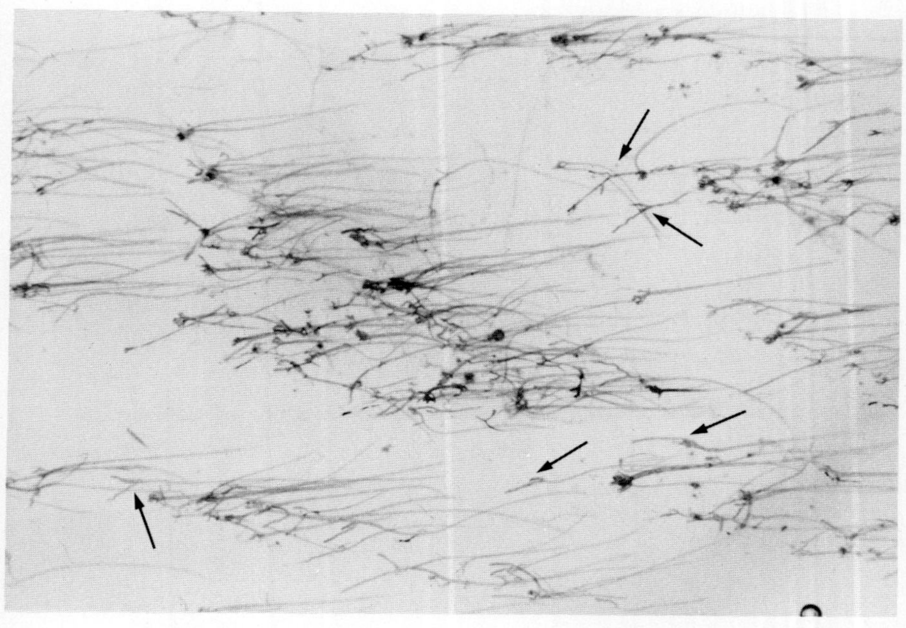

Figure 3. Acetabularia crenulata. Positive phototropism of the stalk. Some clear examples of negative phototropism of the rhizoids are indicated by arrows.

DISCUSSION

The reported results clearly demonstrate that the stalk of A. mediterranea has a positive phototropism. This is in agreement with previous observations[4], but in contrast with the early report of Nasr[2]. Possibly, the stalks of A. mediterranea transplanted by Nasr from the sea to the Zoological Station of Villefranche-sur-Mer were partially calcified and thus unable to show any movement towards light or they were kept in some unsuitable condition, an inadequate light intensity for instance. In our working conditions, the positive phototropism of the growing stalk of A. crenulata was more pronounced than that of A. mediterranea. This

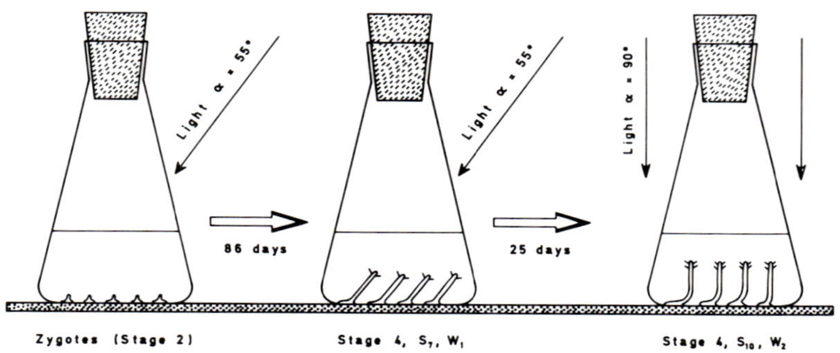

Figure 4. Scheme showing the positive phototropism in Acetabularia crenulata and its capability of reorienting the stalk when light direction changes.

suggests differences between the different Acetabularia species in their phototropic reaction. If we assume that the mechanism responsible for the positive phototropism of Acetabularia is fundamentally similar to that of other algae and of higher plants[9,10,11], the curvature of the stalk should be induced by growth hormones. The concentration of these hypothetical hormones should be higher in the "shaded" side of the stalk with respect to the "lighted" side[9,10].

In both species, the rhizoids grow in direction opposite to the light. At first sight one can ask whether this behavior is due to a negative phototropic reaction (negative phototropism) or to a transverse geotropic reaction (transverse geotropism). In case of a transverse geotropic reaction (as in the brances and leaves of higher plants), the rhizoids should not only grow in the direction opposite to the light, but also in other directions. Moreover, the rhizoids grew longer when the light was at an angle of 55° than under normal illumination (light at 90°). This feature is particularly interesting because it permits a detailed study of morphology and growth of the rhizoids[12]. It is concluded that Acetabularia, like other marine or terrestrial plants, is capable of orienting according to the forces of gravity (geotropism, most evident in nature) and to the light direction (phototropism). Our experimental conditions were suitable for promoting the positive phototropism of the stalk and the negative phototropism of the rhizoids. Under natural conditions, the geotropic reaction is probably the most evident.

ACKNOWLEDGEMENTS

This work was supported in part by the "Fonds de la Recherche Scientifique Fondamentale Collective." We thank Mr. G. Nuyts for his technical assistance, Mr. G. Bas for the photos, Mr. A. Geusens for the graph and Mrs. Jeannine Romeyer-Luyten for typewriting the text. We are indebted to Professor Günther Werz, who kindly provided _Acetabularia crenulata_ plants.

REFERENCES

1. Brachet, J. (1965) Endeavour 24, 155.
2. Nasr, A. H. (1939) Rev. Algol. 11, 347.
3. Feldman, J. (1937) Rev. Algol. 9, 145.
4. Puiseux-Dao, S. (1962) Rev. Gén. Bot. 69-819, 409.
5. Lateur, L. (1963) Rev. Algol. n. s. 1, 26.
6. Lateur, L. and Bonotto, S. (1973) Bull Soc. Roy. Bot. Belgique 106, 17.
7. Bonotto, S. and Kirchmann, R. (1970) Bull. Soc. Roy. Bot. Belgique 103, 255.
8. Vanden Driessche, T. and Bonotto, S. (1969) Biochim. Biophys. Acta 179, 58.
9. Strugger, S. (1962) Biologie I (Botanik), Fischer Bücherei KG, Frankfurt am Main und Hamburg.
10. Muller, W. H. (1977) Botany: A functional Approach, Italian Edition, Piccin Editore, Padova.
11. Seitz, K. (1975) Orientation in space: Plants, Marine Ecology, Otto Kinne Editor, John Wiley & Sons, London, New York, Sidney, Toronto 2, 451.
12. Bonotto, S., Lurquin, P. and Mazza, A. (1976) Adv. Mar. Biol. 14, 123.

ELECTRICAL EVENTS DURING APEX REGENERATION IN *ACETABULARIA MEDITERRANEA*

Friedrich W. Bentrup

Institut für Biologie I der Universität
Tübingen, West Germany

ABSTRACT

Regeneration of a new apex by anucleate posterior stalk segments cut from *Acetabularia mediterranea* is accompanied by the development of a longitudinal bioelectric field and spontaneous action potentials at the site of regeneration, as has been shown previously.

Experimental control of the morphogenetic event via changes of the electric field and the ionic milieu of the segments suggests that the plasmalemma is involved in the initiation of apex regeneration. Evidence is presented, however, that neither of the observed bioelectric signals *per se* is an indispensible link in the initiation process.

INTRODUCTION

Localized cell growth is a common morphogenetic mechanism in plants, particularly lower plants. Examples are the growing tips of fungal hyphae, of algal filamentous thalli and rhizoids, of moss protonemata and pollen tubes. In several cases, transcellular electric fields have been shown to exist, notably in the apical cell of the Cladophoracean *Pithophora*[1], the hyphal tip of *Neurospora*[2], the zygote of the Fucacean *Pelvetia*[3], the anucleate posterior stalk segment of *Acetabularia*[4], and the pollen tube of *Lilium*[5]. In the three algae quoted, the electric field is oriented so that the generated electric current (taken as flow of positive charge) flows acropetally, that is, leaves the cell at the growing apical region in *Pithophora* and *Acetabularia*, and enters the growing region in *Pelvetia* (as well as in *Neurospora* and *Lilium*).

The most plausible origin of such fields which range between 0.01 and 0.1 V/cm, is a transcellular gradient of the membrane potential. To assess a causal relationship between the electrical and the morphogenetic event, we have studied the regeneration of a new apex anlage on anucleate posterior stem segments (PSS) of A. mediterranea first described by Hämmerling[6]. A PSS more or less loses its original cell polarity if kept 5 days in the dark; light then elicits polar growth with 2-3 days. Figure 1 shows both the regenerating

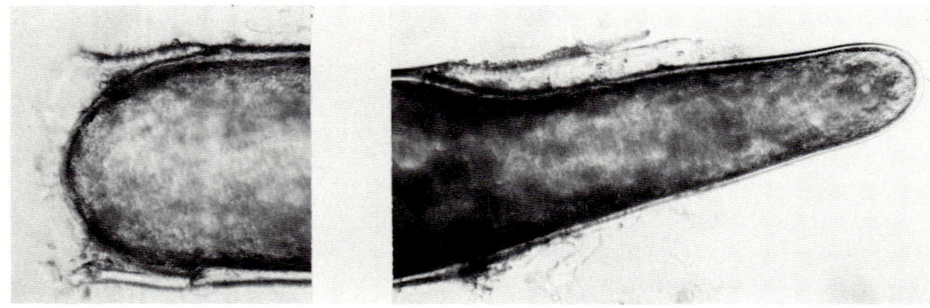

Figure 1. Non-growing basal (left) and regenerating apical end (right) of an anucleate posterior stalk segment (PSS) of Acetabularia mediterranea after 7 days of development. 10 x magnification. From [15].

and the non-growing end of a typical segment of A. mediterranea from our laboratory. The size of the PSS makes it possible to monitor the electrical activity separately at both ends; also any transcellular voltage and current can be controlled by external circuitry. Furthermore, individual ends of a PSS can be easily subjected to different ionic milieus and to known ion concentration gradients. Another point of advantage is that the general electrophysiological properties of the Acetabularia plasmalemma are relatively well understood[7,8].

MATERIAL AND METHODS

12-18 mm long developing PSS of A. mediterranea were mounted across a partition separating two compartments of a plexiglass chamber. For details of all techniques involved see Novák and Bentrup[4]. The medium was TRIS-buffered (pH 8.0) natural seawater with added nitrate, phosphate and soil extract (Erdschreiber). In ion gradient experiments, artificial seawater was used, where the regular K^+ concentration of 10 mM was shifted to 3 and 30 mM, respectively, by replacing KCl with NaCl. The Cl^- concentration was lowered from 550 mM to 30 mM by exchange with sulfate. The segments developed under 10 mW/m^2 of fluorescent white light at 25° C.

RESULTS AND DISCUSSION

Steady transcellular electric fields

About 30 hours after the onset of development the *a priori* variable longitudinal electric field of a PSS attains a steady polarity. The membrane potential at the growing end is about 5-10 mV above its average value of -170 mV[4]; this is indicated by the background level of U_{AC} in Figure 2.

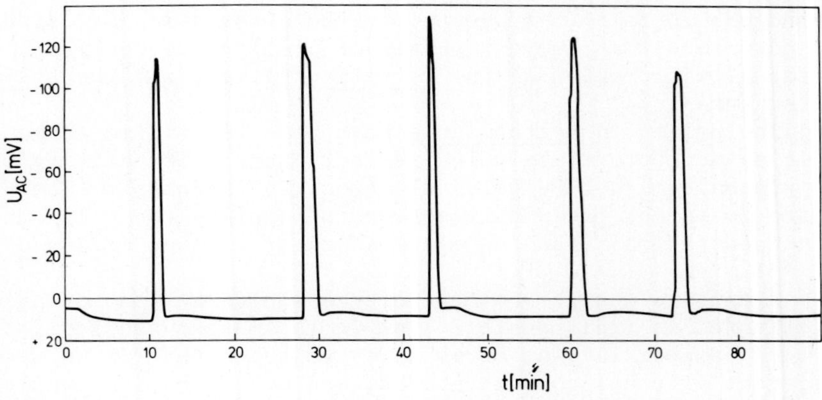

Figure 2. Bioelectric events in regenerating anucleate posterior stalk segments of Acetabularia mediterranea. The extracellularly recorded voltage U_{AC} indicates that the presumptive apex (region A) is steadily hyperpolarized by about 10 mV and periodically depolarizes, i.e. fires action potentials. From [4].

Due to the high electrical resistance between experimentally separated ends of a PSS, the electric current driven by such a field is only about 0.3 nA, that is, 1000 times less than in the control where the PSS is shunted by the surrounding seawater. (In this latter case the field drops almost entirely across the cytoplasm, the current being limited by the cytoplasmic resistivity.) Therefore, initiation and early stages of development of a new apex seems not to depend upon the normal amount of current flow. (Later stages of apex development apparently do[9].) Moreover, PSS subjected to an external control voltage in the culture medium of, say, 10 mV again grow at the end where the membrane potential is increased, although the controlling current _enters_ this region[4]. Obviously, apex initiation can be triggered electrically, but is not unequivocally related to the sign and size of the current passing the membrane at the growing region.

Spontaneous electrical pulses

As early as 8 hours after onset of development the presumptive apex may start to generate trains of some 30-80 spontaneous voltage pulses (or current pulses under voltage-clamp), which are superimposed upon the transcellular electric field and occur at an average frequency of 0.08 min^{-1}. Figure 2 shows a 70 min-period of a representative segment. A morphogenetic role is suggested by the observation of Jaffe and coworkers that current pulses of similar frequency arise at the growing region of the _Pelvetia_ zygote[3], and the _Lilium_ pollen tube[5].

The pulses in _Acetabularia_ have been identified as metabolic action potentials which reflect changes in activity of the plasmalemma's ATP-fueled electrogenic ion pump[8]. The action potential presumably serves to regulate the cellular K^+ concentration[10], and is accompanied by a large efflux of Cl^- [11].

Again, to assess whether this metabolic action potential constitutes an indispensible link in the morphogenetic process of apex initiation we have subjected the PSS to different external concentrations, and concentration gradients, of K^+ and Cl^-. Present results indicate no firm correlation between the site of apex initiation and the action potential. Firstly, in low (30 mM) Cl^- seawater action potentials arise, even simultaneously, at _both_ ends as shown by Figure 3. This particular segment fired 79 action potentials during the recorded period of 18 hours after onset of development; thereof 49 action potentials arose at the presumptive apex, 30 at the basal end.

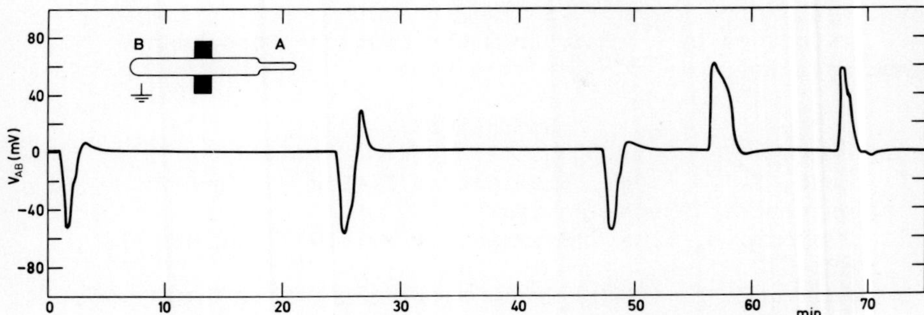

Figure 3. Action potentials from an anucleate posterior stalk segment of Acetabularia mediterranea exposed to seawater of low (30 mM) chloride. The negative-going spikes arise at the regenerating end A, the positive-going spikes at the grounded end B. The graph shows six action potentials fired during a 70 min-period by a segment 11 hours after the onset of development. From [15].

Secondly, in a 3/30 mM K^+ concentration gradient the events are clearly separated: regeneration is preferentially initiated in the low K^+, but the action potentials preferentially arise at the end of the PSS in the high K^+ milieu. A preliminary set of data is given in ref. 12. Unfortunately, the effect of ion gradients upon regeneration is complicated by the existence of a variable residual cell polarity in the PSS of A. mediterranea.

CONCLUSIONS

The experimental analysis of the electrical events accompanying apex initiation in anucleate posterior stalk segments (kernlose Hinterstücke) of A. mediterranea reveals that neither the steady transcellular electric field and the electric current it may drive, nor the metabolic action potential appear to be indispensible elements of the primary morphogenetic process. It seems reasonable to assume that both electrical and morphogenetic events are derived from a common functional pattern developed by the plasmalemma and its immediate vicinity. The external electrical or ionic control of the morphogenetic event indicates a causal chain linking this event to membrane functions.

Hypothetical growth mechanisms producing localized cell wall expansion and synthesis involve electrophoretically moved cytoplasmic vesicles fusing with the membrane at the growing region[13], or localized proton injection from the membrane into the cell wall[14].

Supported by a grant from the Deutsche Forschungsgemeinschaft.

REFERENCES

1. Lund, E. J. (1947) Bioelectric Fields and Growth. Texas University Press, Austin.
2. Slayman, C. L. and Slayman, C. W. (1962) Science 136, 876-877.
3. Jaffe, L. F. (1966) Proc. Natl. Acad. Sci. U.S.A. 56, 1102-1109.
4. Novák, B. and Bentrup, F. W. (1972) Planta (Berl.) 108, 227-244.
5. Weisenseel, M. H., Nuccitelli, R. and Jaffe, L. F. (1975) J. Cell Biol. 66, 556-567.
6. Hämmerling, J. (1934) Biol. Zbl. 54, 650-665.
7. Gradmann, D. (1975) J. Membrane Biol. 25, 183-208.
8. Gradmann, D. (1976) J. Membrane Biol. 29, 23-45.
9. Novák, B. and Sironval, C. (1975) Plant Science Letters 5, 183-188.
10. Mummert, H. and Gradmann, D. (1976) Biochim. Biophys. Acta 443, 443-450.
11. Gradmann, D., Wagner, G. and Gläsel, R. M. (1973) Biochim. Biophys. Acta 323, 151-155.
12. Christ-Adler, M. and Bentrup, F. W. (1976) Planta (Berl.) 129, 91-93.
13. Jaffe, L. F., Robinson, K. R. and Nucitelli, R. (1974) Ann. N. Y. Acad. Sci. 238, 372-389.
14. Bentrup, F. W. (1974) Ber. Deutsch. Bot. Ges. 87, 215-221.
15. Christ-Adler, M. and Bentrup, F. W. unpublished data.

IS THE NUCLEUS INVOLVED IN THE BLUE LIGHT MEDIATED PHOTOMORPHOSES IN *ACETABULARIA MEDITERRANEA*?

R. Schmid and H. Clauss

Institut für Pflanzenphysiologie und Zellbiologie
Freie Universität
Berlin, West Germany

SUMMARY

Nucleate and anucleate cells of *Acetabularia mediterranea* grown in red and blue light have been compared with respect to CO_2 fixation, synthesis and degradation of starch, and the content of soluble sugars. From their identical behavior it has been concluded that the nucleus does not interfere directly with the blue light induced photomorphogenesis. Changes in the morphology, size and nucleic acid content of the nucleus in red light may be due to the diminished metabolic activity of the cells. The content of the "morphogenetic substances" in the cytoplasm increases in red light as shown by enucleation experiments.

INTRODUCTION

The morphogenesis of *Acetabularia* is controlled by light[1]. Normal growth and morphogenesis is maintained only in blue light[2,3,4]. On the other hand under red light conditions the growth rate of *Acetabularia mediterranea* and *Acetabularia crenulata* is strongly reduced. At the same time there are changes in the metabolic activities: in contrast to cells grown either in white or in blue light, in red light the rate of photosynthesis decreases while the starch content per cell rises. When cells are transferred to continuous blue light again, the growth rate and photosynthetic intensity increase and the starch is degraded rapidly.

Since the genetic information for morphogenesis is located in the nucleus[5], but realized in the cytoplasm, the question arises whether or not the nucleus is involved in these blue light dependent events. On the basis of preliminary evidence, Clauss concluded that these events were not under nuclear control[6]. Vettermann, however, considered that the blue light driven morphogenesis in Acetabularia was controlled by the nucleus[7]. Several papers on other organisms have been published[8-11] reporting an increase of RNA synthesis within a few minutes of blue light irradiation and it has been proposed that RNA synthesis is the reason for the intensified protein synthesis in blue light[9].

These contradictory conclusions from Acetabularia and other species made us reexamine in more detail the influence of the nucleus upon some of the blue light dependent reactions in Acetabularia. In these studies, the behavior of the nucleus itself was taken into consideration. Some of our results will be presented here.

MATERIALS AND METHODS

Acetabularia mediterranea was grown under standard conditions[5]. For the experiments, cells of selected stalk length (15-18 mm, 25-30 mm) and cells reduced to a stalk length of 15 mm were used. Cells were enucleated either before or at the end of red light treatment by amputation of the rhizoids which had been ligated previously[1]. Amputation at the end of the irradiation with red light had to be carried out at least two days before the transfer to blue light in order to exclude interference with regeneration processes.

The red and blue light sources have been described previously[12]. In both light regimes, continuous light of equal quantum flux densities was used ($1.85 \cdot 10^{-9}$ Einstein $\cdot$ $cm^{-2} \cdot sec^{-1}$). The temperature was 22 ± 0.5° C.

To measure the rate of photosynthesis the cells were allowed to carry on photosynthesis in white light (15,000 Lux) over a period of 15 minutes in Erd-Schreiber medium, containing 1 µCi and 2 µCi $NaH^{14}CO_3$ per ml, respectively. Subsequently the cells were washed in distilled water and lyophilized.

Cells were fractionated as previously described[13], and counted either in a methane flow counter or in a liquid scintillation counter.

Measurements on the nuclei were carried out after isolation in the medium developed by Berger et al.[14] with the addition of 3.5% formaldehyde. The length and the width of the nuclei were determined directly and volumes calculated assuming rotation ellipsoids[15]. The nuclei were subsequently stained in chrome alum/gallocyanine[16] and embedded in glycerin-jelly. The nucleic acid content was determined cytometrically on a Zeiss scanning microscope photometer.

RESULTS

I. Metabolic activities of nucleate and anucleate cells in red and blue light

Anucleate cells do not differ from nucleate ones in red light as far as morphogenesis is concerned. Their growth rate is reduced and their stalk tip is altered in a manner characteristic of red light treatment[12]. As in nucleate cells, growth and whorl formation can be induced by blue light. While resumption of growth and whorl formation is close to 100% in cells enucleated in red light two days before blue light irradiation, it decreases to only 10-20% if the anucleate cells are held for 17 days in red light. This is in accordance with the fact that anucleate cells cultivated in white light have only a reduced growth capacity after this time.

Parallelling the decrease in growth, the rate of photosynthesis in red light is falling in the same way in nucleate and anucleate cells (Table 1). Upon irradiation with blue light the rate of photosynthesis (rate of CO_2-fixation) increases again (Fig. 1). In anucleate cells, there is a

TABLE 1

Total CO_2-fixation and incorporation of ^{14}C into starch in nucleate and anucleate cells after 20 days in blue or red light

	total fixation		incorporation into starch	
	red light	blue light	red light	blue light
nucleate	1940	11130	87	1530
anucleate	1220	7850	60	1150

Cells of 25-30 mm stalk length were enucleated two days before irradiation with red or blue light. After 20 days in blue light 50% of the nucleate cells and 25% of the anucleate cells had formed caps. There was no cap formation in red light. Data are given in dpm/cell.

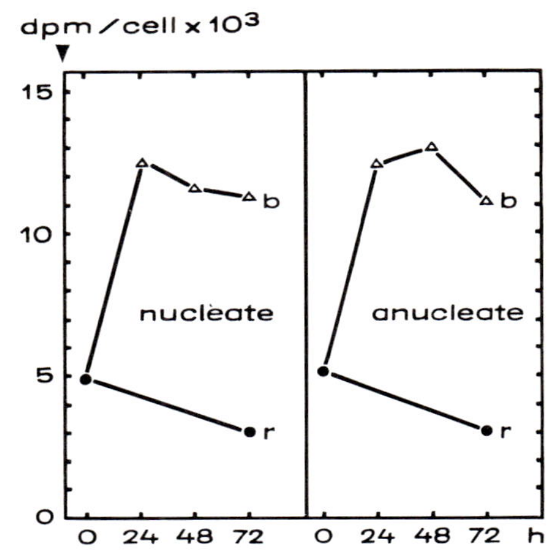

Figure 1. Total $^{14}CO_2$-fixation rates in nucleate and anucleate cells in blue light after 14 days of red light pre-irradiation. Before red light treatment the cells were reduced to 15 mm stalk length. After 12 days in red light they were enucleated and transferred to blue light two days later. Δ—Δ: incorporation rates in blue light (b); ●—●: red light controls (r). Abscissa: time in blue light; ordinate: ^{14}C-carbon fixed during 15 min.

dependency of the rate of fixation on the period after enucleation. In cells enucleated two days before irradiation with blue light the rate of photosynthesis upon induction is almost identical with the rate in nucleate cells, while it is markedly lower in cells enucleated 17 days before blue light irradiation (Fig. 2). In both cases, however, the fixation rate of the blue light induced cells is two to three times higher than in the red light controls.

After 15 minutes of photosynthesis, over 90% of the ^{14}C fixed is found to be in the ethanol-water soluble fraction; this fraction follows the kinetics of total fixation.

It is typical for Acetabularia mediterranea growing in blue light that the soluble sugars (fructose, sucrose and insulin) increase continuously, while the amount of starch grows only slightly during the same interval. In cells irradiated with red light the results are reversed. Here the content of soluble sugars remains constant, while the starch increases manyfold. If blue light is given, again the starch accumulated in red light is rapidly degraded[6,13]. Enucleated cells behave in a similar manner (Fig. 3). There are, however, differences between nucleate and anucleate cells: in anucleate cells the starch content increases again after the second day of blue light. In nucleate and anucleate cells

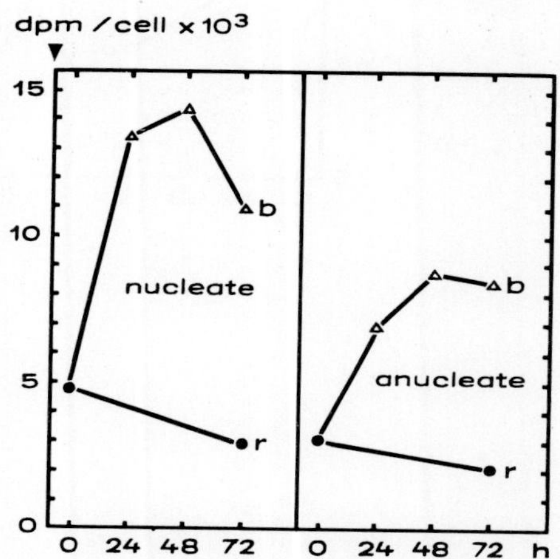

Figure 2. Total $^{14}CO_2$-fixation rates in nucleate and anucleate cells in blue light after 17 days of red light pre-irradiation. Cells of 25-30 mm stalk length were enucleated two days before red light treatment. Δ—Δ: incorporation rates in blue light (b); ●—●: red light controls (r). Abscissa: time in blue light; ordinate: total fixation during 15 minutes.

alike the total amount of soluble sugars increases upon blue light irradiation (Fig. 4)

Coincident with the decrease in the rate of photosynthesis, the rate of starch synthesis (incorporation of ^{14}C) diminishes in red light (Table 1). In contrast to total fixation, the rate of the starch synthesis in blue light increases continuously up to the end of the experiment (Fig. 5). It should be noted that in some of the experiments, the rate of starch synthesis in anucleate cells exceeds that of nucleate ones.

Figure 3. Changes of the starch content in nucleate and anucleate cells in blue light after pre-irradiation with red light. Conditions, see Fig. 2. △—△: starch content in blue light (b); ●—●: red light controls (r). Abscissa: time in blue light; ordinate: µg starch per cell.

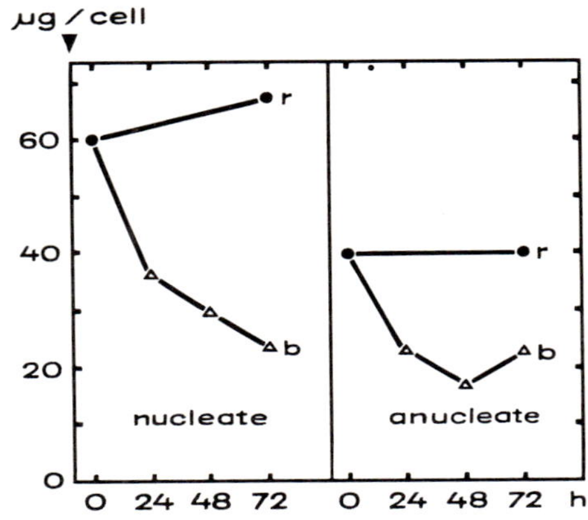

Figure 4. Accumulation of soluble sugars in nucleate and anucleate cells in blue light after pre-irradiation with red light. The cells were reduced to 15 mm stalk length one day before red light irradiation. After 15 days the cells were placed under the blue light. Enucleation was carried out two days before blue light induction. △—△: soluble sugar contents in blue light (b); ●—●: red light controls (r). Abscissa: time in blue light; ordinate: µg fructosans per cell.

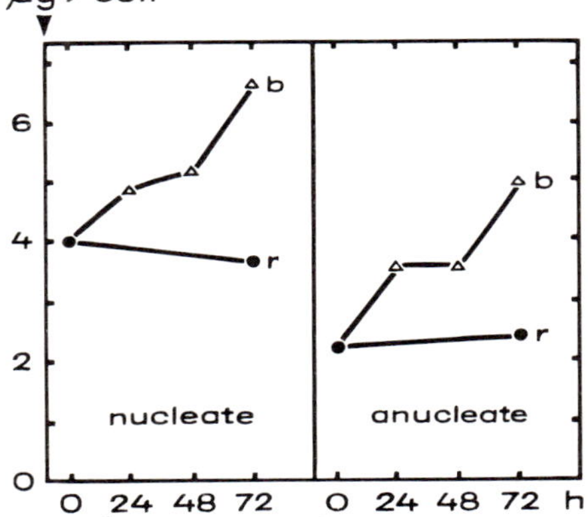

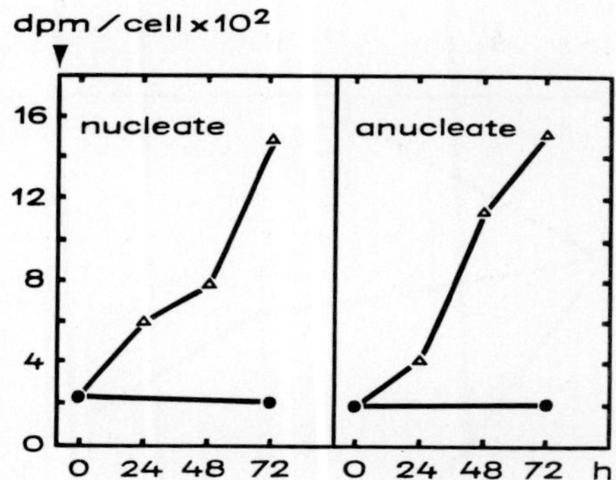

Figure 5. Incorporation of ^{14}C into starch in nucleate and anucleate cells in blue light after pre-irradiation with red light. Conditions, see Fig. 1. Δ—Δ: incorporation rates in blue light (b); ●—●: red light controls (r). Abscissa: time in blue light; ordinate: ^{14}C-carbon fixed into starch over 15 minutes of incorporation.

II. Behaviour of the nucleus in red and blue light

a. Morphology, nuclear volume and nucleic acid content

The nuclei of cells cultivated in blue light resemble those in white light[15,17]. They contain more or less worm-like nucleoli (Fig. 7 A). In contrast to the situation in blue light the nuclei of cells kept in red light alter in a characteristic manner (Fig. 7 B, C). The nucleoli first assume a spherical shape, their outer zone being stained more intensively with gallocyanine as are the worm shaped nucleoli (cf. 7). Later, they form large aggregates with a spongy appearance. At the same time the nuclear volume decreases in red light (Fig. 6). The small nuclei with one compact nucleolus, typical for dark grown cells (Fig. 7 D) can be found only to a very small extent after six weeks in red light.

In predarkened cells (11 days darkness) containing small nuclei the nuclear size increases in blue light as well as in red light. This increase in the nuclear volume is suppressed

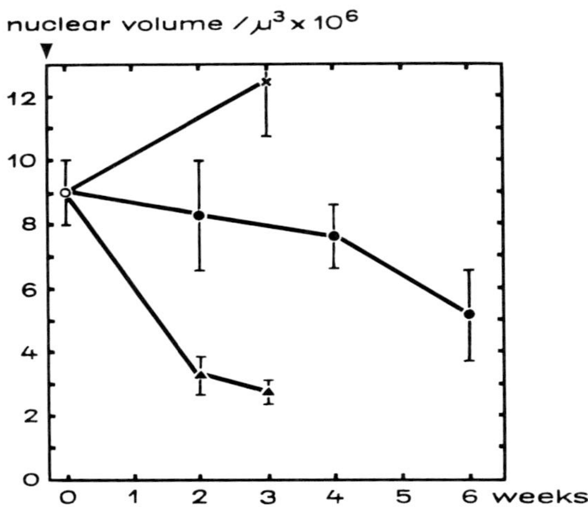

Figure 6. Changes in the nuclear volumes of cells treated with red or blue light or with darkness.

Before the beginning of the experiment the cells were cut down to 5 mm stalk length.

X—X: blue light; ●—●: red light; ▲—▲: darkness. Abscissa: time after onset of the experiment; ordinate: volume of the nuclei.

Figure 7 (opposite page). Appearance of the nuclei under different conditions of irradiation.

A: in blue light
B: after one week of red light
C: after three weeks or red light
D: after two weeks in darkness

in the presence of DCMU (3-(3,4-dichlorphenyl)-1,1-dimethylurea), an inhibitor of photosynthesis (Table 2).

Under all conditions of light quality used (white, blue and red light, and darkness) the nuclear volume is correlated with the nucleic acid content of the nucleus (Fig. 8).

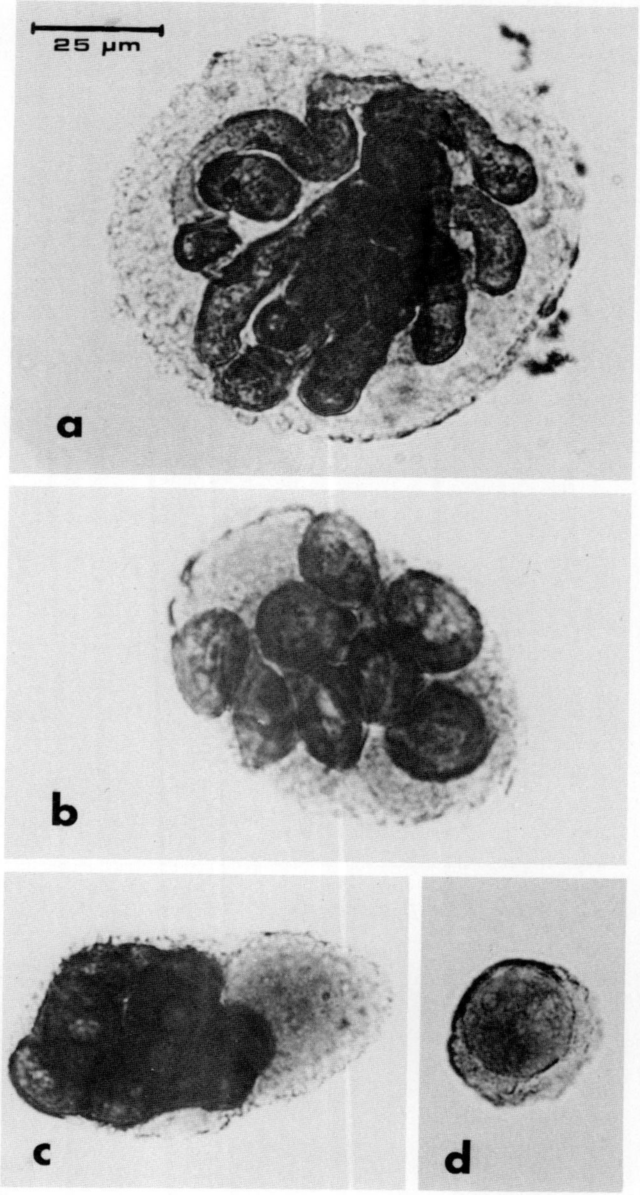

25 μm

a

b

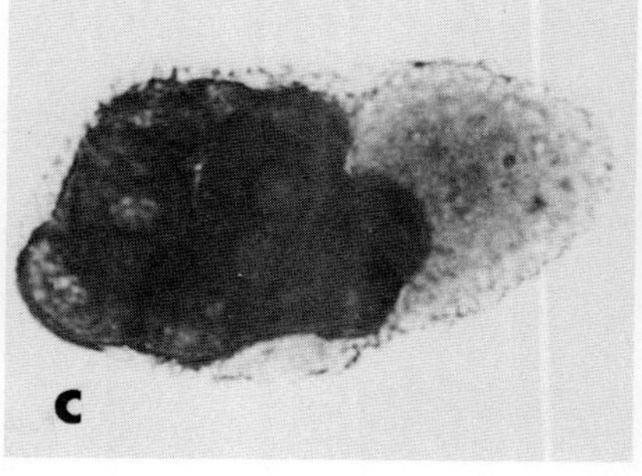

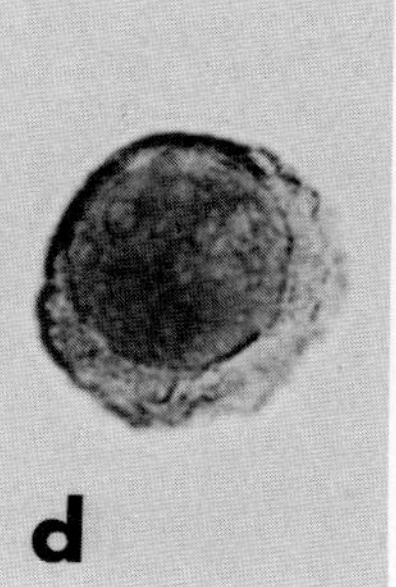

TABLE 2

Effect of DCMU on stalk length, nuclear volume and nucleic acid content of the nucleus in red and blue light after 11 days in darkness

		nucleus	
treatment	stalk length mm	volume $\mu m^3 \cdot 10^6$	nucleic acid content relative
11 days darkness	10.5	4.2±0.6	43 ± 9
+7 days darkness	10.5	3.1±0.7	31 ± 5
+7 days red light	11.9	6.4±1.5	74 ±11
+7 days red light with DCMU	10.7	3.1±0.7	34 ± 5
+7 days blue light	18.1	8.6±0.6	91 ±16
+7 days blue light with DCMU	10.8	4.6±1.7	59 ±14

Cells "shortly before cap formation" were cut down to 10 mm and darkened for 11 days. After the dark period the cells either remained in darkness or were placed for 7 days under red or blue light with or without DCMU (10^{-6} M).

Figure 8. Correlation between the volume and nucleic acid content of the nuclei in relation to blue and red light and darkness. ●: red light; X: blue light; ▲: darkness. Abscissa: nuclear volume; ordinate: relative nucleic acid content of the nuclei.

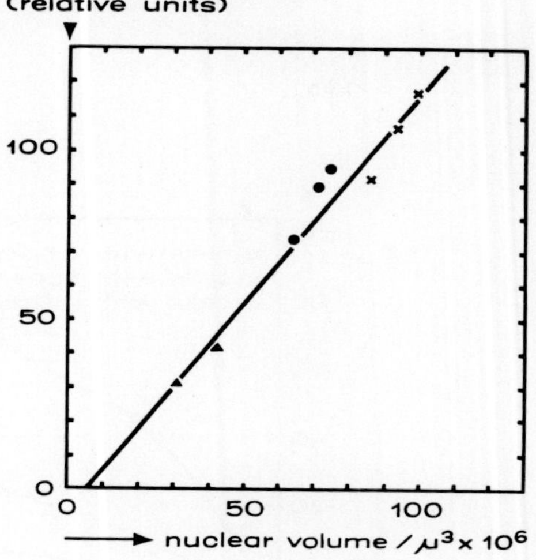

b. Indications for the production of "morphogenetic substances" in red light

In order to get information about the metabolic activity of the nucleus with respect to the production of "morphogenetic substances"[18] under normal red light conditions, we placed nucleate cells cut down to 5 mm stalk length (original stalk length > 30 mm) into red light immediately after cutting. After different times in red light the cells were enucleated and transferred to blue light. 17 days later the cells with whorls, caps, and rhizoids (see Fig. 10) were counted (red light controls did not grow). With increasing time in red light the capability of the anucleate stalks rises (Fig. 9). Similar experiments of Haemmerling and Haemmerling[19] on darkened cells show that the morphogenetic capacity of the stalk increases at first, but later declines.

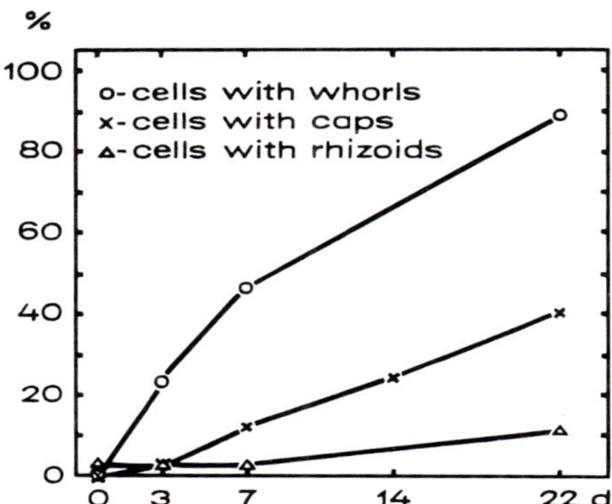

Figure 9. Changes in the morphogenetic capacity within the stalk during irradiation with red light.

Cells of the stage "shortly before cap formation" were reduced to a stalk length of 5 mm and placed under red light immediately. Upon different irradiation times the cells were enucleated by amputation of the rhizoid and the anucleate parts were allowed to grow under blue light. After 17 days each the percentage of cells with whorls (o), caps (X), and rhizoids (Δ) was determined. The percentage of the cells with whorls includes the cells with caps, since the cap formation was always preceeded by whorl formation. An anucleate cell with regenerated rhizoid is shown in Figure 10. Abscissa: time in red light; ordinate: percentage of cells with whorls, caps, and rhizoids after 17 days of blue light.

DISCUSSION

The possibility of inducing the photomorphoses examined, i.e. induction of growth, degradation of accumulated starch, increased starch synthesis, and CO_2-fixation in blue light following red light treatment, even in 17 day old anucleate cells appears to show that nuclear gene activation is not directly involved. Thus the control of these processes in Acetabularia is definitely located in the cytoplasm.

In cases of differences in the behavior of nucleate and anucleate cells, as for instance in starch content and the

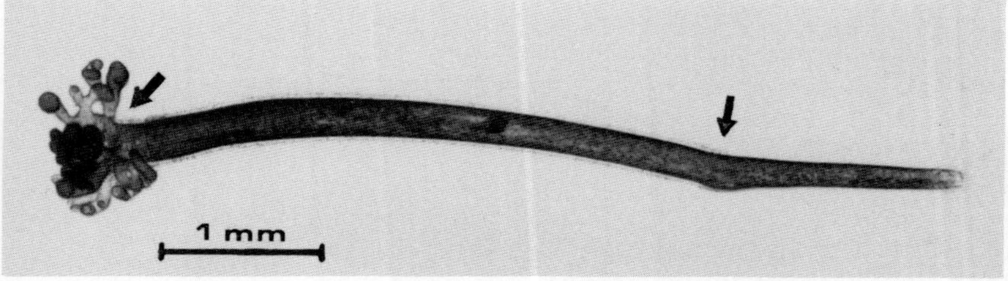

Figure 10. Anucleate cell with regenerated rhizoid.
Note the different thickness of the cell wall of the regenerated parts and the original stalk piece (between arrows).

incorporation into starch after blue light induction, these are most likely due to anucleate conditions (cf. 20) which interfere with the processes induced by blue light.

On the basis of the results presented, including unpublished results, the situation in Acetabularia can be interpreted as follows: Growth processes are induced by blue light (even after total inhibition of photosynthesis by DCMU). The degradation of starch is a consequence of these growth processes (source-sink relation). Whether the increase in the rate of photosynthesis is due to starch degradation or whether additional de novo syntheses of protein are necessary for the activation of the photosynthetic apparatus is not yet known. In any case, the involvement of chloroplast information can be excluded, since rifampicin has no inhibiting effect. On the other hand, the participation of protein synthesis on 80S ribosomes, as indicated by inhibitor experiments (Clauss, unpublished) is essential.

Experiments on Chlorella and Euglena, however, apparently

show a stimulation of the synthesis of rRNA and tRNA within a few minutes after blue light irradiation following red light treatment[9-11]. Schrott and Rau[21] found a blue light driven synthesis of poly-A containing RNA in Fusarium aquaeductuum. These results strongly suggest a participation of transcription of genetic information. The direct involvement of such processes into the blue light induced responses studied in Acetabularia can be excluded as discussed above.

It is difficult at present to evaluate these discrepancies for several reasons. Up to now the blue light absorbing pigment has not been isolated and it is unknown, therefore, whether the pigment involved is identical in all cases. Furthermore, since the primary processes in the blue light mediated responses are not known it is possible that there are different modes of action in the different species or even different responses in the same organism, as discussed for phytochrome action[22].

Changes in the size and the nucleic acid content of the nucleus of Acetabularia under different light regimes and the stimulated RNA accumulation in blue light (Schmid, unpublished) also indicate an influence of light quality on nuclear metabolism. In our present view, however, this seems to be an indirect effect, reflecting a higher metabolic activity of the blue light irradiated Acetabularia cells. This opinion is supported by the fact that the nuclear volume and nucleic acid content after predarkening does not increase in light in the presence of DCMU.

In spite of the reduction of the nuclear volume in red light, the nucleus is still releasing "morphogenetic substances"[18] as may be seen by the increasing morphogenetic capabilities of enucleated stalks derived from nucleate cells kept in red light (Fig. 9). Apparently, the nuclei of cells kept in red light are still producing "morphogenetic substances" even after three weeks under red light conditions (or red light stabilizes the "morphogenetic substances" already present in the cytoplasm) in contrast to cells kept in darkness[19]. This fact clearly shows that the amount of "morphogenetic substances" is not the rate limiting factor for growth processes under red light as suggested by Vettermann[7].

REFERENCES

1. Beth, K. (1953) Z. Naturforsch. 8 b, 334-342.
2. Richter, G. (1962) Naturwiss. 49, 238.
3. Clauss, H. (1963) Naturwiss. 50, 719.
4. Terborgh, J. W. (1965) Nature 207, 1360-1363.
5. Haemmerling, J. (1963) Ann. Rev. Plant Physiol. 14, 65-92.

6. Clauss, H. (1970) in: Biology of Acetabularia (Brachet, J. and Bonotto, S. eds.) Academic Press, 177-191.
7. Vettermann, W. (1973) Protoplasma 76, 261-278.
8. Raghavan, V. (1968) Planta 81, 38-48.
9. Steup, M. (1975) Arch. Microbiol. 105, 134-151.
10. Steup, M. (1975) Plant Physiol. 57 suppl., 118.
11. Cohen, D., Schiff, J. A. (1976) Arch. Biochem. Biophys. 177, 201-216.
12. Clauss, H. (1968) Protoplasma 65, 49-80.
13. Clauss, H. (1972) Protoplasma 74, 357-379.
14. Berger, S., Niemann, R., Schweiger, H.-G. (1975) Protoplasma 85, 115-118.
15. Stich, H. (1951) Z. Naturforsch. 6 b, 319-326.
16. Einarson, L. (1932) Am. J. Pathol. 8, 295.
17. Werz, G. (1962) Planta 57, 636-655.
18. Haemmerling, J. (1934) Roux' Arch. Entwicklungsmech. 131, 1-81.
19. Haemmerling, J. and Haemmerling, Ch. (1959) Planta 52, 516-527.
20. Zetsche, K., Braendle, E. P. O., Streicher, K. (1972) in: Biology and Radiobiology of Anucleate Systems. II. Plant Cells (Bonotto, S., Goutier, R., Kirchmann, R., Maisin, J. R. eds) Academic Press, 239-258.
21. Schrott, E. L., Rau, W. (1977) submitted for publication.
22. Mohr, H. (1972) Lectures on Photomorphogenesis, Springer-Verlag.

<u>ACETABULARIA</u> <u>MEDITERRANEA</u> AS A MODEL FOR STUDIES OF CELLULAR MECHANISMS REGULATING HORMONAL RECEPTIVITY

Bourgeois, P., Baeckelandt, P.,
Henry, P.-E. and Legros, F.

Laboratoire de Physiologie et de Physiopathologie
Université Libre de Bruxelles
Brussels, Belgium

SUMMARY

When *Acetabularia* cells are grown for 7 to 10 days in darkness in plain sea water, the number of insulin receptors increases. Depression of cell receptivity in darkness in the presence of actinomycin D or cycloheximide (10 μg/ml) confirms that synthesis of hormonal receptors is related to nuclear activity and intracellular protein synthesis.

Algae have been cultured in darkness for 10 days in fructose, glucose and o-methyl-glucose at concentrations growing to 100 mg/100 ml.

1. Culture in increasing concentrations of fructose leads to a rapid depression of insulin receptivity. The level of fructosans stored in the chloroplasts remains constant whatever the exogenous fructose concentration. On the contrary, metabolic release of CO_2 increases for cells cultured in growing concentrations of fructose.

2. The level of fructosans increases for glucose concentrations from 0 to 20 mg/100 ml in the culture medium. From 20 to 100 mg/100 ml, the level of fructose reserve material remains constant, although the cell receptivity to insulin keeps on decreasing.

3. O-methyl-glucose is poorly metabolized by *Acetabularia*. When incorporation of this methyl derivative into fructosans reaches a plateau, cell receptivity to insulin stops to decrease. It is concluded that the metabolic activity of the cell induces a signal stimulating nuclear activity and protein synthesis. This influences the binding of insulin to cellular receptors.

INTRODUCTION

It is generally accepted that permeative and metabolic effects of insulin are promoted by binding to the plasma membrane of the target cells[1,2]. Over the last years there has been an increasing body of data suggesting that receptors fluctuate by changing their affinity for the polypeptide hormone or their concentration on target cells[3-6].

The binding of insulin is deeply depressed in purified plasma membranes of fat cells[7], heart muscle[8] and liver[9] from genetically obese mice. When obsese mice are fasted for 24 hours or 40 hours, insulin binding increases by 2 to 3-fold in cardiac muscles and liver membranes[8,10]. These data suggest that cell metabolism may influence hormonal receptivity.

It must be noted that the culture requirements of animal cells restrict the study of the relationship between hormonal receptivity and metabolism at the cellular level. Animal cells must be grown in media containing a well-defined concentration of glucose and other metabolites, in the presence of adult and fetal sera containing insulin. These conditions limit the possibilities of inducing metabolic modifications by introducing variations in the culture medium.

It has been demonstrated that insulin stimulates the oxygen consumption of *Acetabularia mediterranea* grown in darkness[11]. This overall metabolic effect is accompanied by attachment of the hormone to protein receptors at the level of the plasma membrane and of intracellular organites[12]. Binding of insulin to *Acetabularia* plasma membrane increases during culture in darkness, i.e. when the cell utilizes the metabolic substrates synthesized during the autotrophic phase of its life[13]. This increase is not observed for anucleate fragments, suggesting a direct relationship between nuclear activity and the concentration of fixed insulin molecules.

The increase of insulin binding does not occur when *Acetabularia* is cultured in darkness in the presence of glucose or fructose added to sea water[14]. This seems to indicate that exogenous addition of metabolic substrates synthesized in autotrophic conditions inhibits the intracellular mechanisms leading to increased cell fixation of insulin in darkness.

These results indicate the value of *Acetabularia mediterranea* as a cellular model for the study of metabolic influences on cell receptivity. *Acetabularia* presents biological characteristics permitting a more detailed approach to the cellular mechanisms leading to modification of the concentration of insulin receptors. *Acetabularia* is a unicellular organism, grown in sea water, i.e. in a simple and well-defined ionic medium. In autotrophic conditions, no exogenous substrate is needed. In darkness, the cell utilizes the chloroplastic reserve material. This material is made of polymers of fructose called fructosans; other soluble carbohydrates are found such as glucose and saccharose[15]. Utilization of these carbohydrates ensures a survival of several weeks in dark conditions. Addition of various concentrations of hexoses to sea water influences the cell metabolism. Relationships may be established between the metabolic reserve of the cell, addition of hexoses to sea water and variations of cell receptivity to insulin.

The present report aims at determining the origin and nature of the intracellular mechanisms leading to the induction of membrane receptors to an animal hormone, insulin.

MATERIALS AND METHODS

Algae are cultured for 0 to 10 days in darkness in sea water with and without addition of actinomycin D or cycloheximide (10 µg/ml), and fructose, glucose or o-methylglucose at concentrations ranging from 0 to 100 mg/100 ml. During this culture period, _Acetabularia_ cells are transferred every day to new sterile flasks containing the same solution in order to minimize bacterial contamination and to maintain the concentration of hexoses or antibiotics throughout the experiment.

Insulin binding

After different periods of culture in various media, cells are incubated for 20 minutes in 40 ml sea water containing ^{125}I-insulin (^{125}I-iodinated insulin in HCl solution, pH 3; Sorin, specific radioactivity: 3.5 mCi/mg; 85% to 90% of radioactivity is attributed to immunologically active insulin molecules). The concentration of ^{125}I-insulin in the incubation solution is 2.10^{-9}M.

After a 20 minute incubation in solutions containing radioiodinated insulin, cells are removed from the radioactive medium and rinsed for 10 minutes in plain sea water. Previous results indicate that a 20 minute incubation ensures a maximal cell labeling[12].

Radioactivity is measured on 25 cell samples. Counting of radioactivity bound to whole cells is an appropriate index of receptivity, as indicated by previous work[12,13]. Other 25 cell samples are homogenized with a Turmix blender in 1 ml sea water and centrifuged at 70g for 2 minutes[16]. The supernatant is filtered on bolting silk in order to separate fragments of membrane remaining in this fraction. It may be considered that the pellet thus obtained contains cell membranes, while the supernatant is enriched with cytoplasmic material. Crude membrane and cytosol extracts are separated and counted.

In order to compare results obtained with cells incubated in different solutions or with algae of various size and from different genotypic cultures, results are expressed as a ratio between CPM bound to *Acetabularia* and CPM counted in 1 ml of the corresponding radioiodinated medium.

All results are corrected for "non-specific" binding by substracting CPM fixed to *Acetabularia* in the presence of ^{125}I-insulin 2.10^{-9}M and an excess (10^{-6}M) of native non-radioactive insulin.

Measurements of reserve material

Chloroplasts from 10 algae are isolated at 4° C following the method described by Goffeau and Brachet[16]. Cell homogenization is performed with a Turmix blender in 1 ml of mannitol 0.4M, $MgCl_2$ 0.02M, phosphate buffer 0.06M, pH 6.9.

Homogenates are centrifuged at 200g for 1 minute and the membrane-containing pellet is discarded. The supernatant is centrifuged at 1000g for 5 minutes.

The green pellet is resuspended in 1 ml buffer medium. This suspension is centrifuged two additional times at 1000g for 5 minutes.

The reserve material of *Acetabularia* has been isolated following the method described by Vanden Driessche and Bonotto[17,18]. 1 ml of absolute ethanol at 4° C is added to the chloroplastic pellet. The precipitate thus obtained is washed several times with absolute ethanol by centrifugation at 1000g for 5 minutes. When the pellet is absolutely white, alcohol is evaporated by vacuum dessication for 15 hours.

The reagent used for fructose measurement is a solution of 150 mg resorcinol in 100 ml concentrated HCl. 9 ml of this solution are diluted in 100 ml of concentrated HCl. 2 ml of this reactive mixture are added to the *Acetabularia* reserve pellet in the presence of 1 ml acetic acid. After boiling at 90° C for 5 minutes, the fructose reserve material is rapidly measured spectrophotometrically at 485 nm.

Studies of the metabolization of exogenous fructose

25 algae are incubated at 20° C for 4 hours in 3 ml sea water containing fructose 1 mg/100 ml and 50 µCi/ml D-U-^{14}C fructose. Liberated $^{14}CO_2$ is trapped in 0.4 ml Hyamine phosphate (Packard) for 10 minutes and radioactivity is counted in 15 ml Instagel (Packard). Reserve material is isolated as indicated above. The white pellet is diluted in 1 ml distilled water and radioactivity is measured in 15 ml Instagel. Results are expressed as nM of fructose

metabolically used as $^{14}CO_2$ and as nM of fructose stored by 1 g of algae during 1 hour.

RESULTS

1. Effect of actinomycin D and cycloheximide on cell receptivity to insulin

Cycloheximide (10 µg/ml) has been added to Acetabularia cells during 7 days of culture in darkness. Table 1 indicates a significant decrease of insulin binding to whole cells

TABLE 1

Fraction	Actinomycin D	Cycloheximide
Whole cells	37.2%	28.3%
Membrane extracts	20 %	31.9%
Cytosol fraction	51.2%	15.4%

Percent of inhibition of ^{125}I-insulin binding to whole cells, crude membrane extracts and cytosol fraction after a 7 day dark incubation in actinomycin D or cycloheximide (10 ug/ml).

and specifically to their plasma membrane.

The same treatment with actinomycin D (10 µg/ml) sharply depresses total insulin fixation to samples of 25 cells, binding to plasma membranes as well as cytoplasmic incorporation of the hormone.

It is known that at the concentration of 10 µg/ml, actinomycin inhibits ribonucleic acid synthesis in Acetabularia mediterranea. The main effect of actinomycin is a reduction of ribosome and mRNA formation, alteration of nuclear morphology and a loss of nuclear enzymatic activity[15]. Cycloheximide sharply inhibits protein synthesis of Acetabularia[19]. The inhibitory action of both actinomycin D and cycloheximide on cell receptivity to insulin agrees with observations of Legros et al[13] showing the absence of increased receptivity in anucleate fragments incubated in darkness.

2. Measurements of fructosan reserve material

Fructosan reserve material of 10 algae was measured for 0 to 13 days of culture in darkness. Figure 1 indicates a rapid fall of fructosans stored in the chloroplasts during the first five days of dark culture.

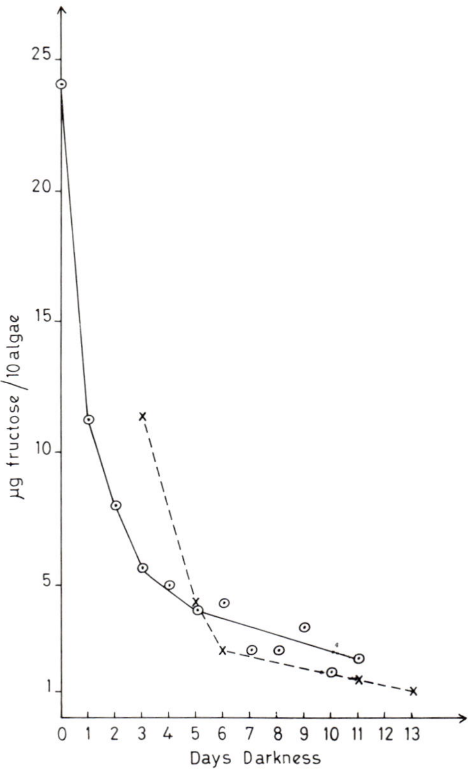

Figure 1. Fructose reserve material measured during incubation in darkness in two different cultures of Acetabularia mediterranea

It is observed (Fig. 2) that daily consumption of fructose is very important during the fifth to eighth first days of dark growing. For longer periods of dark incubation, the metabolic use of fructosans remains very weak.

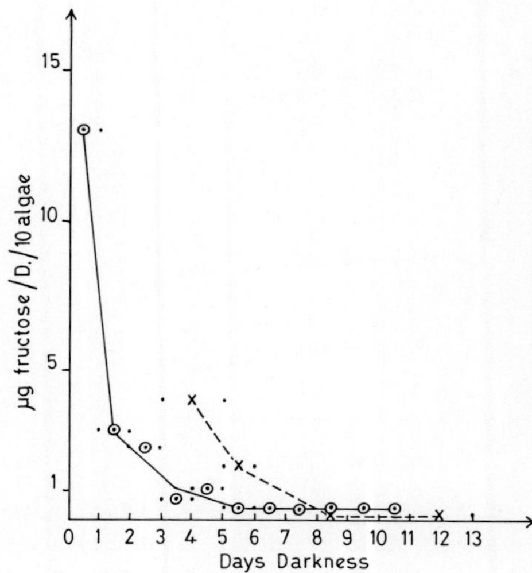

Figure 2. Daily consumption of fructose in two different cultures of Acetabularia. Ordinate: ug of fructose utilized by 10 algae during 1 day. Abcissa: days of culture in darkness.

3. Effect of incubation in fructose on insulin receptivity and on the level of reserve material

Acetabularia cells are cultured in darkness in the presence of fructose concentrations ranging from 0 to 100 mg/100 ml. After 10 days, fixation of ^{125}I-insulin 2.10^{-9}M is measured. The level of fructosan stored in the chloroplasts remains constant at all concentrations of fructose added, as indicated in Figure 3.

It is shown (Fig. 3) that insulin binding to 25 cells increases when algae are grown in sea water for 10 days in darkness, as compared to cell receptivity of Acetabularia grown in 12 hours light/12 hours dark conditions. This confirms previous observations of Legros et al[13].

When fructose is added to sea water, cell receptivity

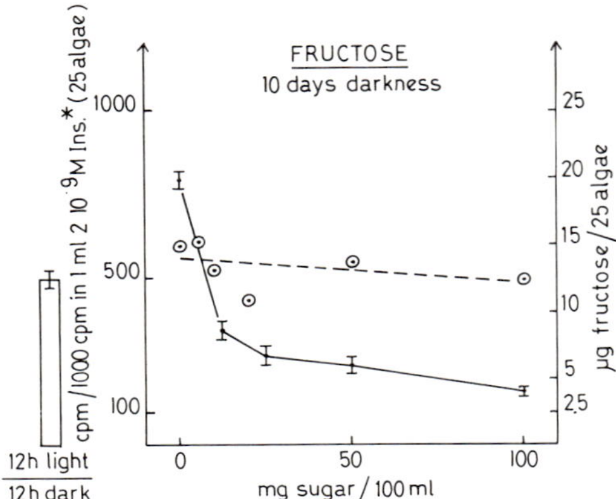

Figure 3. Receptivity to insulin (•——•——•) and level of stored fructosans (⊙---⊙---⊙) measured in 4 cm long cells incubated for 10 days in darkness in the presence of fructose concentrations ranging from 0 to 100 mg/100 ml. Receptivity is expressed as CPM "specifically" bound to 25 cells per 1000 CPM counted in 1 ml of $2x10^{-9}M$ radioiodinated insulin diluted in the incubation medium (n=8). Incubation time is 20 minutes. Fructose stored in the chloroplastic reserve material is expressed as ug/25 algae (n=4). Column on the left represents fixation of insulin to 25 cells of the same culture grown under 12 hour light/12 hour dark conditions (n=8).

decreases and, the values being even lower than the insulin binding capacity of algae grown in 12 hour light/12 hour dark conditions. Decrease of cell receptivity is particularly important at concentrations ranging from 0 to 12.5 mg/100 ml. The level of insulin binding decreases more slowly for fructose concentration from 12.5 mg/100 ml to 100 mg/100 ml.

Figure 4 indicates that the decrease of insulin binding to Acetabularia cells occurs for short periods of incubation in fructose. When cells are grown in fructose at concentration of 100 mg/100 ml, decrease of insulin binding is significant after 2 days.

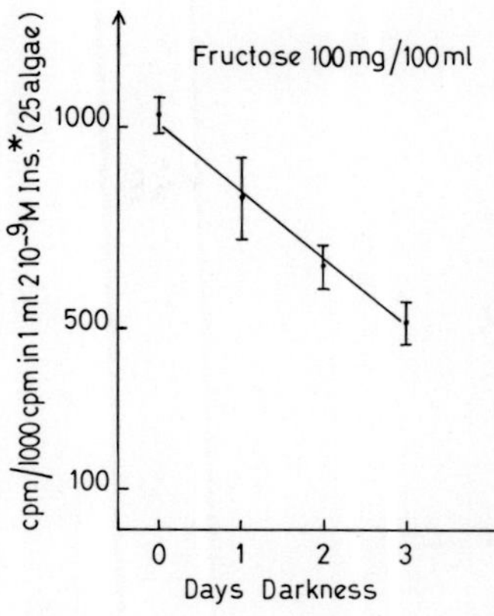

Figure 4. Decrease of insulin binding to 25 algae (4 cm long) grown for 0 to 3 days in darkness in the presence of fructose 100 mg/100 ml. Incubation time in ^{125}I-insulin is 20 minutes (n=8).

4. Metabolization of fructose after 10 days in darkness

Acetabularia cells are cultured for 10 days in darkness in the absence and in the presence of fructose at concentrations of 10 mg/100 ml and 100 mg/100 ml. They are incubated for 4 hours in sea water containing 1 mg/100 ml fructose and 50 mμCi/ml D-U-^{14}C fructose.

Figure 5 (overleaf). Metabolic utilization of ^{14}C-fructose by 25 algae (4 cm long). Cells are cultured in darkness in fructose concentrations of 0, 10 and 100 mg/100 ml. After 10 days, they are incubated for 4 hours in fructose 1 mg/100 ml and 50 muCi/ml ^{14}C-fructose. Radioactivity of the reserve fructosans is measured and results are expressed as uM of fructose incorporated into the chloroplastic reserves of 1 g algae during 1 hour (___.___.___.___). The quantity of fructose metabolically used as $^{14}CO_2$ is given as 1 g of cells and 1 hour incubation (--------) (n=4).

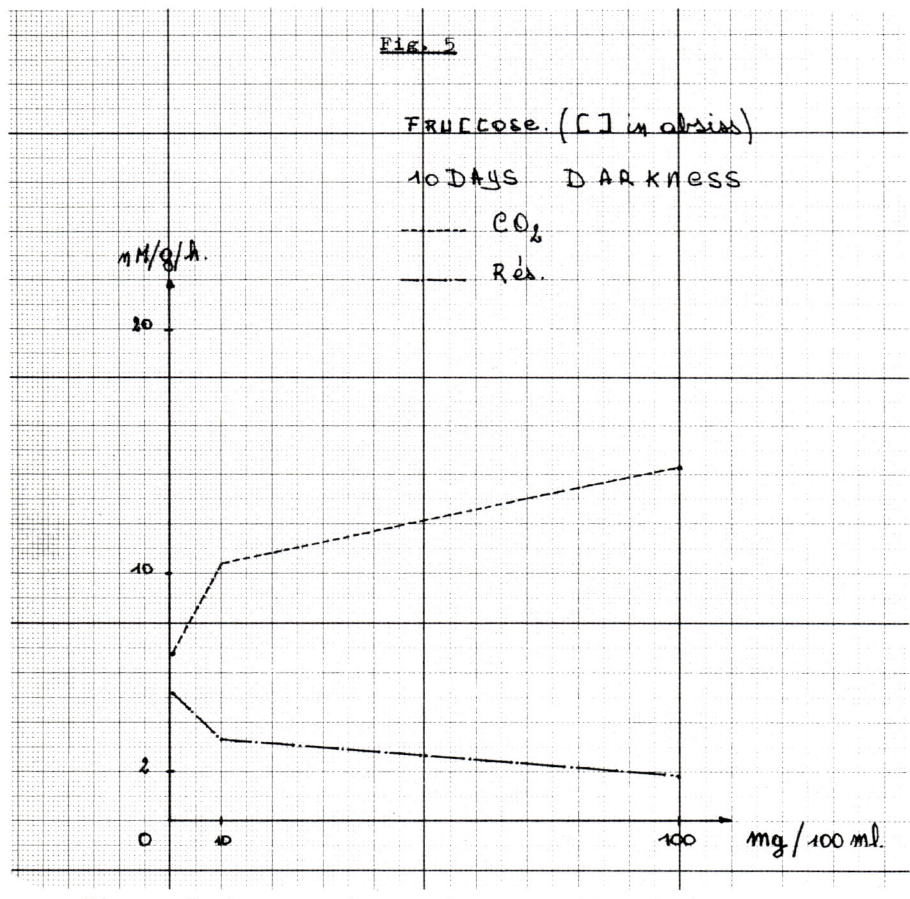

Figure 5 shows an increasing capacity of the algae to metabolize fructose into $^{14}CO_2$ when they are previously grown in increasing concentrations of the hexose. On the contrary, the incorporation of ^{14}C-fructose into chloroplastic fructosans decreases in the same experimental conditions in the presence of growing concentrations of fructose.

The storage of fructose after 10 days of dark culture in plain sea water may be considered as the maximal value of hexose incorporation into chloroplastic fructosans. A 10 day incubation in fructose 10 mg/100 ml is sufficient to reduce carbohydrate incorporation into chloroplastic reserve material.

5. Effect of glucose on insulin receptivity and on the level of the reserve material

The same culture conditions as those described for fructose have been applied in the presence of glucose concentrations ranging from 0 to 100 mg/100 ml.

A 10 day addition of glucose in concentrations increasing from 0 to 20 mg/100 ml promotes a rise in fructose stored in the chloroplasts. For concentrations of 20 to 100 mg/100 ml, the level of fructose reserve material remains constant (Fig. 6). It may be supposed that the enzymatic equipment involved in incorporation of glucose into chloroplastic fructosans is saturated for an exogenous concentration of glucose of about 20 mg/100 ml.

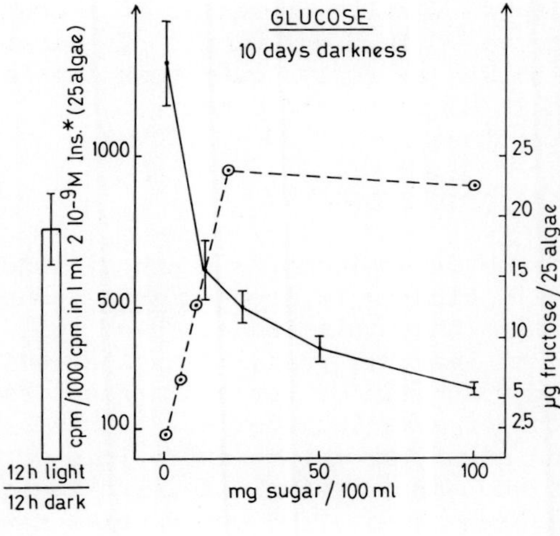

Figure 6. Insulin receptivity (——·——·——) and level of stored fructosans (⊙---⊙---⊙) measured in 2 cm long cells incubated for 10 days in darkness in the presence of glucose concentrations growing from 0 to 100 mg/100 ml. Receptivity is expressed as CPM "specifically" bound to 25 cells per 1000 CPM counted in 1 ml of ^{125}I-insulin $2.10^{-9}M$. Labeling time is 20 minutes (n=8). Fructose stored in the chloroplasts is expressed as ug/25 algae (n=4). Column on the left represents binding of insulin to 25 cells of the same culture grown in 12 hour light/12 hour dark conditions (n=8).

Figure 6 also indicates a continuous decrease of insulin receptivity of cells incubated in growing concentrations of glucose. For an exogenous glucose concentration of 12.5 mg/100 ml, insulin receptivity is inferior to hormonal binding measured for algae cultured in 12 hours light/12 hours dark conditions.

6. Effect of o-methyl-glucose on insulin receptivity and on the level of the reserve material

Acetabularia cells are grown for 10 days in concentrations of o-methyl-glucose varying from 0 to 100 mg/100 ml.

Figure 7 shows that the capacity of the cells to incorporate o-methyl-glucose into chloroplastic fructosans is rather limited. This incorporation reaches a plateau for an o-methyl-glucose concentration of 10 mg/100 ml. The level of reserve material increase is significantly less important than the values recorded for glucose. Animal cells are unable to metabolize o-methyl-glucose, although insulin stimulates its transport into the cytoplasm. When comparing incorporation of increasing concentrations of glucose and its methyl derivative into chloroplastic fructosans, it clearly appears that conversion of o-methyl-glucose into fructose is much more limited than it is in the case for glucose.

The cell receptivity to insulin decreases at a concentration of o-methyl-glucose of 12.5 mg/100 ml. It remains relatively constant, although slightly lower than levels recorded for culture in 12 hours light/12 hours dark conditions, for concentrations up to 100 mg/100 ml.

DISCUSSION

The inhibitory effects of actinomycin D and cycloheximide on the increase of insulin binding to *Acetabularia* induced by culture in darkness confirm that this induction of cell receptivity is related, at least in part, to nuclear activity. It may be concluded that synthesis of hormonal receptors starts from a stimulation of genetic material.

The question arises about the nature and origin of the signal stimulating this nuclear activity. A first indication may be found in the measurements of fructose reserve material during increasing periods of incubation in darkness. Previous results of Legros et al[13] have demonstrated a net increase of insulin binding to the plasma membrane after dark culture periods ranging from 7 to 10 days. At that time, the fructosans have undergone their rapid and quantitatively important decrease. It is observed that when the level of stored fructosans strongly decreases and daily variations become insignificant, insulin binding to the cells is increasing.

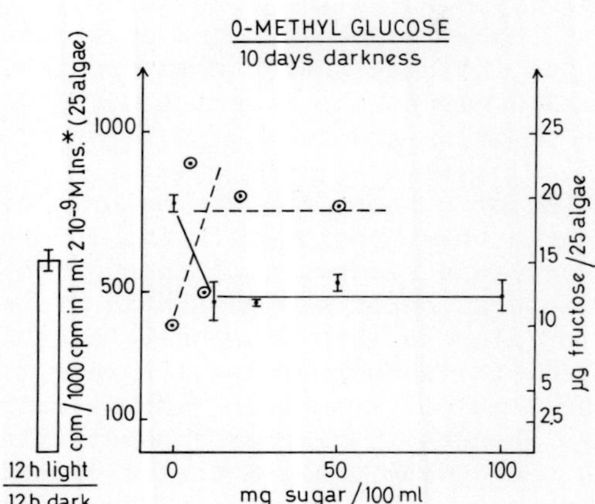

Figure 7. Receptivity to insulin (·——·——·) and level of stored fructosans (⊙---⊙---⊙) measured in 3.5 long cells incubated for 10 days in darkness in the presence of o-methyl-glucose increasing from 0 to 100 mg/100 ml. Receptivity is expressed as CPM specifically bound to 25 cells per 1000 CPM counted in 1 ml of radioiodinated insulin 2.10^{-9}M. Labeling time is 20 minutes (n=8). Fructose stored in the chloroplastic reserves is expressed as ug/25 algae (n=4). Column represents fixation of insulin to 25 cells of the same culture grown in 12 hour light/12 hour dark conditions (n=8).

Two hypotheses may be made from these experimental results. Firstly, a drop in stored fructosans in 24 hours dark conditions (comparable in the alga to heterotrophic fasting), promotes an intracellular signal which stimulates genetic activity coding for insulin receptors synthesis.

Secondly, fructosan utilization in the metabolism of Acetabularia diminishes during culture in darkness. This induces a signal which stimulates nuclear activity.

Variation of cell receptivity to insulin in the presence of fructose and the metabolization of this hexose show that fructose incorporation into stored fructosans remains constant for carbohydrate concentrations of 1 to 100 mg/100 ml. A 4 hour incubation in ^{14}C fructose of cells grown for 10 days in increasing concentrations of non radioactive hexose confirms this constant incorporation into reserve material. On the other hand, fructose metabolization, measured by $^{14}CO_2$ release, becomes more important when fructose concentration in the 10 day dark incubation medium increases. In the same conditions, the number of insulin receptors decrease for fructose concentrations varying from 0 to 100 mg/100 ml. The hormonal receptivity even falls below values recorded for algae grown in 12 hours light/12 hours dark conditions.

These results indicate that the metabolic capacity of reserve utilization may be the signal leading to the stimulation of nuclear activity and to the increase of cell receptivity.

Incorporation of glucose and its methyl derivative into fructosans supports this hypothesis. The incorporation of glucose into fructosans reaches a plateau which presumably corresponds to saturation of the enzymatic system ensuring transformation of glucose into fructose. When this system becomes saturated, the number of insulin receptors is still decreasing. The level of fructosan reserve material being constant despite changes in glucose concentration (from 20 to 100 mg/100 ml), these data confirm that a dynamic, metabolic signal, rather than a static one, i.e. the level of the reserve, induces the insulin receptivity.

O-methyl-glucose is known to be non-metabolizable by animal cells. In Acetabularia, its incorporation into reserve fructosans is limited. Recent unpublished data indicate that its utilization (measured by $^{14}CO_2$ release from ^{14}C-o-methyl glucose) is very weak, when compared to glucose or fructose. It is shown that the decrease of insulin receptivity is blocked at o-methyl-glucose concentrations corresponding to the maximal incorporation of this metabolite derivative into fructosans.

All these data strongly suggest that the metabolic consumption of reserve material leads to a signal inducing nuclear activity and increase of cell receptors to insulin.

Experimental studies presented in this report provide a contribution to discussions concerning variations in cell sensitivity to insulin. Two hypotheses exist. The first one suggests that impairment of hexose assimilation must be related to a decreased affinity and/or receptivity of hormonal receptors[20]. It has also been assumed that this impairment is related to a defect of intracellular enzymatic systems[21].

The relationship between Acetabularia receptivity to insulin and metabolic activity of this unicellular organism grown in darkness indicates that these two hypotheses might not be mutually exclusive. The data presented here indicate that intracellular signals would relate general enzymatic activity and/or precise enzymatic capability corresponding to particular steps of metabolism to synthesis of protein receptors for insulin.

ACKNOWLEDGEMENTS

We express our gratitude to Professor J. Brachet who allowed us to use cells from the *Acetabularia* culture of his laboratory.

This work has been supported by a grant from the "Fonds de la Recherche Scientifique Médicale" (Contract 3.455.75).

REFERENCES

1. Cuatrecasas, P. (1969) Proc. Nat. Acad. Sci. USA 63, 450-457.
2. Freychet, P., Roth, J. and Neville, D. M. Jr. (1971) Proc. Nat. Acad. Sci. USA 68, 1833-1837.
3. Kahn, C. R. (1975) in Methods in Membrane Biology (Korn, E. D., ed), pp 81-146, Plenum Press, New York and London.
4. Freychet, P. (1975) Diabète et Métabolisme 1, 57-68.
5. Livingston, J. N., Cuatrecasas, P. and Lockwood, D. H. (1974) J. Lipid Res. 15, 26-32.
6. Olefsky, J. M. and Reaven, G. M. (1974) J. Clin. Invest. 54, 1323-1328.
7. Freychet, P., Laudat, M. H., Rosselin, G., Kahn, C. R., Gorden, P. and Roth, J. (1972) FEBS letters 25, 339-342.
8. Forgue, M. E. and Freychet, P. (1975) Diabetes 24, 715-723.
9. Kahn, C. R., Neville Jr., D. M., Gorden, P., Freychet, P. and Roth, J. (1972) Biochem. Biophys. Res. Commun. 48, 135-142.
10. Soll, A. H., Kahn, C. R. and Neville Jr., D. M. (1975) J. Biol. Chem. 250, 4702-4707.
11. Legros, F. and Conard, V. (1973) Hormone Res. 4, 107-113.
12. Legros, F., Uytdenhoef, P., Dumont, I., Hanson, B., Jeanmart, J., Massant, B. and Conard, V. (1975) Protoplasma 86, 119-134.
13. Legros, F., Hanson, B., Dumont, I., Jeanmart, J. and Conard, V. (1975) in Molecular Biology of Nucleocytoplasmic Relationships (Puiseux-Dao, S., ed), pp 299-304, Elsevier Scientific Publishing Company.
14. Bourgeois, P., Baeckelandt, P., Legros, F. and Conard, V. (1975) Arch. Internat. Physiol. Bioch. 83, 619-623.
15. Puiseux-Dao, S. (1975) Acetabularia and Cell Biology, Logos Press Ltd.
16. Goffeau, A. and Brachet, J. (1965) Biochim. Biophys. Acta 95, 302-313.

17. Vanden Driessche, T. and Bonotto, S. (1968) Arch. Internat. Physiol. Bioch. 76, 205-206.
18. Vanden Driessche, T. (1972) in Radiobiology of Anucleate Systems. II. Plant Cells (Bonotto, S., ed), pp 53-73, Academic Press, New York.
19. Brachet, J. (1973) De l'Embryologie Expérimentale à la Biologie Moléculaire (Wolff, E., ed) Dunod, Paris.
20. Freychet, P. (1976) Diabetologia 12, 83-100.
21. Czech, M. (1976) J. Clin. Invest. 57, 1523-1532.

THE PRESENCE OF AN AUXIN-LIKE SUBSTANCE IN *ACETABULARIA* AND ITS RELATION TO GROWTH AND MORPHOGENESIS

Thérèse Vanden Driessche and Viviane Delegher

Laboratoire de Cytologie et d'Embryologie Moléculaires
and
Laboratoire de Physiologie Végétale
Université Libre de Bruxelles
Brussels, Belgium

SUMMARY

The presence of an auxin-like substance is demonstrated in *Acetabularia mediterranea*. The methanol extract of the algae was chromatographed on paper using an isopropanol; ammonium hydroxide; water solvent. The chromatogram was divided in 20 bands which were assayed for activity. One particular band is characterized as follows:

1. It has a Rf of 0.35-0.40, which is close to that of reference indolacetic acid (IAA) when chromatograms are run in parallel and identical with it when the extract is co-chromatographed.
2. It has a biological activity comparable to that of reference IAA as estimated by the *Arena* coleoptile assay[1].
3. It fluoresces in UV light on chromatograms and the fluorescence spectra in methanol and ethanol are similar to that of reference IAA.

This auxin-like substance binds to membranes (as ascertained by biochemical methods and by autoradiography); this binding is inhibited by puromycin but not by actinomycin D.

We propose that this auxin-like substance has a biological significance: binding of exogenous IAA is hindered by morphactins, which are specific inhibitors of IAA intracellular movement and which, in *Acetabularia*, interfere with growth and morphogenesis. This inhibition of IAA binding has been determined both biochemically and by autoradiography.

INTRODUCTION

The regulation of morphogenesis in algae and more specifically in unicellular algae has been much investigated with respect to the role of nucleic acids and protein synthesis[2-11] but the control by plant growth substances has been subjected to only a few investigations.

The effects of exogenous IAA and NAA (naphtaleneacetic acid) on the morphogenesis of _Acetabularia_ have been examined by Dao[12] and Thimann and Beth[13] who have shown that IAA promotes elongation of the stalk (at 10^{-5} and 10^{-6} M) and increases the rate of cap formation and the final number of caps in a population (IAA 10^{-4} and NAA 10^{-5} M).

However, the metabolic state of the algae (i.e. as influenced by the season when the algae are taken from nature) and the quality of the medium influence the response[11,13,14]. The latter observation is consistent with the recent findings on the effects of nutrients on development and morphogenesis in plants[15-19], although it has been previously used as an argument against the existence of IAA in _Acetabularia_.

NAA acts in a very similar way as IAA[13]. Both hormones are more effective at higher concentrations in accelerating cap formation rather than stimulating elongation. Their effects are antagonized by 2,3,5-triiodobenzoic acid.

The auxins promote growth and cap formation in both whole and anucleate algae. However, as Thimann and Beth[13] have demonstrated, the isolated rhizoid behaves differently from the stalk, being inhibited rather than stimulated by auxins. From the irregular and limited effects of plant hormones on _Acetabularia_, (notably the dependence on the quality of the medium) and from the lag required in order to obtain visible effects, Puiseux-Dao[11] concluded that IAA is not likely to play a role in growth and differentiation in _Acetabularia_.

Tandler[20,21] has reported the presence of indole-containing compounds in _Acetabularia_. He stated that the compounds were not free in the cell but either bound or in crystalline form. These crystals are regularly seen in electron micrographs of _Acetabularia_ (Fig. 1), and are thought to be a complex of indol and proteins. It seemed desirable to ascertain whether or not auxins are actually present in _Acetabularia_.

In order to ascertain the physiological significance of this substance in _Acetabualaria_, the binding of labelled IAA has been examined both by biochemical analysis and by autoradiography in control and morphactins-treated algae. Morphactins, specific inhibitors of IAA intracellular movement, are known to interfere with growth and development of _Acetabularia_[22].

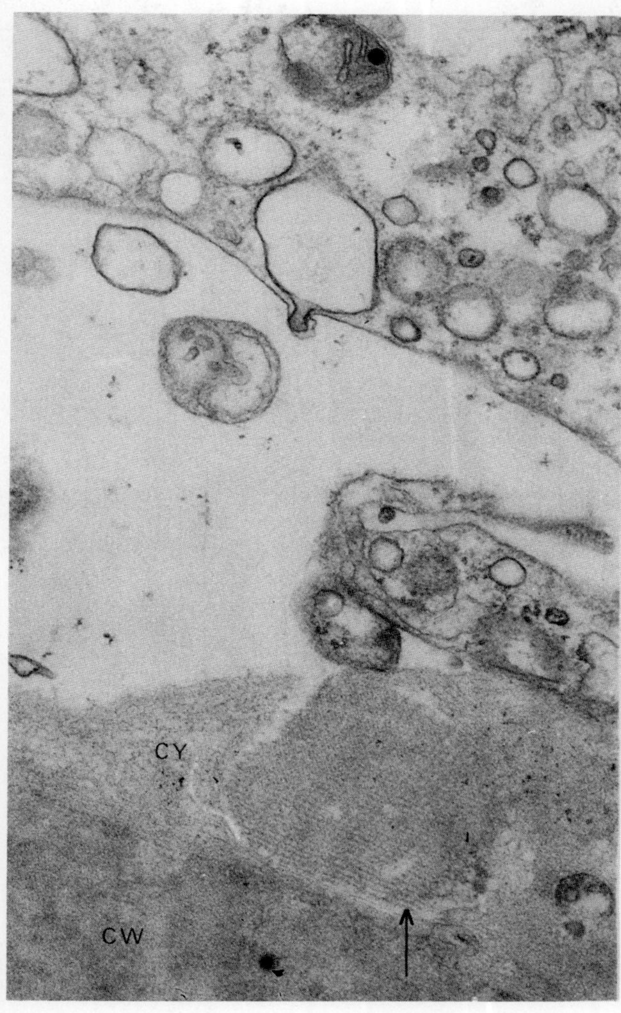

Figure 1. Indole crystal in the cytoplasm of Acetabularia (arrow). (courtesy of Dr. M. Boloukhere.) cw: cell wall cy: cytoplasm. magnification x 60,000.

MATERIALS AND METHODS

Culture

The algae are cultivated in enriched sea-water at 20° C in light-dark cycles of 12 h light, 12 h dark as previously described[23]. The light is given by daylight tubes (Phytor ACEC) and the intensity is of approximately 1200 lux at the level of the flasks.

Determination of auxin-like substances

The methods of extraction, chromatography and the biological assays have been described by Nitsch and Nitsch[1] and modified by Delegher[24].

In summary, the material was extracted in 3 steps: first, extraction of intact algae with cold methanol, two more extractions with cold methanol following homogenization. The extract was evaporated to dryness. The residue was resuspended in a small volume of methanol and submitted to ascendent chromatography on Whatman paper (3 MM). The solvent was isopropanol/ammonium hydroxide/water: 80/0.1/19.9. The paper was cut out in 20 bands, perpendicular to the migration direction of the solvent. Each band was incubated for 20 h with 10 mesocotyls of *Avena*. (The Brighton variety of *Avena sativa* was used pre-soaking 1 h, culture on filter paper about 65 h.) The sensitivity of the test is 5.10^{-4} μg for IAA.

The fluorescence spectra were recorded both in methanol and ethanol with reference IAA using a Perkin Elmer MPF3 spectrophotometer[25]. The sensitivity of the fluorescence test is 5 μg/ml. Reference IAA and IAN (indolacetonitrile) were obtained from Sigma (USA).

Determination of the binding of labelled IAA

3-Indolyl acetic acid-{I-^{14}C} (Amersham) with a specific activity of 52 mCi/mM (270 μCi/mg) was used. The *Acetabularia* were incubated for 60 min. in 1.0 or 2.0 ml of culture medium to which was added 2-5 μCi of a solution of IAA 10^{-4} to $5x10^{-6}$ M. After a 4 h chase in the culture medium, the algae were homogenized according to Goffeau and Brachet[26]. The membranes and largest chloroplasts were sedimented at 480 g for 5 min. The sediment was allowed to stand first at 37° C in either NCS (Amersham) or Soluene 300 (Packard) for at least 24 h, then at room temperature until the material was entirely digested. It was transferred to scintillation vials with Omnifluor and counted in a Packard spectrophotometer. Counts were automatically corrected for quenching.

Autoradiography was performed according to Ficq[27] on sections of *Acetabularia* fixed by freeze-substitution after the incubation and chase procedure described above. Fixed material was embedded in paraffin and sectioned with a refrigerated microtome. The grains were counted under the microscope with the aid of a reticle so that the cytoplasm along 2500 μm of cell wall was considered. Alternatively the grains were counted on photographs at which time the whole photograph was considered. Control and treated cells in the morphactins experiments were counted in the same way. Puromycin was obtained from the Nutritional Biochemicals

Corporation and Actinomycin D (in pure form) was a gift from Merk, Sharpe and Dohme. Morphactins were kindly provided by Merk, Darmstadt and contained 80% 2-chloro-9-hydroxyfluorene-9 carboxylic methylester (IT 3456), ca. 20% 9-hydroxyfluorene-9-carboxylic methylester and a small amount of 2,7-dichloro-9-hydroxyfluorene-9 carboxylic acid methylester. The action of the first compound is known to be the strongest in biological tests[28]. The morphactins were dissolved in the culture medium.

EXPERIMENTAL RESULTS

Isolation of auxin-like substances

Eight experiments have been carried out on samples of algae weighing from 0.5 to 2.9 g (fresh weight). The UV fluorescence of the material eluted from the chromatograms was assayed in each case. The biological test was carried out in 4 experiments. The latter is more sensitive than the former, since it is positive with material extracted from 0.5 g of fresh weight for which no UV fluorescence was detectable.

One representative histogram is given in Figure 2. The histograms indicate the length of the *Avena* mesocotyl in mm as a function of the Rf of the chromatographically fractionated extract. Confidence intervals are shown on both sides of the base line[24]. The statistically significant stimulating effect of the substance migrating with an Rf of 0.35-0.45 is shown by the shaded area. The Rf of reference IAA and IAN, run on parallel chromatography, are 0.3-0.4 and 0.7-0.8 respectively.

In Table 1 are given the Rf values obtained in the different experiments. In experiments 5 and 6 a larger quantity of material was used, which enlarges the area containing the biologically stimulating substance. The presence of an inhibitory substance migrating with an Rf of 0.0-0.3 is suggested; however, it is seen only at high concentration (initial weight 1.0 g).

In experiment 8, reference IAA was co-chromatographed with the extract. Only one fluorescent band appears with an Rf of 0.39-0.45, which is the position of the extract when chromatographed alone. This indicates that, in the extract, IAA migrates with a higher Rf. However, no color developed with the Salkowski reagent.

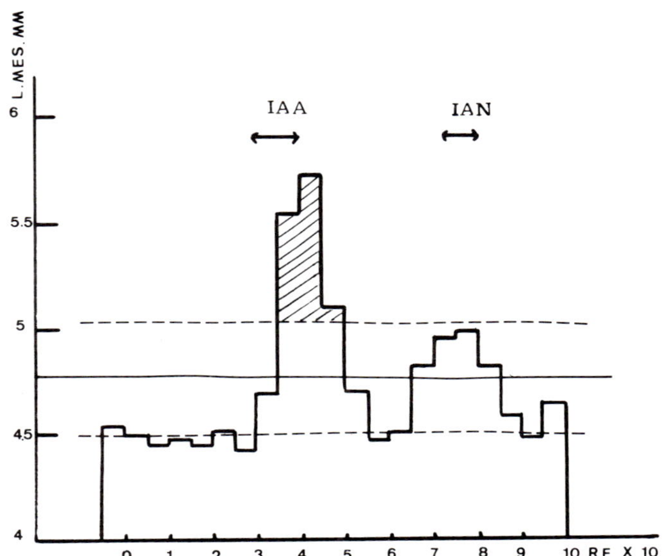

Figure 2. Biological activity in the Avena first internode bioassay of Acetabularia methanolic extract. Position of pure IAA and IAN are indicated.

Fluorescence spectrum

The excitation spectra of reference IAA and of the chromatographed Acetabularia extract were taken in both methanol and ethanol (emission at 340 nm) (Fig. 3). The spectrum of the Acetabularia extract was recorded with an amplification factor of 10 relative to the IAA solution (10 μg/ml).

The absorbance peaks of extract and reference IAA occured at very close positions in both methanol and ethanol. The ratios of the optical densities at the peaks have been calculated (Table 2).

TABLE 1

Chromatography experiments

Exper. No.	Quantity of material used for extraction (g)	Rf of the IAA-like substance	Rf of the reference IAA (parallel chromatograph)	Rf of reference IAA (co-chromatograph)	Biological test	UV fluorescence
1	0.5	0.35–0.45	0.30–0.40		+	–
2	0.5	0.35–0.45	0.30–0.40		+	–
3	1.0	0.40–0.50	0.30–0.40		+	+
4	1.1	0.40–0.45	0.30–0.40			+
5	2.9	0.40–0.50	0.30–0.40			+
6	2.0	0.40–0.50	0.30–0.40			+
7	1.0	0.39–0.45	0.30–0.40			+
8	0.7	0.35–0.45	0.30–0.40	0.39–0.45	+	+

TABLE 2

Fluorescence excitation spectra (emission 340 nm)

In methanol						
Wave-length (nm)	Optical density at				Ratios of the OD	
	230	235	280	288	a $\frac{280}{230}$	b $\frac{288}{230}$
IAA 10 μg/ml	0.072		0.832	0.855	11.555	11.97
Chromatographed extract of <u>Acetabularia</u> value at the peak	0.037	0.047	0.188	0.160	4.00	3.40

In ethanol

Wave-length (nm)	Optical Density at 230	235	285	288	Ratios of the OD a $\frac{285}{230}$	b $\frac{288}{230}$
IAA 10 μg/ml	0.080		0.775	0.802	9.69	10.025
Chromatographed extract of Acetabularia value at the peak	0.060	0.065	0.208	0.208	3.47	3.47

Optical density at the peaks. The sensitivity was adjusted to 10 for reference IAA and 100 for the extract. For the extract, the OD values used for the ratio are those of the peak.

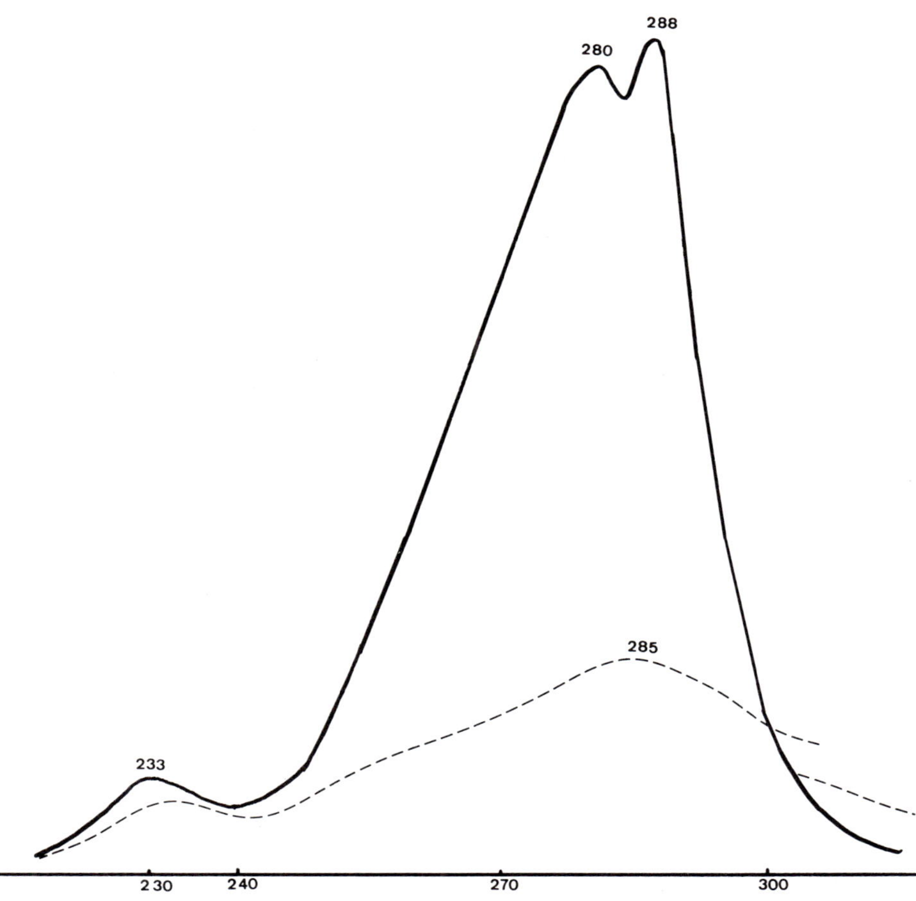

Figure 3 (opposite page). Fluorescence excitation spectrum in ethanol (emission at 340 nm).

Solid line, reference IAA 10 ug/ml (sensitivity 10).

Dotted line, Acetabularia extract (sensitivity 100).

Binding of labelled IAA

Five experiments have been carried out and are reported in Table 3. In experiment 1 and 2, the algae have been individually cut into two parts of equal length. The apical part is very narrow near the apex and has thin hair whorls. The basal part is much larger in diameter and includes all the rhizoidal outgrowths. Binding of labelled IAA is approximately 5 times higher in the latter than in the former; the area of membrane might be 5 times greater in this segment, but is difficult to estimate. In experiments 3, 4 and 5, apical parts only 13 or 15 mm in length were considered. Large differences between the experiments were observed in the binding. In all cases, however, a considerable amount of IAA becomes attached to the membranes, since, after the chase, the label remains in the sediment fraction of the homogenized *Acetabularia*.

The binding is equally evident on the autoradiograms: silver grains are visible in the cytoplasm (Fig. 4).

In order to determine the effects of puromycin (20 μgm/ml) and actinomycin D (3-5 μgm/ml) on the binding, algae were treated with inhibitor for 19 h and then incubated with labelled IAA in presence of the inhibitor. The results are reported in Table 3 (experiments 6, 7 and 8). It is clear that puromycin strongly inhibits the binding of IAA to the membrane fraction of *Acetabularia*, reducing the radioactivity to 30-50% of that of the controls.

Actinomycin D either has no inhibiting effect (experiments 7 and 8) or it increases the binding of IAA (experiment 6). Both drugs were used at concentrations known to affect the morphogenesis of Acetabularia[29,30].

Effect of morphactins on the binding of labelled IAA

The incorporation of labelled IAA was examined in the presence of morphactins (20 μg/ml) in parallel with the controls described above. Except in experiment 3 (Table 3), a decrease of labelling is observed. The decrease is more accentuated in the apical part than in the rhizoidal part of the algae. A few individuals of each case were kept for autoradiography and the results confirmed with this method. Grain counting shows that in spite of a large variability

TABLE 3

Binding of ^{14}C-IAA by *Acetabularia* and effects of morphactins, puromycin and actinomycin D (incubation with labelled IAA, 60 min., chase, 4 h)

Experiment	Mean length of algae (mm)	Part of alga or apical length	Duration of drug treatment in days (d) or hours (h)	^{14}C-IAA in membrane fraction						
				Control	Morphactins		Puromycin		Actinomycin D	
				dpm	dpm	% of controls	dpm	% of control	dpm	% of control
1	31	apical	4 d	4893	2257	46				
		basal	4 d	22234	16396	74				
2	16	apical	4 d	2992	1780	59				
		basal	4 d	17482	16049	92				
3	19	13 mm	38 h	770	937	122				
4	20	15 mm	38 h	1113	932	84				
5	21	15 mm	91 h	555	238	43				
			115 h		206	37				
6	22	whole	19 h	749			315	42	1607	215
7	24	whole	19 h	4800			2280	47.5	4824	101
8	22	whole	19 h	4595			1385	30	5024	109

between regions, morphactins reduce the IAA binding in Acetabularia (Table 4, Figs. 4 and 5).

TABLE 4

Counts of silver grains from autoradiograms

Slide number	Control (a)	Morphactins-treated (b)	Ratio a/b
1	27	18	1.5
2	76	42	1.8
3	2300	540	4.0
4	34	11	3.1
5	87	15	5.8
6	22	9	2.4

In slides 1-3 the grains have been counted with a reticle.
In slides 4-6 the grains have been counted on photographs.

DISCUSSION AND CONCLUSIONS

Methanol extraction yielded a biologically active substance which is either free in the cell or bound in a labile way. When chromatographed in parallel experiments, this substance migrates at a slighty higher Rf than commercial IAA; but this is attributable to some substance present in the extract, since in co-chromatography, the biologically active substance and reference IAA are superimposed. Such a difference is frequently observed.

The substance could be IAA or a closely related compound. This would agree with Tandler's observation[21] that the cytoplasm of Acetabularia when fixed with Carnoy's ethanol-chloroform-acetic acid mixture and extracted with ethanol in the dark for at least three weeks reacts positively to all indole tests including Salkowski's. The UV fluorescence

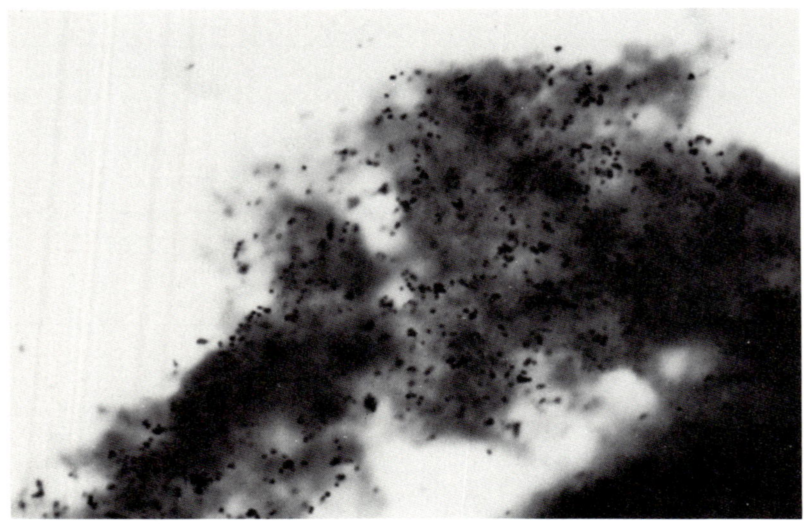

Figure 4. Autoradiogram of cell labelled with ^{14}C-IAA. x 1000.

assay gave positive results only on chromatograms heavily loaded with the extract.

The absence of color development with Salkowski's reagent is probably due to the small amount of the reacting substance in the algae. Tandler did not encounter this limitation in his chromatographic analysis of the alkaline hydrolyzate of Acetabularia since his exhaustive ethanol extraction method yielded sufficient quantities of indole compounds bound in the indole crystals which are so abundant in Acetabularia. A significant role for these crystals is suggested by the recent work of Kuraishi[31] who has shown that synthesis of IAA readily occurs in Avena from indole compounds. Thus Acetabularia might be endowed with a regulatory mechanism that enables it to adjust the IAA level rapidly.

On linear chromatography, Tandler obtained one spot migrating as IAA, but resolved it into two adjacent spots by two-dimensional chromatography. Both spots were positive to Ehrich and Salkowski reagents and thus were probably of indole nature. Tandler[21] pointed out that hydrolyzates of ethanol-extracted maize and pea root yielded a larger number of indole compounds than Acetabularia.

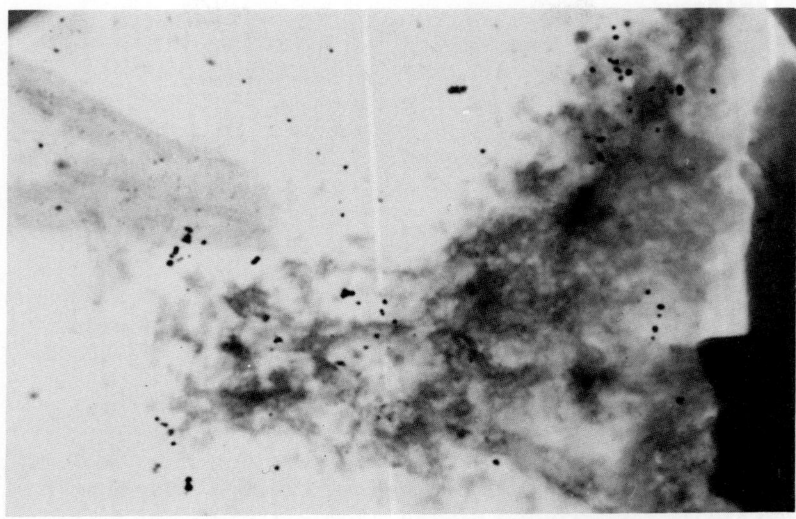

Figure 5. As Figure 4, but morphactins-treated alga (20 ug/ml, 3 days). x 1000.

The excitation fluorescence spectra of Acetabularia extract correlates well with that of reference IAA in both ethanol and methanol. These spectra show that indeed the extract contains a compound of indolyl nature. They do not allow discrimination between tryptophan and IAA, but the amino acid migrates on the chromatogram with an Rf of 0.18-0.20 whereas the active component of the extract had an Rf value of 0.35-0.45.

Thus, three lines of evidence, the Rf value of the particular fraction, its biological activity and its UV fluorescence excitation spectra, suggest that Acetabularia contains an auxin-like substance.

From the observed effects of IAA on growth and morphogenesis of Acetabularia (see Introduction) and the opposite effects of morphactins[22], the auxin-like substance has been presumed to play a role in growth and development of the alga. Exogenous IAA binds onto the membrane fraction of Acetabularia: if IAA could not bind onto the membranes, any biological role would be doubtful since the way in which active IAA induces morphogenesis involves its attachment to the plasma-membrane[32]. Labelled IAA becomes bound to the membrane fraction of Acetabularia, sedimenting with the largest chloroplasts; the variability between experiments is due to differences in age of the algae and also presumably to differences between cultures (Table 3, experiments 4 and 5). Figure 5 shows that labelled IAA is retained on cytoplasmic structures after the intensive and repeated washing of the sections involved in the method. The binding of IAA or its penetration into the cell involves proteins of short life time since *Acetabularia* cells pretreated with puromycin for 10 hours bound only one third to one half as much labelled IAA as the controls. Actinomycin D has little effect (Table 3, experiments 7 and 8), showing that no *de novo* synthesis of RNA is required in short term experiments. The increased binding observed in experiment 6 is similar to the results occasionally obtained with other materials and attributed to a stabilization of mRNA, on the basis of parallel experiments with cordycepin[33]. The fact that puromycin, a p-methoxy-phenylalanin, which binds to the phenylalanine tRNA inhibits the binding of IAA but not actinomycin D (which is a poly-peptide containing a phenoxazin), argues against totally nonspecific binding.

A more specific way to approach the possible biological role of the substance was to examine whether or not morphactins interfere with this binding since it is known that they inhibit growth and morphogenesis of the alga[22]. These fluorenol compounds have been found (in all cases except one) to reduce the labelling of the *Acetabularia* membrane fraction with radioactive IAA, suggesting that indeed the auxin-like substance is implicated in the development and differentiation of *Acetabularia*.

ACKNOWLEDGEMENTS

We are very grateful to Pr. H. Chantrenne for the discussions he had with one of us (T. VdD). We are indebted to Mr. A. Magnusson for his help with the fluorescence spectrum recordings and to Dr. B. Cairns for kindly improving the English of the text. We thank Miss M. Hayet and Mr. L. Lateur for technical assistance.

REFERENCES

1. Nitsch, J. P. and Nitsch, C. (1956) Plant Physiol. 31, 94.
2. Brachet, J. (1963) Nature 199, 714.
3. Brachet, J. (1965) Acad. Roy. Belge cl. Sc. 51, 269.
4. Brachet, J. (1968) Current Topics Devel. Biol. 3, 1.
5. Brachet, J. (1975) Bioch. Physiol. Pflanzen 168, 493.
6. Brachet, J., Denis, M. and de Vitry, F. (1964) Devel. Biol. 9, 398.

7. Brachet, J. and Six, N. (1966) Planta 68, 225.
8. Hämmerling, J. (1934) Wilhelm Roux Archiv. für Entwicklungsmechanik der organismen 131, 1.
9. Hämmerling, J. (1953) Inter. Rev. Cyt. 2, 475.
10. Hämmerling, J. (1963) Ann. Rev. Plant Physiol. 14, 65.
11. Puiseux-Dao, S. (1970) Logos Press 162.
12. Dao, S. (1954) C. R. Acad. Sci. Paris 338, 2340.
13. Thimann, K. V. and Beth, K. (1959) Nature 183, 946.
14. Dao, S. (1956) C. R. Acad. Sci. Paris 243, 1552.
15. Cumming, B. G. and Wagner, E. (1968) Ann. Rev. Plant Physiol. 19, 381.
16. Steward, F. C. and Krikorian, A. D. (1971) Acad. Press 1.
17. Posner, H. (1969) Plant Physiol. 44, 562.
18. Posner, H. (1970) Plant Physiol. 45, 687.
19. Posner, H. (1971) Plant Physiol. 48, 361.
20. Tandler, C. J. (1962a) Naturwiss. 9, 213.
21. Tandler, C. J. (1962b) Planta 59, 91.
22. Vanden Driessche, T. (1974) Protoplasma 81, 323.
23. Lateur, L. (1963) Rev. Algol. 1, 26.
24. Delegher, V. (1963) Ann. Physiol. végét. Univ. Bruxelles 7, 113.
25. Udenfriend, S. (1962) (1969) Acad. Press I, III.
26. Goffeau, A. and Brachet, J. (1965) Biochem. Biophys. Acta 95, 302.
27. Ficq, A. (1955) Experim. Cell Res. 9, 286.
28. Pilet, P. E. V. (1970) Experientia 26, 608.
29. Bonotto, S., Goffea, A., Janowski, M., Vanden Driessche, T. and Brachet, J. (1964) J. Biochim. Biophys. Acta 174, 704.
30. Brachet, J. (1963) Bull. Cl. Sc. Acad. Roy. Belge 49, 862
31. Kuraishi, S. (1976) The 9th Internat. Conf. on Plant Growth Substances 88, 203.
32. Thimann, K. V. (1969) The Auxins. Physiology of plant growth and development Edit. M. B. Wilkins, MacGraw Hill p. 1-45.
33. Grayson, S. and Berry, S. J. (1973) Science 180, 1071.

FLEXIBILITY OF A CELL WALL PROTEIN FROM *ACETABULARIA*

H. Hasko Paradies, Lüder Göke, and Günther Werz

Fachbereich Biologie
Freie Universität Berlin
Berlin, West Germany

ABSTRACT

Aqueous solutions of a cell wall protein from *Acetabularia* were studied by means of small angle X-ray scattering in solution. The experimentally determined molecular weight was 14,000 daltons, the radius of gyration was found to be 46.3 Å. The geometrical description of an oblate or prolate ellipsoid could not be applied to this protein. Therefore, the possibility that the protein was shaped like a coil was investigated and a persistence length of 16.2 Å was determined.

INTRODUCTION

Although Wiessner in 1888 [1] deduced from histochemical reaction that plant cell walls are alive, containing proteinaceous material, this remained a matter of controversy until Preston[2], Lamport[3] and others[4,5,6] unequivocally showed that proteins are constitutional components of plant cell walls. Cell wall proteins have subsequently been investigated thoroughly, and it has been found that they are very heterogeneous. Cell walls contain several classes of proteins or polypeptides that are demonstrable by using different methods (e.g. extraction by weak or strong solvents, hydrolysis with acids or bases, digestion by enzymes). Although this kind of classification is somewhat artificial, it has shown that the cell wall proteins differ in their molecular properties and in their relationships to the other cell wall constituents, especially to the matrix and the fibrillar polysaccharides.

On the basis of today's knowledge it seems to be justified to divide plant cell wall proteins into two preliminary groups: group one, which contains those proteins (e.g.

extensine) that are primarily associated with the structural component of the cell walls, the polysaccharides[7,8,9]; group two, which contains proteins (e.g. peroxidases, hydrolases) that are present temporarily or constantly in the cell wall but not so intimately associated with the structural components[10].

In spite of several uncertainties concerning the true nature of cell wall proteins or polypeptides, two main aspects of cell wall protein function have crystallized from work during the past: a) intercellular communication (e.g. controlling and/or possibly modifying substances during transport through the intermicellar space of the cell wall), and b) morphogenesis of plant cells (e.g. formation of polysaccharides and determination of their spatial distribution). In this paper we will refer to the latter aspect.

It has been shown that the shape of a plant cell is intimately related to variations in its cell wall protein composition and, because proteins are gene-coded, these relationships seem to be fundamental for cell wall and cell morphogenesis. How do cell wall proteins work? Their role is not well understood, not only because of difficulties in acquiring some kind of well defined protein components but also due to the lack of a suitable hypothesis for the polysaccharide-protein interaction during cell wall morphogenesis.

Because of the great amount of relatively homogeneous polysaccharides that are built up during the life of a plant cell one might suggest the existence of some kind of elementary protein unit related to polysaccharide formation and cell wall morphogenesis. The relationship of cell wall proteins to cell wall and cell morphogenesis may be best established by using a unicellular organism like *Acetabularia* which possesses defined morphogenetic stages, like those of stalk and cap formation. Moreover, *Acetabularia* has been shown to contain stalk and cap cell wall polypeptides both of which, although differing somewhat in detail, possess large amounts of the amino acids alanine, glycine, glutamic and aspartic acids, suggesting a fairly rigid protein or polypeptide configuration[11] which may be important for structural purposes.

In the following we describe first approaches to the determination of *Acetabularia* cell wall protein structure by means of biochemical and X-ray procedures. On this basis we investigate the possible existence of a cell wall protein unit responsible for the formation of similar polysaccharide units as cell wall precursors.

In this investigation we have undertaken a study of the small angle X-ray patterns of a cell wall protein isolated from the green alga *Acetabularia*. The experiments were performed in aqueous solution at low ionic strength to obtain detailed information about i) the influence of buffer constitutents on the conformation, and ii) the flexibility of the cell wall protein in solution.

MATERIAL AND METHODS

The cell wall protein from Acetabularia (Polyphysa) cliftonii was isolated as described by Göke et al.[12]. The protein was purified by means of chromatography on a Sephadex G-25 column (2 x 50 cm) in 2 M acetic acid, containing 0.1 M KCl. Normally, the protein elutes as a single peak in the void volume and consists of dimers and trimers of the cell wall protein. Further purification can be achieved by Bio Gel A-0.5 m column chromatography in moderate salt solutions at pH 7.2. The molecular weight of the protein was estimated by analytical polyacrylamide gel electrophoresis according to Hedrick and Smith[13]. Amino acid determination, diffusion coefficient and sedimentation constant under various conditions, e.g. ionic strength, were performed as described by Paradies et al.[14,15].

Small angle X-ray scattering measurements

Diffraction measurements were performed using a medium resolution Kratky camera, nickel filtered CuK_α-radiation (water cooled, rotating anode, GX 13, Elliott-Marconi, U.K.), an experimental arrangement already described by Paradies and Franz[16] and Paradies et al.[12]. The settings of the Kratky camera, including slit width, resulted in a theoretical resolution of approximately 1000 Å. The scattered intensities were placed on an absolute scale by comparison with the scattering from a calibrated Lupolene platelet, according to Kratky et al.[18].

RESULTS

Experimental parameters

The radius of gyration of 46.3 Å for the protein was obtained according to the law of Guinier[19] for sufficiently small scattering angles (see Appendix).

The intercepts of different concentrations are extrapolated to infinite dilution, yielding (I_o/c_o) from which the molecular weight of the scattering particle can be calculated (see Appendix).

For filled, elongated particles the radius of gyration of the cross section, R_c, can be determined from the slope of the linear portion of a plot of $\ln(hI/c)$ vs. h^2 (see Appendix). Moreover, applying Luzzati's theory[20] for rod-like particles, we were able to show that the cell wall protein in 0.1 M KCl,

0.01 M CH_3COOK, pH 5.5, behaves as a rod[14] with molecular dimensions of L = 175 Å and D = 10 Å. Data obtained at the smallest angles for three concentrations of the cell wall protein at pH 5.5 and low ionic strength (0.005 M CH_3COOK, pH 5.5) are shown in a Guinier plot in Figure 1. A plot of log (hI/c) against h^2 is shown in Figure 2, while Figure 3 documents the uninterpretable concentration dependence of

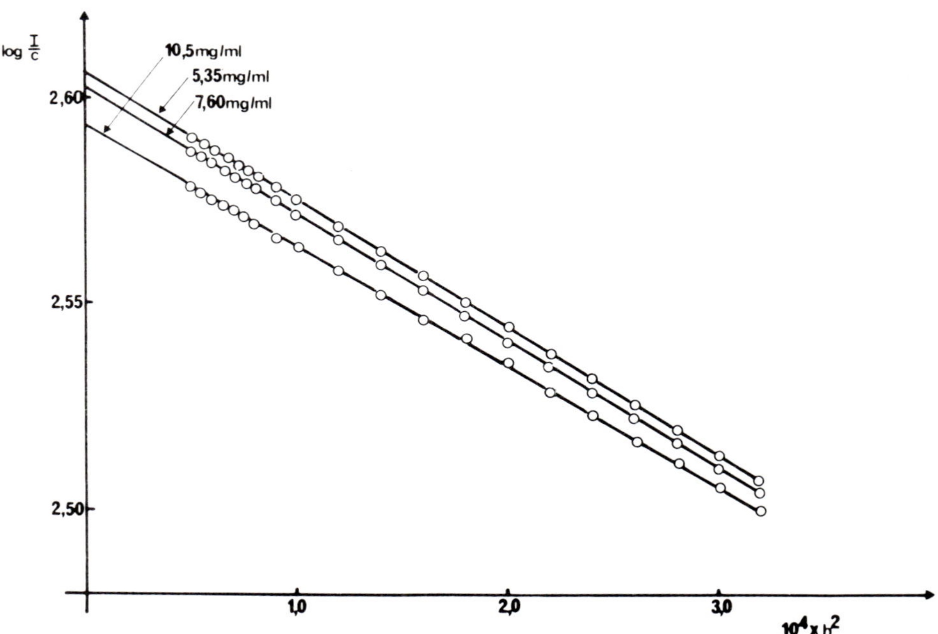

Figure 1. Guinier plot of the data at smallest angles for three concentrations of the cell wall protein.

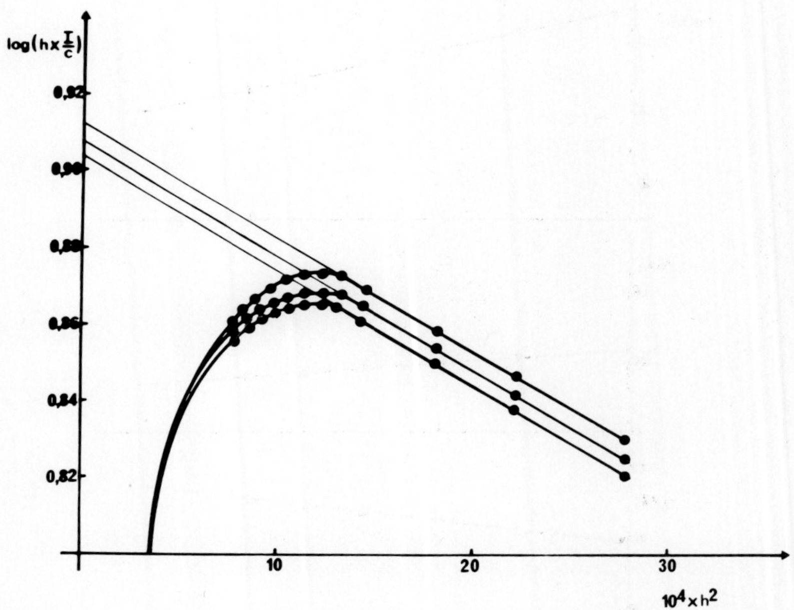

Figure 2. Plot for determining the radius of gyration of the cross section. Concentrations are in inverse order to those shown in Figure 1.

these intercepts and slopes. Extrapolation to infinite dilution yields M = 14,800, R = 46.3 Å, and R_c = 9.9 Å. The volume of the scattering particle was determined by making use of the invariant term, A, according to Porod[21,22] to be 4.75×10^4 $Å^3$ (see Appendix). The average area of the cross-sectioned surface, S_c, is 215.0 Å. The surface per unit volume, S, is 0.412 A^{-1} [16] and the total surface area per molecule is 1.95×10^4 $Å^2$.

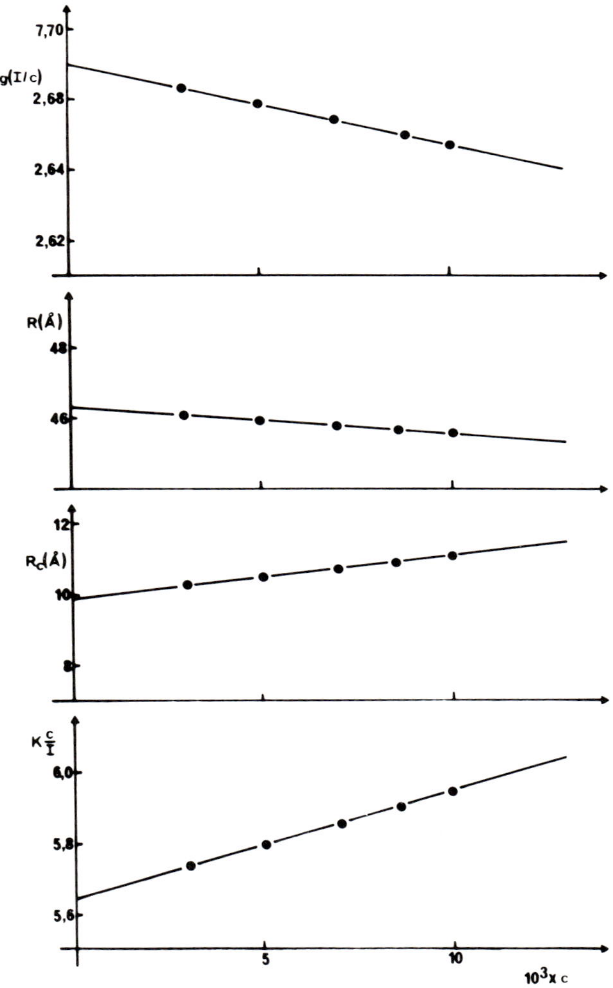

Figure 3. Concentration dependence of several experimental parameters extrapolated to infinite dilution.

In contrast to our measurements of the cell wall protein at high ionic strength in 0.1 M KCl [15] we were not able to find a scattering equivalent for any particular geometrical scattering body at low ionic strength. The experimental volume of $V = 4.75 \times 10^4$ Å^3 is much larger than the dry volume of the protein of 2.15×10^4 Å^3. This large swelling ratio suggests an open coil form. A comparison of the observed radius of gyration of R = 46.3 Å with the radius of gyration of 17.4 Å of a sphere having the observed volume, V, and the radius of gyration of 39.5 Å of a rod with L = 170.0 Å and D = 10.0 Å indicates that the equivalent scattering particle must be quite anisotropic. The same conclusions can be reached concerning the two cross-sectional radii of gyration, R_c = 9.9 Å and that of a circular cross section area, S_c = 5.9 Å. Comparisons of the experimental scattering curve, plotted as log I vs. log h, with corresponding plots of normalized intensities, calculated for particles with particular shape and various axial ratios, e.g. long thin rods or discs, show that the cell wall protein under these experimental conditions cannot be described as a cylinder, rectangular prism, etc. No equivalent particle could be found that is compatible with all the experimental parameters obtained at a 0.005 M KCl concentration at pH 5.5. These findings are also true for experiments performed at pH 7.2 in 0.01 M Tris-HCl, containing 0.005 M KCl, 0.01 M $MgCl_2$.

Therefore, we examined the possibility that the cell wall protein from *Acetabularia* under these conditions exists as an open coil using as a model the worm-like chain with finite persistence length. The degree of flexibility of the polypeptide chain of the cell wall protein seems to be very sensitive to environmental conditions, e.g. ionic strength, pH, temperature and divalent cations.

The mass per unit length, $\bar{w}$, of a coiling chain is calculated to be 39.5 g/(mol · Å). The contour length of the chain, $L = M/\bar{w}$, is found to be 375.0 Å.

A chain with finite persistence length will undergo a transition with increasing scattering angle from coil behavior, $I \sim h^{-2}$, to rod-like behavior, $I \sim h^{-1}$. This implies that the persistence length can be evaluated from the h-value at which this transition occurs. This is illustrated in Figure 4 that shows a plot of $h^2 \cdot I$ against h for the cell wall protein at low ionic strength. The function is observed to rise to a horizontal plateau which corresponds to the $I \sim h^{-2}$ region and to be followed by an increasing value of $I \sim h^{-1}$, the rod-like domain. The persistence length, a, is then calculated to be 16.2 Å. Hence, according to this model the cell wall protein can be described as a chain of L/a = 373/16.2 = 23 persistence lengths, each consisting of 6.5 residues. The root mean square chain displacement length,

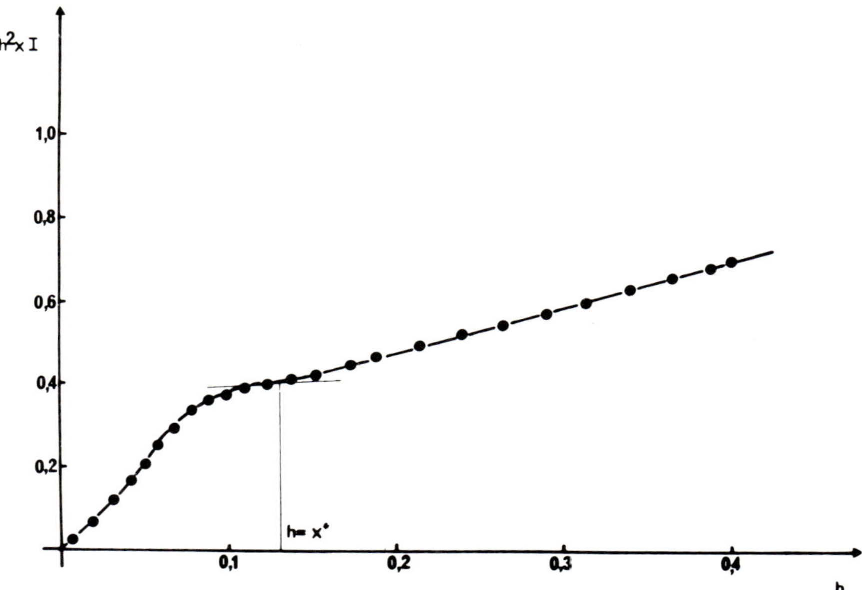

Figure 4. Plot of small angle data to determine the persistence length.

$(\bar{r})^{\frac{1}{2}}$, for such a worm-like chain is calculated to be 107.5 Å (see Appendix). This would correspond to a radius of gyration, R, of 46.8 Å, which agrees quite well with the experimentally determined value of 46.3 Å.

The fact that Figure 4 shows defined coil and rod-like regions and the agreement between the experimental value of R and that of a predicted worm-like chain, with the observed contour and persistence lengths, argue in favor of a coiling form of the cell wall protein in solution under the described conditions.

DISCUSSION

The cell wall protein from Acetabularia behaves in solutions of different strength either as a rod-like molecule with dimensions of L = 170.0 Å and D = 10.0 Å or as a coiled polypeptide chain with a contour length of 375.0 Å and a persistence length of a = 16.2 Å. Since the rod-like particle is stabilized by helicogenic solvents, e.g. hexafluorisopropanol or chloroform, and by high protein concentration, the coiled form of the cell wall protein at low protein concentration may have to do with loosened protein-protein interactions, as was observed in oriented fibers[14]. Moreover, additional verification of the conclusion that the cell wall protein at low ionic strength is coiled can be deduced from the characteristic ratio, $r_o^2/np \cdot lp^2$, where np is the number of residues in the chain and lp = 3.80 Å is the length of the transpeptide unit. The r_o^2-value must be converted for the excluded volume effects and the finite value of np (see Appendix).

The characteristic ratio was found to be 5.2 for the cell wall protein. This is in reasonable accord with a theoretical value of 5.9 predicted by Miller et al.[23] for a random copolymer containing 15% glycine. According to the amino acid composition[14] there are 12 residues of glycine and 15 residues of alanine, equalling 15 percent. This makes a direct comparison of the characteristic ratio of 5.2 with the results of Miller et al.[23] for random L-alanine-glycine-type copolymers possible. However, their conformational calculations[23] were not intended to represent proteins, but homopolypeptides of glycine and alanine and their possible random copolymers. Considering all these factors, the acidic cell wall protein of *Acetabularia* could be behaving like a flexible protein due to its amino acid sequence when influenced by ionic strength.

The basic idea of this investigation of the physical and chemical structure of the cell wall protein was to find a possible stereochemical explanation for the linkage between polysaccharides and proteins within the architecture of the cell wall of *Acetabularia*. Not too much can be said about the details of this linkage because the manner of attachment of the sugar residues to cell wall proteins is still uncertain. All mannan-protein complexes studied so far in this laboratory release a part of the carbohydrate as small oligosaccharides with different chemical composition under $NaBH_4$ reduction or mildly alkaline conditions which promote β-elimination.

REFERENCES

1. Wiessner, J. (1888) Ber. Deutsch. Bot. Ges. 6, 187-195.
2. Preston, R. D. (1952) The Molecular Architecture of Plant Cell Walls. Chapman and Hall, London, 1st Ed.
3. Lamport, D. T. A. (1967) Nature 216, 1322-1324.
4. Crook, E. M. and Johnston, I. R. (1962) Biochem. J. (U.K.) 83, 325-329.

5. Gotelli, I. B. and Cleland, R. (1968) Amer. J. Bot. 55, 907-914.
6. Thompson, E. W. and Preston, R. D. (1966) J. Exp. Bot. 19, 690-697.
7. Lamport, D. T. A. (1970) Ann. Rev. Plant Physiol. 21, 235-270.
8. Lamport, D. T. A. and Miller, D. H. (1971) Plant Physiol. 48, 454-456.
9. Loewus, F. (1973) Biogenesis of Plant Cell Wall Polysaccharides. Academic Press, New York, London.
10. Matile, Ph. (1975) The Lytic Compartment of Plant Cells. Protoplasmatologia, Cell Biol. Monographs, Vol. 1. Springer Verlag, Wien.
11. Chou, P. Y. and Fasman, G. D. (1974) Biochemistry 13, 211-222.
12. Göke, L., Paradies, H. H. and Werz, G. (1974) Biochem. Biophys. Res. Commun. 60, 22-27.
13. Hedrick, J. L. and Smith, A. J. (1968) Arch. Biophys. Biochem. 126, 155-164.
14. Paradies, H. H., Göke, L. and Werz, G. (1977a) J. Membrane Biol. (in press).
15. Paradies, H. H., Göke, L. and Werz, G. (1977b) Arch. Biochem. Biophys. (in press).
16. Paradies, H. H. and Franz, A. (1976) Eur. J. Biochem. 67, 23-29.
17. Paradies, H. H., Zimmer, B. and Werz, G. (1976) Biochem. Biophys. Res. Commun. (in press).
18. Kratky, D., Pilz, I. and Schmitz, P. J. (1966) J. Colloid Interface Sci. 21, 24-34.
19. Guinier, A. (1939) Ann. Physik (Leipzig) 12, 161-237.
20. Luzzati, V. (1960) Acta Crystallograph. 13, 939-942.
21. Porod, G. (1951a) Kolloid-Z. 124, 83-114.
22. Porod, G. (1951b) Kolloid-Z. 125, 51-57.
23. Miller, W. G., Brandt, D. P. and Florey, P. J. (1967) J. Mol. Biol. 23, 67-77.

APPENDIX

The radius of gyration for a homogeneous scattering particle can be obtained at small scattering angles according to

$$\text{(A-1)} \qquad \ln (I/c) = \ln(I_o/c) - (h^2 \cdot R^2/3)$$

with $h = (4\pi/\lambda) \sin \theta$, θ = half of the scattering angle and $\lambda = 1.543$ Å, from the initial slope of a plot $\ln(I/c)$ vs. h^2. The intercepts of different concentrations, c, extrapolated to zero concentration, $(I_o/c)_o$, yields the molecular weight

(A-2) $M = d^2/i_e NP_o \cdot D(\Delta z)^2 \cdot (\frac{I_o}{c})_o$

with i_e = the scattering factor for one electron, N = Avogadro's number, P_o = the intensity of the primary beam, D = sample thickness (cm), Δz = the excess scattering of the solute (protein) of the solvent. For elongated particles we can determine the radius of gyration of the cross section, R_c,

(A-3) $\ln(hI/c) = \ln(HI_o/c) - h^2 \cdot R_c{}^2/2$

by plotting $\ln(hI/c)$ vs. h^2.

The volume of a scattering particle can be determined according to [21,21]

(A-4) $V = 4\pi^2 \cdot I_o/\tilde{Q}$; $\tilde{Q} = \int_o h\tilde{I}dh$

using slit-smeared intensities, $\tilde{I}$. The surface per unit volume, S/V, is $4\nu_1 k_1/\tilde{Q}$ with ν_1 = the volume fraction of the solvent and k_1 the tail end constant of the scattering function[16].

The root mean square displacement (r^2) for a worm-like chain is obtained from

(A-5) $(\bar{r}^2) = 2a(L - a + a \cdot e^{-L/a})$

where L = the length of the polypeptide chain and a = the persistence length.

The dependence of $r_o{}^2$ upon protein concentration (c) can be evaluated by determining the second virial coefficient according to

(A-6) $k(c/I_o) = (1/M) + 2A_1 \cdot c + \ldots..$

A_1 reflects the polyelectrolytic behavior of the protein and the interaction between protein and solvent.

V METHODOLOGY

CULTURE CONDITIONS FOR *ACETABULARIA*

H. G. Schweiger, P. Dehm and S. Berger

Max-Planck-Institut für Zellbiologie
Wilhelmshaven, West Germany

SUMMARY

Up until now, *Acetabularia* cells have been cultured most successfully in Erd-Schreiber medium. Recently, a defined synthetic medium has been found that fulfills the requirements of *Acetabularia* cells to at least the same extent as the undefined Erd-Schreiber medium. Furthermore, cells grow excellently in a flow-through system containing unsupplemented sea-water. This system permits the possibility to study special culture conditions in detail.

Axenic cultures of *Acetabularia* can be prepared by making use of the high resistance of the cysts to different chemical and physical disturbances.

INTRODUCTION

A number of features make *Acetabularia* a well suited organism for cell biology investigations. The possibility of applying cell biology methods has allowed the use of *Acetabularia* not only for studies on nucleo-cytoplasmic interrelationships[1], but also for studies on other fields[2]. However, despite all these advantages, if work on *Acetabularia* is performed in only a few labs, the question arises as to whether this limited utilization of the organism as compared with the possibilities it offers is due to the special difficulties in the culturing of this organism. Indeed, there are a number of reasons which indicate why this may be true. The three major reasons are: The slow growth rate, the inability to grow cells in a defined medium, and, finally, the specific difficulties in growing *Acetabularia* axenically.

In this contribution we will summarize the standard

culture techniques and will report on and discuss the results obtained with an artificial medium.

DIFFERENT SPECIES

One specific advantage of Acetabularia is that a number of related species within the Dasycladaceae can be grown in the lab and are therefore available for experiments[3]. Moreover, the different species can conveniently be kept under similar culture conditions.

CULTURE DISHES

In the simplest case, Acetabularia can be grown in an aquarium. This method has been mainly used for demonstrations. The effect is more pronounced for example if the algae are grown on pieces of wood or shells. Two drawbacks of this method are that the culture conditions are uncontrolled and that the rhizoids intertwine.

Another possibility is to grow the Acetabularia cells in Petri dishes. Petri dishes of 120 mm diameter and 55 mm height are filled with 150 ml of medium, and for example, 50 cells of A. mediterranea, A. crenulata or a similar species are added. The Petri dishes are then covered with a glass lid.

Besides Petri-dishes Erlenmeyer flasks have been used[4]. The flasks which contain 150 ml of medium are sealed with a glass or metal cover or with a cotton plug. Minor disadvantages of the Erlenmeyer flasks in comparison to the Petri dishes could be that the illumination is less defined and that the handling of the plants is more laborious.

Under special conditions, the utilization of glass tubes has proven to be advantageous[5]. Such tubes are suited for growing cells in a flow-through system (Fig. 1). The tubes have a diameter of 20 mm and a length of about 500 mm. The interior of the glass is subdivided with plugs of glass wool to yield compartments with a height of about 10 cm. In each compartment, about 12 cells are kept. If the glass tube is provided with a flow-through jacket, the temperature-dependent growth can be studied in a precise way.

CULTURE MEDIA

We can distinguish between natural or non-defined and synthetic or defined culture media. So far, the non-defined media which have been used to growing Acetabularia are all based on sea-water. Attempts to grow Acetabularia in plain sea-water have been unsuccessful until recently. Although it

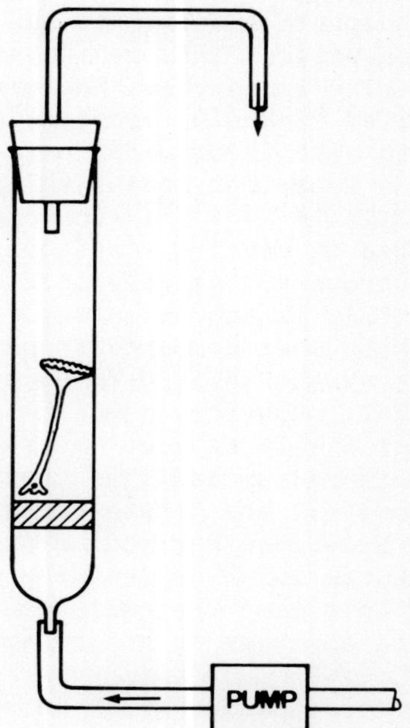

Figure 1. A glass tube for growing Acetabularia cells in a flow-through system.

The interior of the tube contains a plug of glass wool to maintain the cells at a specific position. Depending on the length of the tube and the species grown, more glass plugs might be used to subdivide the tube into several compartments. Sea-water is pumped through the tube at a speed of 15 ml per hour. It exits through a narrow glass tube fitted into a rubber stopper.

is possible to keep Acetabularia cells alive in sea-water, the growth is significantly reduced or even completely stopped within a short time.

More recently it was shown that by means of a flow-through system, good growth results could be obtained even in plain sea-water. Figure 2 and Table 1 show that cells grown in sea-water in the flow-through system exhibit growth rates equally as good or even superior to those of cells maintained in Petri dishes filled with Erd-Schreiber medium. In addition, it is apparent that when the sea-water has passed a distinct number of cells at a given speed it is no longer capable of maintaining an optimum growth rate. It is unlikely that the reduced growth rate results from the release of growth inhibiting material from the cells. It is more probable that this reduced growth rate is due to an exhaustion of essential components of the sea-water.

Under non-flow-through conditions, sea-water which was supplemented with phosphate and nitrate has turned out to be superior to plain sea-water. This medium was described originally by the marine researcher, Schreiber[6], in Helgoland, and is therefore called "Schreiber-medium."

Most experiments described so far on Acetabularia have been performed with a Schreiber-medium which was supplemented with a soil extract (Table 2)[7,8,9]. In this Erd-Schreiber medium first described by Føyn[10], Acetabularia mediterranea, for example, can be grown so that the life cycle is completed in about 120 days. This is approximately a 4- to 5-fold increase in growth rate when compared to natural conditions.

Attempts to use synthetic or defined media have been basically unsuccessful. However, a medium described by Shephard[11] seems most likely to meet the requirements. Cells which are kept in this medium continue growing and are capable of forming caps. However, the growth rates are significantly lower than those in Erd-Schreiber medium and in experiments with anucleate cells the inferior features of this medium become obvious. In this case the cells do not exhibit a normal morphogenesis, and they do not possess the capability of forming a cap.

When searching for a medium which is equivalent to Erd-Schreiber medium, a number of synthetic media were tested in our lab. It was found that a medium described by Provasoli et al.[12] and modified by Müller[13] suffices to meet all requirements (Table 3). The growth rate and morphogenesis of cells cultivated in Müller-medium are easily comparable to those which are obtained in Erd-Schreiber medium (Table 4). Perhaps, the capabilities of this synthetic medium may even be superior to the Erd-Schreiber medium.

TABLE 1

Growth and Cap Formation of A. Mediterranea in Seawater (Flow-through-system; 70 Days)

Tube	Stalk (length; mm)	Cap (diameter; mm)	Cap (%)	Cap with cysts (%)
1	26	8.40	94	78
2	31	7.40	100	66
3	37	5.80	90	36
4	42	5.65	82	28
5	40	4.00	66	22
6	43	2.50	58	4
7	50	0.92	4	-
8	48	0.60	-	-
control (ESM)	45	6.00	78	8

Figure 2 (overleaf). Cap and cyst formation of A. mediterranea in sea-water in a flow-through system.

Cap and cyst formation were followed in eight tubes connected in series through which sea-water was sequentially pumped. Each tube was subdivided into 5 compartments each of which contained 12 cells. Control cells were grown in Erd-Schreiber medium in Petri dishes.

Caps

●——●——● *flow through system*

▲——▲——▲ *Petri dishes*

Cysts

o——o——o *flow-through system*

△——△——△ *Petri dishes*

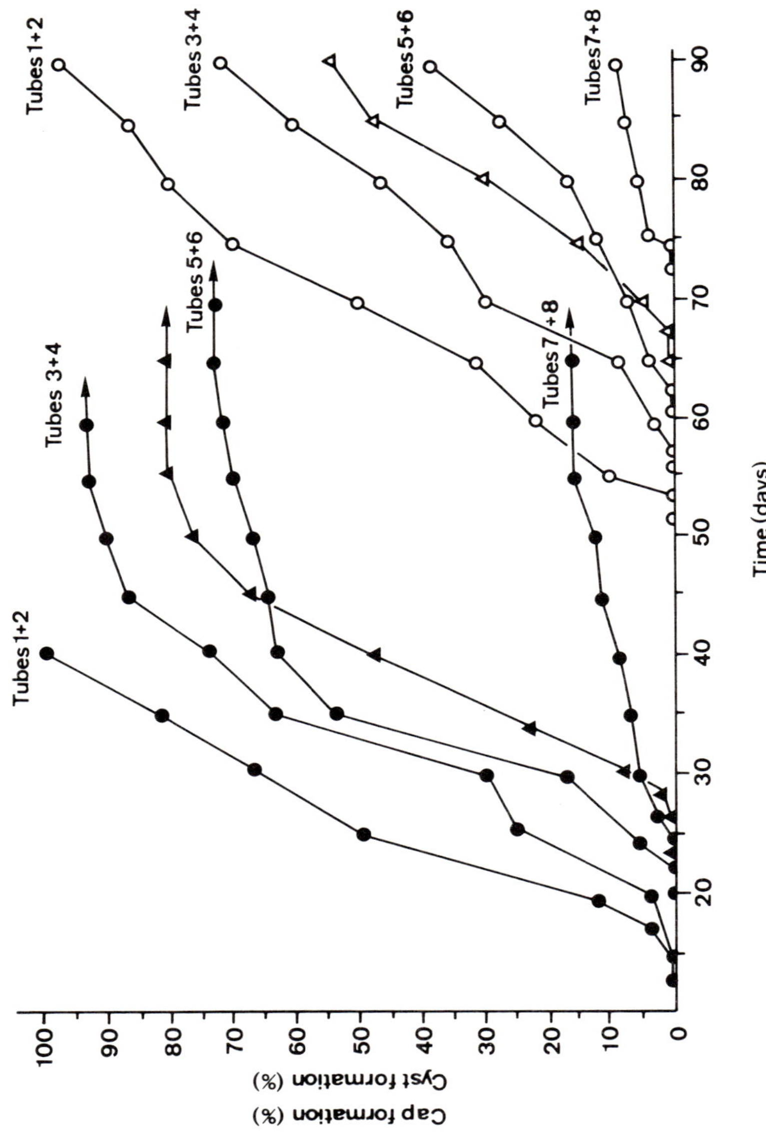
Tubes 1+2
Tubes 3+4
Tubes 5+6
Tubes 7+8
Tubes 1+2
Tubes 3+4
Tubes 5+6
Tubes 7+8
Cap formation (%)
Cyst formation (%)
Time (days)
0
10
20
30
40
50
60
70
80
90
100

TABLE 2

Erd-Schreiber medium

Preparation of soil extract

Autoclave humus-rich, dried, sieved soil for 1 h at 2 atm. and at 125° C. Suspend 100 g of soil in 500 ml sea-water and boil for 2 h. Replenish evaporated water and filter through a paper filter.

Preparation of medium

Mix in the following sequence:

1500 ml sea-water

plus 40 ml nitrate solution ($NaNO_3$; 4 mg/ml)

plus 40 ml phosphate solution ($Na_2HPO_4 \cdot 12\ H_2O$; 0.8 mg/ml)

plus 40 ml soil extract

Sterilize by filtering through nitro-cellulose filters with pore size of first 0.45 µm and then 0.2 µm.

Table 3 (opposite page)

Distilled water is the solvent for all solutions. The individual solutions should be prepared by dissolving the quantity of the dry salts required for the final concentration in sufficient water for solution. After all solutions are mixed, water is added to bring the medium to the designated volume.

$MgCl_2$ and $CaCl_2$ are highly deliquescent. Therefore, they cannot be weighed accurately. The approximate amount of $CaCl_2$ or $MgCl_2$, respectively, should be weighed and dissolved in about 80% of the final volume. The chloride concentration has to be determined by titration with $AgNO_3$ and the solution diluted to the required volume of the desired concentration.

Na_2SiO_3 dissolves in warm water. If the stock solution is acidified to pH 2 with concentrated HCl, the solution is stable and no precipitation occurs in the medium when Na_2SiO_3 is added.

The solutions 10 to 15 tend to precipitate in alkaline medium. Therefore, they should be added in a chelated form. All these chemicals are sufficiently soluble to permit preparation of concentrated stock solutions. Equivalent amounts of stock solutions 10 to 14 are mixed with 2/3 of the final concentration of EDTA and boiled for 5 to 10 min. After cooling to room temperature, the pH is adjusted to 8.0 with NaOH. Fe citrate is dissolved together with the remaining 1/3 of EDTA and boiled for 5 to 10 min. After cooling to room temperature, the pH is adjusted to 7.0 with NaOH.

The chemicals 18 to 22 should be mixed and dissolved together. The pH should be adjusted to 8.0 with NaOH.

A separate stock solution should be prepared of KI. To prevent oxidation the pH should be adjusted to 8.0 with NaOH.

No further pH adjustment is necessary after combination of all chemicals to the final medium.

Vitamins are added to the complete medium immediately before using it.

The medium is sterilized by filtering it through nitrocellulose filter of 0.22 μm pore size.

Table 3

Synthetic medium

Solution No.	Chemical	Final concentration	
1	NaCl	475	mM
2	KCl	9.8	"
3	$MgSO_4$	26.6	"
4	$MgCl_2$	23	"
5	$CaCl_2$	13.5	"
6	$NaHCO_3$	2.4	"
7	$NaNO_3$	1.18	"
8	Na_2HPO_4	140	μM
9	Na_2SiO_3	70	"
10	$ZnCl_2$	14	"
11	$MnSO_4 \cdot H_2O$	3.8	"
12	$Na_2MoO_4 \cdot 2\ H_2O$	0.83	"
13	$CoCl_2 \cdot 6\ H_2O$	0.04	"
14	$CuSO_4$	0.008	"
15	EDTA	53.7	"
16	Fe citrate Fe^{II}	1.2	"
17	Boric acid	32	"
18	NaBr	185	"
19	$SrCl_2 \cdot 6\ H_2O$	14	"
20	$AlCl_3 \cdot 6\ H_2O$	0.21	"
21	RbCl	0.13	"
22	LiCl	0.14	"
23	KI	0.12	"
Vitamin B 12	0.5 μg/1000 ml medium		
Biotin	0.5 " /1000 ml "		
Thiamin HCl	100 " /1000 ml "		

TABLE 4

Comparison of rates of growth of 3 species of *Acetabularia* in Müller medium (MM) and in Erd-Schreiber medium (ES)

Species	Day	Length (mm)		Cells with caps (%)		Diameter of caps (mm)		Caps with cysts (%)	
		MM	ES	MM	ES	MM	ES	MM	ES
A. cliftonii	0	27	27	0	0	0	0	0	0
	90	128	131	98	98	3.6	3.2	89	95
A. mediterranea	0	13	13	0	0	0	0	0	0
	88	44	42	93	90	3.4	3.0	0	0
A. major	0	7	7	0	0	0	0	0	0
	121	79	74	34	30	10.7	10.3	6	5

AXENIC CULTURES

It is difficult to obtain and culture axenic cells for two reasons. On the one hand, it is a problem to completely remove microbial contaminations like bacteria and fungi which normally stick to the algae, without damaging the cells. On the other hand, it is not easy to maintain cells axenically because the growth rate is very low, and, therefore, long culture times are needed. And, finally, the cells have a very low antibiotic activity.

Although laborious, a frequently reproduced and reliable method for obtaining axenic cells is based on the treatment of cysts with a solution of silver protein (Table 5)[14,15].

TABLE 5

Preparation of axenic cysts

Treat cyst bearing caps for 2 h in the dark with 10% silver protein solution (Targesin).
Rinse several times with sterile sea-water to remove silver protein.
Remove cysts from cap rays under sterile working conditions.
Treat cysts for 2 h in the dark with 10% silver protein.
Rinse several times with sterile sea-water to remove silver protein.
While stirring the cysts with a magnetic stirrer, irradiate with UV light at a distance of 19 cm from the light source for 4 to 8 minutes.

During studies on the mutagenic effect on *Acetabularia*, we observed that it exhibits an extraordinary resistance to UV irradiation. This observation resulted in an attempt to remove microbial contaminants by means of UV irradiated cysts. This can be done in a reliable way (Table 5), and the cells so obtained do not exhibit any changes as compared to normal cultures. Nevertheless, one must keep in mind that non-visible genetic changes can occur and that one should not use such cells for experiments over a number of generations.

ACKNOWLEDGEMENT

The authors appreciate the technical assistance of Mr. Horst Kretschmer and the proof reading of Mrs. Rose Zellmer.

REFERENCES

1. Schweiger, H. G. (1976) Handbook of Genetics 5, 451-475.
2. Berger, S. and Schweiger, H. G. (1977) in Handbook of Phycological Methods (Gantt, E., ed.) Vol. II, in press, Cambridge University Press.
3. Berger, S., Sandakhchiev, L. and Schweiger, H. G. (1974) J. Microscopie 19, 89-104.
4. Lateur, L. (1963) Rev. Algolog. 7, 26-37.
5. Schweiger, H. G. and Kretschmer, H. (1975) Protoplasma 83, 179.
6. Schreiber, E. (1927) Wiss. Meeresunters., N. F. Abt. Helgoland 16, 10. Abh., 2-34.
7. Hämmerling, J. (1931) Biol. Zentralbl. 51, 633-647.
8. Beth, K. (1953) Z. Naturforsch. 8 b, 334-342.
9. Schweiger, H. G. (1969) Curr. Top. Microbiol. Immunol. 50, 1-36.
10. Føyn, B. (1934) Arch. Protistenkd. 83, 1-56.
11. Shephard, D. C. (1970) in Methods in Cell Physiol. (Prescott, D., ed.), Vol. 4, pp. 49-69.
12. Provasoli, L., McLaughlin, J. J. A. and Droop, M. R. (1957) Arch. Microbiol. 25, 392-428.
13. Müller, D. (1962) Bot. Mar. 4, 140-155.
14. Gibor, A. and Izawa, M. (1963) Proc. Natl. Acad. Sci. USA 50, 1164-1169.
15. Berger, S. (1967) Doctoral Thesis, University of Cologne.

IMPROVED PROCEDURE FOR PROCESSING OF CIRCADIAN RHYTHM DATA FROM INDIVIDUAL CELLS OF *ACETABULARIA*

H. G. Wallraff, E. Schweiger,
W. L. Cairns, D. Wolff and H. G. Schweiger

Max-Planck-Institut für Verhaltensphysiologie
Seewiesen über Starnberg, West Germany
and
Max-Planck-Institut für Zellbiologie
Wilhelmshaven, West Germany

SUMMARY

A method of curve smoothing and normalization is described for processing the raw data of oscillating oxygen evolution by a single cell of *Acetabularia*. Application of the computerized procedure to the data for the freerunning circadian rhythm enables a better determination of the rhythm parameters of period length and phase, and a more reliable comparison of the rhythm between different individual cells or following perturbation of the circadian rhythm in a single cell. The procedure of data processing is general and can be applied to other systems.

INTRODUCTION

The photosynthetic oxygen evolution of *Acetabularia* cells exhibits circadian oscillations even under constant conditions (Schweiger et al.[1], Sweeney and Haxo[2]). A flow-through method has been developed for continuous recording over several weeks of the oxygen evolution by individual cells or by cell fragments of *Acetabularia*. This method is currently used in investigations of the molecular mechanism of the circadian clock (for references see Schweiger and Schweiger[3]). So far however, the processing of data is less developed than the production of data. This paper describes an improved method of processing the data and as an example applies the procedure to the freerunning rhythms in individual cells of *Acetabularia mediterranea*.

MATERIALS AND METHODS

Cells and Culture Conditions

Acetabularia mediterranea were grown at 20° C under diurnal illumination (10 h light, 2500 lux; 14 h darkness) in Erd-Schreiber medium as has been previously described (Hämmerling[4], Schweiger[5]). Cells were routinely entrained to a light dark cycle (L 0800 - 2000, 2500 lux; D 2000 - 0800) at 20° C for 4 or 5 days before being exposed to constant conditions of temperature (20° C) and illumination (2500 lux). A transfer from Erd-Schreiber medium to sterile 90% filtered sea water was made at the time the cells were placed in the cell chambers of the oxygen monitoring systems.

Oxygen Measurement

Details of the flow-through method for continuous monitoring of O_2 production by individual cells have been described (Mergenhagen and Schweiger[6]). The mV output of the monitor system is proportional to O_2 tension of the medium passing the electrode. Since changes in oxygen tension rather than absolute quantities of oxygen are important in determining the phase and period of the circadian rhythm, the mV output was not converted to absolute values. The output of the flow-through recording system is punched onto paper tape and then processed by use of a digital computer (PDP-11/40, Digital Equipment Corp.).

RESULTS AND DISCUSSION

While in many cases circadian oscillations are obvious in the untreated output (Fig. 1), there are some records in which a rhythmicity is hard to detect (Fig. 2 A). The most prominent disturbing factors are short-term fluctuations and long-term drifts from which the more regular oscillations have to be extracted. This can be done by a sequence of curve smoothing and normalization steps. The steps of this procedure, as applied to the data of Figure 2 A, are shown in Figure 2 B, C and D.

The digital ordinate values of the original output (Fig. 2 A) are designated as $y_{1,i}$ ($i = 1, 2, 3, \ldots, n$), where i is the number of the reading at 30 min intervals. This curve is then smoothed by determining running means according to the equation:

$$y_{2,i} = \frac{1}{2k+1} \sum_{j=i-k}^{i+k} y_{1,j} \qquad (1)$$

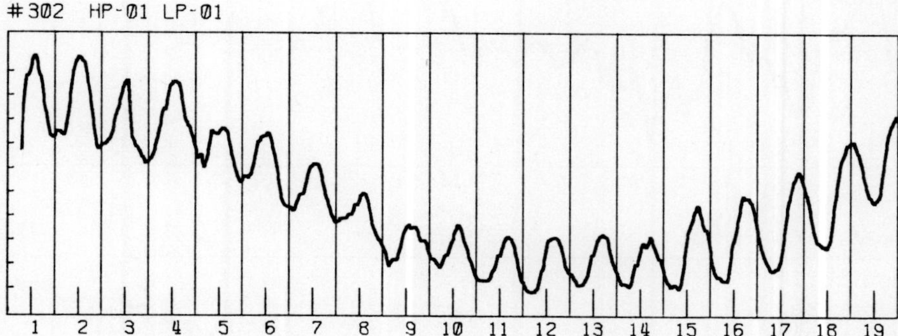

Figure 1. Original data of O_2 evolution by an individual cell (#302) of Acetabularia mediterranea in constant light (LL, 2500 Lux) and constant temperature (20° C). The cell had been kept in a light-dark cycle LD 12 : 12 h and was transferred to LL at 0 h of day 1 (i.e., at end of last dark phase). Time (abscissa) is divided into 24 h days. Scale of the ordinate is relative.

Figure 2 (overleaf). Steps in processing of the original data (A) from Cell #308 (B) after data averaging, (C) after long term drift correction, (D) after amplitude normalization. Scale of the ordinate in A, B and C as in Figure 1; scale steps in D are in units of running s. Further explanations in the text. Time (abscissa) is divided into 24 h days.

In Figure 2 B (prominent curve) the constant k is set to 3 so that the running mean is an average over seven time steps or 3.5 hours. The same procedure, but with a greater time constant (k = 24) reveals the long-term drift (Fig. 2 B, thin curve) which is called $y_{3,i}$. The difference between the two curves,

$$y_{4,i} = y_{2,i} - y_{3,i} \qquad (2)$$

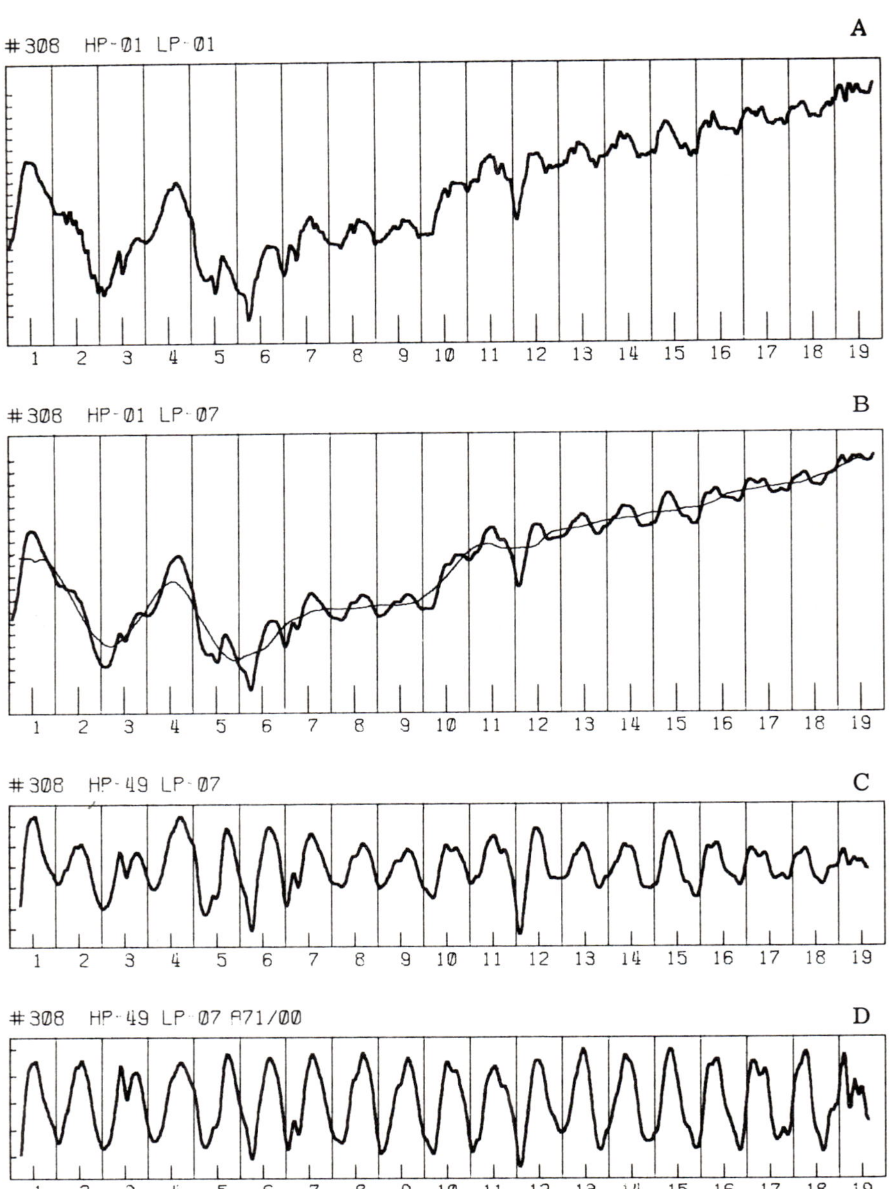
A
#308 HP-01 LP-01
1 2 3 4 5 6 7 8 9 10 11 12 13 14 15 16 17 18 19
B
#308 HP-01 LP-07
1 2 3 4 5 6 7 8 9 10 11 12 13 14 15 16 17 18 19
C
#308 HP-49 LP-07
1 2 3 4 5 6 7 8 9 10 11 12 13 14 15 16 17 18 19
D
#308 HP-49 LP-07 A71/00
1 2 3 4 5 6 7 8 9 10 11 12 13 14 15 16 17 18 19

leads to the drift compensated curve shown in Figure 2 C in which rhythmicity is obvious.

A further step for visual presentation of the data, can be the standardization of the amplitudes. This is done by calculating, over a certain number of time steps, the mean values $\bar{y}_i$ according to formula (1) and, in addition, the corresponding running standard deviations s_i. Then one calculates

$$y_{5,i} = (y_{4,i} - \bar{y}_i)/s_i \qquad (3)$$

The resulting curve, with k = 35, is shown in Figure 2 D.

Details of the derived curves are dependent on the respective time constants, k, selected during the procedure. Within reasonable limits however, there is negligible influence on the most important parameters of circadian periodicity, i.e., period length τ and phase φ.

The data in Figure 2 D are conveniently converted to another diagramatic form exhibiting time of day along the abscissa and the days in vertical columns. This kind of presentation is commonly used in demonstrating locomotor activity of animals (see, e.g., Hoffmann[7], Pittendrigh and Daan[8]). In Figure 3 the raw data from Figures 1 and 2 A are shown after having been processed by the above procedures. The difference in quality between the two records is much less pronounced than in Figures 1 and 2 A, and it can easily be determined that the period length for one cell is longer (Fig. 3 A) and for the other cell shorter (Fig. 3 B) than 24 hours.

With these methods of data processing it is possible to obtain an immediate impression of the circadian behavior of an individual <u>Acetabularia</u> cell and of the variability of this behavior within a given cell and between different cells. This is illustrated (Fig. 4 A-C) by three long time records of freerunning rhythms in individual cells kept under identical and constant conditions. A detailed analysis of these long time experiments reveals some striking peculiarities (e.g., Fig. 4 B day 42; Fig. 4 A day 46). In each case one must consider the possibilities of disturbances of the rhythmic behavior of the cells and of irregularities in the measuring method. The flow-through method for recording the oxygen evolution over long periods is a potent tool in studying the circadian rhythm mechanism, and the methods of processing data will further improve the usefulness of this method.

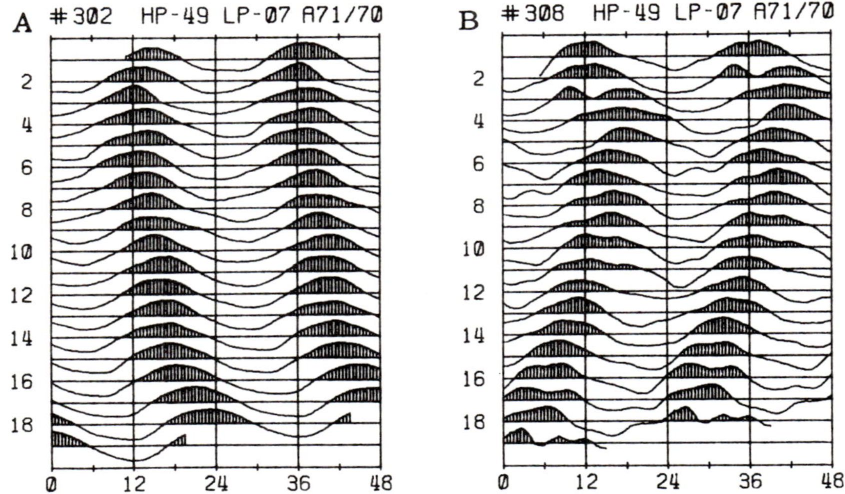

Figure 3. The processed data for cell #302 (A, raw data shown in Fig. 1) and for cell #308 (B, raw data shown in Fig. 2 A). Time in days (ordinate downward) and in hours per every two days (abscissa). Days are drawn twice, i.e., second day is repeated as first day in the following line. Ordinates per day are relative and correspond to those shown in Figure 2 D. Areas between the mean and curve above the mean are hatched.

Figure 4 (opposite page). Examples of freerunning rhythm in three cells of Acetabularia mediterranea. All plants were kept under identical constant conditions (LL, 2500 Lux; 20° C). They had been transferred from LD 12 : 12 to LL at 0 h of the first day. Note that period length τ varies between about 20 h (parts of #367) and 27 h (parts of #371). See Figure 3 for further explanation.

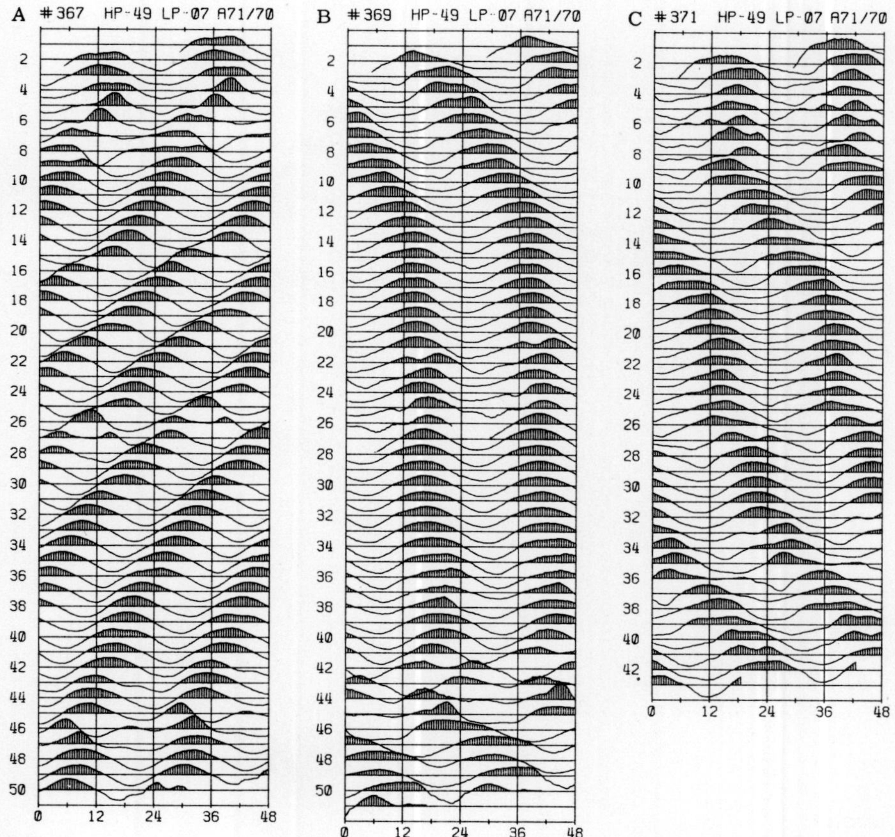
A #367 HP-49 LP-07 A71/70
B #369 HP-49 LP-07 A71/70
C #371 HP-49 LP-07 A71/70
2
4
6
8
10
12
14
16
18
20
22
24
26
28
30
32
34
36
38
40
42
44
46
48
50
0
12
24
36
48

ACKNOWLEDGEMENTS

We wish to thank Mrs. M. Berthel for her technical assistance in collecting of the experimental data.

REFERENCES

1. Schweiger, E., Wallraff, H. G. and Schweiger, H. G. (1964) Science 146, 658-659.
2. Sweeney, B. M. and Haxo, F. T. (1961) Science 134, 1361-1363.
3. Schweiger, H. G. and Schweiger, M. (1977) Int. Rev. Cytol., in press.
4. Hämmerling, J. (1963) Ann. Rev. Plant Physiol. 14, 65-92.
5. Schweiger, H. G. (1969) Curr. Top. Microbiol. Immunol. 50, 1-36.
6. Mergenhagen, D. and Schweiger, H. G. (1973) Exptl. Cell Res. 81, 360-364.
7. Hoffmann, K. (1955) Z. vergl. Physiol. 37, 253-262.
8. Pittendrigh, C. S. and Daan, S. (1976) J. Comp. Physiol. 106, 223-252.

Index

G

H

I

L

M

N

P

R

S

T

U

X

Z

A
B 7
C 8
D 9
E 0
F 1
G 2
H 3
I 4
J 5